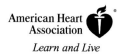

American Heart
Association
Learn and Live

The AHA Clinical Series

SERIES EDITOR ELLIOTT ANTMAN

Novel Techniques for Imaging the Heart

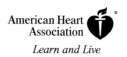

American Heart Association

Learn and Live

The AHA Clinical Series

SERIES EDITOR ELLIOTT ANTMAN

Novel Techniques for Imaging the Heart

Cardiac MR and CT

EDITED BY

Marcelo F. Di Carli, MD, FACC, FAHA
Chief of Nuclear Medicine/PET
Director of Noninvasive Cardiovascular Imaging
Brigham and Women's Hospital
Associate Professor of Radiology and Medicine
Harvard Medical School
Boston, MA

Raymond Y. Kwong, MD, MPH, FACC
Director, Cardiac Magnetic Resonance Imaging
Cardiovascular Division
Department of Medicine
Brigham and Women's Hospital
Assistant Professor of Medicine
Harvard Medical School
Boston, MA

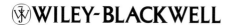

WILEY-BLACKWELL

A John Wiley & Sons, Ltd., Publication

This edition first published 2008, © 2008 American Heart Association
American Heart Association National Center, 7272 Greenville Avenue, Dallas, TX 75231, USA
For further information on the American Heart Association:
www.americanheart.org

Blackwell Publishing was acquired by John Wiley & Sons in February 2007. Blackwell's publishing programme has been merged with Wiley's global Scientific, Technical and Medical business to form Wiley-Blackwell.

Registered office: John Wiley & Sons Ltd, The Atrium, Southern Gate, Chichester, West Sussex, PO19 8SQ, UK

Editorial offices: 9600 Garsington Road, Oxford, OX4 2DQ, UK
The Atrium, Southern Gate, Chichester, West Sussex, PO19 8SQ, UK
111 River Street, Hoboken, NJ 07030-5774, USA

For details of our global editorial offices, for customer services and for information about how to apply for permission to reuse the copyright material in this book please see our website at www.wiley.com/wiley-blackwell

Library of Congress Cataloging-in-Publication Data
Novel techniques for imaging the heart : cardiac MR and CT / edited by Marcelo Di Carli, Raymond Kwong.
    p. ; cm. – (AHA clinical series)
    Includes bibliographical references.
    ISBN 978-1-4051-7533-3
    1. Heart–Magnetic resonance imaging.   2. Heart–Tomography.   I. Di Carli, Marcelo F.   II. Kwong, Raymond Y.
III. American Heart Association.   IV. Series.
    [DNLM: 1. Heart Diseases–diagnosis.   2. Magnetic Resonance Imaging–methods.   3. Tomography, X-Ray
Computed–methods. WG 210 N937 2008]
    RC683.5.M35N68 2008
    616.1'207548–dc22

                                                                                              2008027413

ISBN: 9781405175333

A catalogue record for this book is available from the British Library.

Set in 9/12 pt Palatino by Aptara® Inc., New Delhi, India
Printed and bound in Singapore by Markono Print Media Pte Ltd

1   2008

Contents

PART III Advanced Applications of CT and CMR Imaging

A companion CD-ROM with video clips is included at the back of the book

Contributors

Editors

Marcelo F. Di Carli, MD, FACC, FAHA

Noninvasive Cardiovascular Imagining Program
Departments of Radiology and Medicine (Cardiology)
Boston, MA, USA

Raymond Y. Kwong, MD, MPH, FACC

Department of Medicine (Cardiovascular Division)
Brigham and Women's Hospital
Boston, MA, USA

Contributors

Suhny Abbara, MD

Assistant Professor
Harvard Medical School
Director Cardiovascular Imaging Section
Director of Education
Cardiac MR/PET/CT Program
Department of Radiology
Massachusetts General Hospital
Boston, MA, USA

Rahul Aggarwal, MD

Department of Internal Medicine (Cardiology Section)
Wake Forest University Health Sciences
Winston-Salem, NC, USA

Hiroshi Ashikaga, MD, PhD

Laboratory of Cardiac Energetics
National Heart, Lung, and Blood Institute
Bethesda, MD, USA

Leon Axel, PhD, MD
Department of Radiology
NYU Langone Medical Center
New York, NY, USA

George A. Beller, MD
Department of Medicine (Cardiovascular Division)
University of Virginia Health Sciences Center
Charlottesville, VA, USA

Colin Berry, BSc, PhD, FRCP
Division of Intramural Research (Cardiovascular Branch)
National Heart, Lung, and Blood Institute
National Institutes of Health
Bethesda, MD, USA

David A. Bluemke, MD, PhD, FAHA
Clinical Center
National Institutes of Health
Bethesda, MD, USA

Robert O. Bonow, MD
Division of Cardiology
Northwestern University Feinberg School of Medicine
Chicago, IL, USA

James C. Carr, MD
Department of Radiology
Northwestern University
Chicago, IL, USA

Robert R. Edelman, MD
Department of Radiology
Northwestern University Feinberg School of Medicine
Evanston Northwestern Healthcare
Evanston, IL, USA

Mario J. Garcia, MD, FACC, FACP
Cardiovascular Imaging Center
Mount Sinai Hospital
New York, NY, USA

Bernhard L. Gerber, MD, PhD, FESC
Department of Cardiology
Cliniques Universitaires St.-Luc
Brussels, Belgium

Ahmed M. Gharib, MD
Diagnostic Radiology and NHLBI
National Institutes of Health
Bethesda, MD, USA

Ilan Gottlieb, MD
Johns Hopkins University
Baltimore, MD, USA

Rory Hachamovitch, MD, MSc
Los Angeles, CA, USA

Henry R. Halperin, MD, MA
Department of Medicine (Division of Cardiology)
Johns Hopkins Hospital
Baltimore, MD, USA

Riple J. Hansalia, MD
Cardiovascular Imaging Center
Mount Sinai Hospital
New York, NY, USA

W. Gregory Hundley, MD, FACC, FAHA
Department of Internal Medicine (Cardiology Section) and Radiology
Wake Forest University Health Sciences
Winston-Salem, NC, USA

Mannudeep K. Kalra, MD
Cardiovascular Imaging Section
Department of Radiology
Massachusetts General Hospital
Harvard Medical School
Boston, MA, USA

Theodoros D. Karamitsos, MD, PhD
Oxford Centre for Clinical Magnetic Resonance Research
John Redcliffe Hospital
University of Oxford
Oxford, UK

Philip J. Kilner, MD, PhD
CMR Unit
Royal Brompton Hospital
London, UK

Danny Kim, MD
Department of Radiology
NYU Langone Medical Center
New York, NY, USA

Han W. Kim, MD
Department of Medicine
Duke University Medical Center
Durham, NC, USA

Raymond J. Kim, MD
Departments of Medicine (Cardiovascular Division) and Radiology
Duke University Medical Center
Durham, NC, USA

Dara L. Kraitchman, VMD, PhD
Russell H. Morgan Department of Radiology and Radiological Science
Johns Hopkins University
Baltimore, MD, USA

Christopher M. Kramer, MD
Departments of Medicine and Radiology (Cardiovascular Imaging Center)
University of Virginia Health System
Charlottesville, VA, USA

Susan H. Kwon, MD
Fellow in Cardiovascular Imaging
Cardiovascular Imaging Section
Department of Radiology
Brigham and Women's Hospital
Harvard Medical School
Boston, MA, USA

Robert J. Lederman, MD
Division of Intramural Research (Cardiovascular Branch)
National Heart, Lung, and Blood Institute
National Institutes of Health
Bethesda, MD, USA

Debiao Li
Department of Radiology (Biomedical Engineering)
Northwestern University
Chicago, IL, USA

Peter Libby, MD
Department of Medicine (Division of Cardiovascular Medicine)
Brigham and Women's Hospital
Harvard Medical School
Boston, MA, USA

João A.C. Lima, MD
Johns Hopkins University
Baltimore, MD, USA

Xin Liu
Department of Radiology
Northwestern University
Chicago, IL, USA

Elliot R. McVeigh, PhD
Laboratory of Cardiac Energetics
National Heart, Lung, and Blood Institute
Bethesda, MD, USA

Federico E. Mordini, MD
Department of Medicine
Department of Radiology
Northwestern University Feinberg School of Medicine
Evanston Northwestern Healthcare
Evanston, IL, USA

Saman Nazarian, MD
Department of Medicine (Division of Cardiology)
Johns Hopkins Hospital
Baltimore, MD, USA

Elsie T. Nguyen, MD
Department of Radiology
Toronto General Hospital
University Health Network
Toronto, ON, Canada

William O. Ntim, MB, ChB, FACC, FACP
Department of Internal Medicine (Cardiology Section), and Radiology
Wake Forest University Health Sciences
Winston-Salem, NC, USA

Amit R. Patel, MD
Department of Medicine (Cardiovascular Imaging Center)
University of Virginia Health System
Charlottesville, VA, USA

Roderic I. Pettigrew, PhD, MD
NIBIB
National Institutes of Health
Bethesda, MD, USA

Geoffrey D. Rubin, MD
Department of Radiology
Stanford Medical Center
Stanford, CA, USA

Michael Salerno, MD, PhD
Duke Cardiovascular Magnetic Resonance Center
Duke University Medical Center
Durham, NC, USA

Joseph B. Selvanayagam, DPhil, FRACP, FESC
Department of Cardiovascular Medicine
Flinders Medical Centre
Adelaide, Australia

Matthias Stuber, PhD
Radiology, Medicine, Electrical and Computer Engineering
Johns Hopkins University
Baltimore, MD, USA

Allen J. Taylor, MD
Cardiology Service
Walter Reed Army Medical Center
Washington, DC, USA

Humberto Wong
Department of Radiology
Stanford Medical Center
Stanford, CA, USA

Henry Wu
Cardiovascular Division
Department of Medicine
Brigham and Women's Hospital
Boston, MA, USA

Preface

The field of Cardiovascular Imaging has witnessed dramatic advancement over the past decade, enhanced by emerging new technologies such as multi-detector CT and MRI. Recent technological advances (e.g., emergence of multi-detector CT, high field MRI) have enabled high quality imaging of coronary and cardiac anatomy and myocardial physiology. As a result, cardiac CT and MRI are no longer research tools that are restricted to the domains of University hospitals. This is the good news. The bad news is that there is now an enormous gap between the growth of these technologies for diagnosis and management of patients with heart disease, and the unmet knowledge base obtained by cardiologists and radiologists lacking clinical experience in performing and interpreting these procedures. Although only a handful of teaching programs are offering specialized training in cardiac CT and MRI currently, it is expected that educational resources in this regards will grow rapidly in response to the mounting clinicians interests in parallel with the increasing clinical roles of these technologies. For example, the American College of Cardiology, and the American College of Radiology have recognized the growing importance of imaging in cardiovascular medicine, and are debating specific ways of incorporating cardiac imaging as a distinct area within their respective training programs.

The handful of books on cardiac CT and MRI are almost exclusively dedicated to advances in technology with limited discussion of where these tests might fit in a patient-centered testing strategy. Those books were designed to illustrate the possible applications of these technologies in cardiology, and not to provide the trainee or imaging specialist a systematic approach to the complexities of cardiac imaging. *Novel Techniques for Imaging the Heart: Cardiac MR and CT* is intended to narrow the above-referenced gap between technology and clinical knowledge base. The objective is to provide Cardiology and Radiology trainees, as well as imaging and medical specialists with, the most current and clinical entity-based information, regarding the roles of CT and MRI in the evaluation of patients with known or suspected cardiovascular disease.

To this end, we have assembled a multi-disciplinary and authoritative group of clinical and imaging experts from Cardiology, Radiology, and Nuclear Medicine to provide a systematic, practical, and in-depth approach to imaging with CT and CMR, as well as correlative imaging technologies. With such a novel conception behind the design of this textbook, together with over 130 figures and tables, it is our hope that its content will remain current in an era of rapid technical and scientific evolution.

Part I includes the fundamentals of imaging with CT and CMR. In addition, this section also includes chapters on contrast agents used in CT and CMR imaging, strategies to reduce radiation dose with CT, and general safety considerations regarding CMR imaging.

Part II is entirely devoted to clinical applications of cardiac CT and CMR. This section is organized by disease entities and it includes comprehensive reviews on the role of CT and CMR in coronary artery disease, heart failure including the evaluation of myocardial viability and differential diagnosis of cardiomyopathies, pre-operative risk evaluation, and valvular heart disease. It also includes a discussion on the emerging role of these imaging modalities prior to interventional electrophysiology. This section also contains reviews on the emerging role of hybrid imaging, and a discussion on the relative merits of CT and CMR relative to more established technologies such as SPECT imaging and Echocardiography. Finally, this section also includes comprehensive reviews of the evidence supporting the potential role of CT and CMR for diagnosis of pre-clinical atherosclerosis and risk assessment.

Part III provides comprehensive reviews of technical innovations and advanced applications of CT and CMR for evaluating CAD, cardiac mechanics, and for guiding cardiac interventions. This section also provides a leap-forward view at the emerging role of these technologies in molecular imaging including reviews on imaging of the vulnerable plaque and cell therapy.

We would like to acknowledge the dedication and the professionalism of our technical staff in CT and MRI and of our advanced imaging fellows and trainees. We are also grateful for the expert editorial assistance of Maggie Meitzler, who has tolerated our frequent requests for changes which we believe had improved the readers' experience. Finally, we would also like to acknowledge the editor of the AHA books series, Elliott Antman, for his relentless support and his encouragement during the production of this book.

Forewords

The strategic driving force behind the American Heart Association's (AHA) mission of reducing disability and death from cardiovascular disease and stroke is to change practice by providing information and solutions to health care professionals. The pillars of this strategy are knowledge discovery, knowledge processing, and knowledge transfer. The books in the AHA Clinical Series, in which *Novel Techniques for Imaging the Heart: Cardiac MR and CT* is included, focus on high-interest, cutting-edge topics in cardiovascular medicine. This book series is a critical tool that supports the AHA mission of promoting healthy behavior and improved care of patients. Cardiology is a rapidly changing field and practitioners need data to guide their clinical decision making. The AHA Clinical Series serves this need by providing the latest information on the physiology, diagnosis, and management of a broad spectrum of conditions encountered in daily practice.

Rose Marie Robertson, MD, FAHA
Chief Science Officer, American Heart Association

Elliott Antman, MD, FAHA
Director, Samuel A. Levine Cardiac Unit, Brigham and Women's Hospital

Imaging the cardiovascular system has always been an essential approach to the accurate diagnosis of cardiovascular disease. In recent years, the field of cardiovascular imaging has expanded greatly, with evolving methodologies rapidly gaining their place in the diagnostic armamentarium as technologies improve and their application to diagnostics and prognostics is supported by clinical evidence.

In this highly authoritative text, Marcelo Di Carli and Raymond Kwong have compiled a first-rate overview of noninvasive imaging techniques and their application to cardiovascular disease. While the emphasis of this book is on cardiac computed tomography and magnetic resonance imaging, the application of hybrid imaging approaches that utilize these two increasingly common modalities, such as positron emission tomography with computed tomography, is also reviewed and put in appropriate clinical context.

The technical aspects of these imaging modalities is thoroughly reviewed early in the text, but another key strength of the presentation is in the direct application of the techniques to specific clinical situations. For example, Salerno and colleagues provide a superb overview of the application of these modalities to evaluating the patient with left ventricular dysfunction, and Kilner reviews the application of cardiac magnetic resonance to the assessment of blood flow and valvular heart disease. These chapters are notable for their clarity, comprehensive review of the topics, and practicality in patient management. In addition to these chapters of clinical immediacy, several chapters are also included that focus on advanced applications of these methodologies to promising areas not yet ready for clinical application, such as imaging coronary atheromata, stem cell imaging, and imaging myocardial mechanics.

The text is notable not only for its authoritative approach to this rapidly growing field, but also for the quality of the images contained within it. The examples of imaging studies are particularly well-reproduced, highlighting the information that one can glean from them and their practical importance in patient management.

Novel Techniques for Imaging the Heart is well suited for anyone with a serious interest in cardiovascular imaging, from full-time cardiovascular imagers to clinicians wishing a deeper understanding of these growing technologies. A rich treasure trove of very helpful information is contained within its cover that, in my view, is essential for anyone wishing to keep current with this rapidly expanding, important field of cardiovascular medicine.

Joseph Loscalzo, M.D., Ph.D.
Hersey Professor of the Theory and Practice of Medicine
Harvard Medical School
Chairman, Department of Medicine
Physician-in-Chief
Brigham and Women's Hospital
Boston, Massachusetts

👁 Video clips on CD-ROM

A companion CD-ROM is included at the back of the book

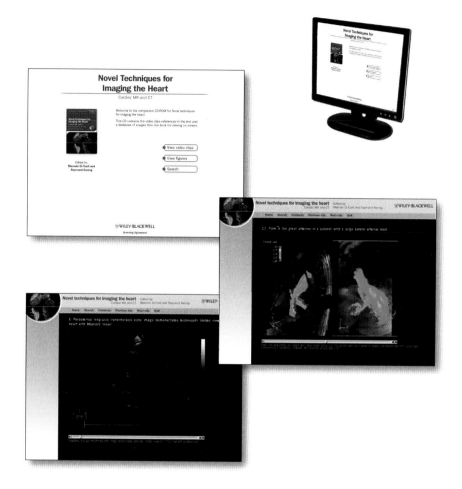

The CD includes:

A searchable database of figures from the book
A searchable database of video clips
All video clips are referenced in the text where you see this icon

PART I

General Considerations and Fundamentals of Imaging

Chapter 1

Principles of CT and MRI

Leon Axel and Danny Kim

X-ray computed tomographic (CT) imaging and magnetic resonance imaging (MRI) are relatively new methods for imaging the cardiovascular system. Although both methods can be used to produce high-quality tomographic (cross-sectional) images of the heart and vascular system, and there are some parallels in the underlying mathematics of the image reconstruction used for the two imaging methods, the basic physical principles of the two methods are quite different. In addition, they have different relative strengths and weaknesses. In this chapter, we will briefly review the basic concepts and principles of cardiovascular imaging with CT and MRI as a background for the more specialized chapters to follow.

Cardiac CT Basics

Cardiac CT imaging, predominantly involving coronary computed tomographic angiography (CTA) imaging, has emerged in importance with the development of multidetector CT scanning technology and slip-ring technology [1]. These technologies allow noninvasive imaging of the body in greater detail with faster speed and higher temporal resolution. For cardiac imaging, this timing is critical because the anatomic structures of interest in the heart are very small and the heart is constantly moving. This section will review the technological advances that have brought cardiac imaging into prominence as an important tool in the evaluation of cardiac disease.

Novel Techniques for Imaging the Heart, 1st edition. Edited by M. Di Carli and R. Kwong.
© 2008 American Heart Association, ISBN: 9-781-4051-7533-3.

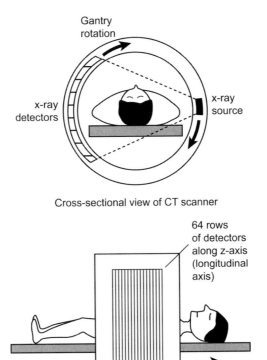

Cross-sectional view of CT scanner

Longitudinal view of CT scanner
(64-slice CT scanner)

Fig. 1.1 Schematic of the principles of cardiac CT image acquisition.

Physical Principles of CT Imaging

At present, a 64-slice multidetector CT scanner is the standard configuration used in cardiac CT examinations [1]. Newer developments, such as the dual-source CT scanner and the volume CT scanner, have been recently introduced and will likely supplant 64-slice multidetector CT as the future standard (see also discussion in Chapter 21). Nevertheless, this section will review 64-slice multidetector CT technology because it is the most commonly used device today. This configuration involves a rotating gantry that houses an x-ray source and multiple rows of x-ray detectors, located opposite each other (Figure 1.1). For a 64-slice multidetector CT scanner, x-ray transmission data are acquired simultaneously at 64 levels along the bore of the gantry, or z-axis. As the patient passes along the axis of the scanner on a moving table, the gantry rotates around the patient. While the gantry rotates, x-ray beams pass through the patient and data are collected at the detectors regarding the amount of attenuation of the x-ray beam that occurs along each projection. Because the patient and gantry are both moving, the projection data are collected in a helical or spiral manner to cover the volume of interest. From this projection data, mathematical algorithms are used to reconstruct cross-sectional images of the body based on attenuation values of the different tissues. The *pitch* is defined as the table travel per complete rotation of the gantry divided by the x-ray beam width. Thus, a pitch between zero and one implies overlap of the projections, whereas a pitch greater than one implies gaps in the projections. The pitch is generally selected prior to the scan and based on the patient's heart rate. For faster heart rates, a higher pitch is applied. However, if the pitch is too high for a given heart rate, there will be gaps in the data set, decreasing image quality. As discussed in Chapter 3, if the pitch is too low for a given heart rate, the scan time, and consequently breath hold time, is unnecessarily increased along with the radiation dose.

The spatial resolution of the images is determined by the image matrix size, the detector height and geometry, and the reconstruction algorithm. Because a volumetric data set is acquired, images can be reconstructed at different slice thicknesses. The lower limit of slice thickness will correspond to the height of a single row of detectors. Thicker slices can be reconstructed by combining thinner slices. The average current 64-slice multidetector CT scanner has detector heights ranging from 0.5 to 1.25 mm. The average spatial resolution is approximately $0.4 \times 0.4 \times 0.4$ mm.

The temporal resolution of the images is determined by the gantry rotation speed and the reconstruction algorithm. For example, a partial scan reconstruction algorithm can decrease the temporal resolution to half the gantry rotation time. This technique uses $180°$ of data in parallel geometry to reconstruct the whole image. Another algorithm called multisegment reconstruction can decrease the temporal resolution by using data from more than one cardiac cycle to reconstruct the images. The resulting temporal resolution will depend on the heart rate. The average current 64-slice multidetector CT scanner has gantry rotation times ranging from 0.33 to 0.42 sec. The average temporal resolution ranges from 83 to 210 msec.

Image Reconstruction Principles

Electrocardiogram (ECG)-gated data acquisition for cardiac CT examinations is necessary to reduce cardiac motion artifact and improve temporal resolution [2,3]. There are two primary methods of ECG gating. One method is prospective ECG triggering, in which data are acquired at a predefined point during the cardiac cycle, also known as a "step-and-shoot" technique. In this method, sequential axial slices are acquired through the heart. As discussed in Chapter 3, the advantages of this method include speed and a lower radiation dose. However, one disadvantage of this method is the dependency upon a regular heart rate. Variability in the heart rate will result in data acquisition at different points along the cardiac cycle, producing misregistration artifacts. Another disadvantage is the lower z-axis resolution, secondary to the slice-by-slice acquisition rather than a volumetric acquisition.

The second method is retrospective ECG gating, in which data are acquired throughout the entire cardiac cycle. In this method, data acquired at specified points during the cardiac cycle are extracted to reconstruct the images. Two types of reconstruction algorithms can be applied. In one type, data can be extracted at a specified fraction of the R–R interval. For instance, image reconstruction can be performed at 10% intervals of the R–R interval from 0% to 90%. In another type, an absolute time interval before or after the R peak can be used, rather than a fraction, to reconstruct the images. In this manner, multiple image data sets are produced that allow the viewing of the cardiac anatomy during all phases of the cardiac cycle [2]. In addition, functional analysis can be performed by visualizing the data sets of the beating heart in a dynamic or cine form to evaluate systolic and diastolic function [2]. One advantage of the retrospective ECG gating method is the ability to edit the ECG reference points to adjust data acquired during an irregular or ectopic beat. Another advantage is the isotropic resolution of the data set, secondary to the volumetric data acquired. The disadvantage of this method is a higher radiation dose. However, there are strategies, such as ECG-triggered dose modulation, that can be used to reduce the total dose. By reducing the tube output during systole, when there is more cardiac motion and anatomical imaging is less useful, the total dose can be reduced without sacrificing data needed for functional analysis. Radiation dose considerations and strategies to reduce it are discussed in more detail in Chapter 3.

Image Contrast and Contrast Agents

Most cardiac CT examinations will require administering an intravascular contrast agent ("contrast") to perform a complete examination. Contrast administration serves several functions. First, it allows identification of the vessels and delineates their endoluminal anatomy [4]. In coronary CTA examinations, contrast opacification of the lumen is required to determine the presence and degree of luminal stenosis secondary to atherosclerotic plaque. Without the presence of contrast, the blood pool, vessel wall, and noncalcified atherosclerotic plaque will have similar attenuation values, preventing accurate assessment of the vessel lumen. Contrast also opacifies the cardiac chambers, allowing identification of space-occupying lesions such as intraluminal masses or thrombus. Opacification of the lumen also allows functional analysis of the ventricles. The ventricular volumes can be determined in both systole and diastole to calculate an ejection fraction. Contrast also perfuses the soft tissues, demonstrating their enhancement patterns. For example, the enhancement pattern of the myocardium can assist differentiation of normal myocardium from scarred myocardium, which might occur following a myocardial infarct. Thus, contrast administration is an important element of the cardiac CT examination.

There are several contrast agents available for cardiac CT examinations. These contrast agents are water-soluble and contain high concentrations of iodine. The high x-ray absorption by the contrast agent attenuates the x-rays from the CT scanner to a greater degree than soft tissues but less than bone. On a CT image, the contrast will appear as a shade of gray depending upon its concentration. The radiodensities of structures in a CT image are measured in Hounsfield units, where water is set to the value zero. Soft tissues have Hounsfield values of approximately 40 to 80, and bone has a Hounsfield value of approximately 1000. The contrast within the vessel lumen has values ranging from 100 to 400, depending upon concentration and volume. For a more detailed discussion on the clinical use of contrast agents in cardiac CT, please refer to Chapter 2.

Imaging Protocol

Patient preparation is an essential step in any imaging protocol. Patients are instructed to remain NPO for three hours prior to the examination and refrain from caffeine intake. After obtaining patient history and informed consent, vital signs are recorded. If necessary, beta-blockers are administered to lower the heart rate. Beta-blockers may be relatively contraindicated in patients with asthma, aortic stenosis, heart block, or severe left ventricular dysfunction. After achieving an adequate heart rate, the patient is placed supine on the CT table. Patients must be able to lie on their back for the duration of the examination, which typically ranges from 5 to 20 min. For a coronary CTA examination, a large-bore intravenous catheter is inserted into a large arm vein, preferably an antecubital vein. This large-bore catheter is necessary to accommodate the high rate of contrast infusion, ranging from 2 to 6 cc/sec. ECG leads are placed on the patient's chest to acquire an ECG tracing. The decision to perform prospective or retrospective ECG triggering gating should be made after considerations of the advantages and disadvantages of each method discussed previously and the type of CT scanner available. To facilitate the visualization of small-caliber coronary arteries, nitroglycerin is generally administered at the start of the examination if there are no contraindications [4]. After obtaining a scout image of the thorax to identify anatomic landmarks, a coronary calcium scan (i.e., without IV contrast) may be performed to determine the calcified atherosclerotic burden. An extremely elevated calcium score or proximal and clumped distribution of the calcium can render the coronary CTA unable to be interpreted and preclude contrast administration. Once this scan is completed, the coronary CTA portion of the examination can be performed. A typical coronary CTA protocol for a 64-slice CT scanner is outlined in Table 1.1.

Image Display and Analysis

An advanced three-dimensional (3D) workstation is essential for analyzing the image data set accurately and efficiently. Multiple post-processing techniques, including bi-orthogonal projections, maximum intensity projections (MIPS), curved planar reformations, and surface- or volume-rendered displays can be used to evaluate the anatomy of interest [3]. For coronary CTA examinations,

Table 1.1 Typical Coronary CTA Examination Protocol: 64-Slice Multidetector CT

Coronary Calcium Scan	
Scan Parameters	
Range	Tracheal bifurcation to the bottom of the heart
Voltage (kV)	120
Effective current (mA)	310
Slice collimation (mm)	1.2
Slice width (mm)	3
Pitch	0.2
ECG gating	Prospective
Coronary CTA	
Patient Preparation	
NPO	3 hours prior to exam
Beta-blockade*	Metoprolol PO (50–100 mg) 1 hour prior to exam
	5 mg IV prn (20 mg total maximum)
Nitroglycerin†	0.4 mg SL
IV catheter	18 gauge (preferably in antecubital fossa)
Scan Parameters	
Range	Tracheal bifurcation to the bottom of the heart
Voltage (kV)	120
Effective current (mA)	700–900
Detector collimation (mm)	0.6
Slice thickness (mm)	0.75
Pitch	0.2 (0.18 for heart rate < 50 bpm)
Rotation time (sec)	0.33 (0.37 for heart rate < 50 bpm)
Reconstruction interval (mm)	0.5
ECG gating	Retrospective or prospective

* Use with caution in patients with asthma, aortic stenosis, atrioventricular block, or severe left ventricular dysfunction.
† Recent use of PDE5-selective phosphodiesterase inhibitors (sildenafil, tadenafil, and vardenafil) for treatment of erectile dysfunction is a contraindication.

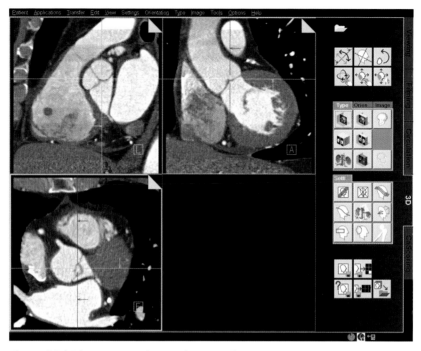

Fig. 1.2 Multiplanar image reformats from a cardiac CT data set.

these techniques assist with the identification of the coronary anatomy, the detection of atherosclerotic disease, and the diagnosis of any significant stenosis [3]. A screenshot of a 3D workstation display is shown in Figure 1.2.

A four-dimensional (4D) analysis can be performed when image data are acquired over the entire cardiac cycle. The 3D data set can be visualized as a dynamic or cine motion display. This dynamic capability allows the evaluation of cardiac function in addition to the cardiac anatomy. Left ventricular wall motion can be assessed. For instance, patients with significant stenosis of the LAD might demonstrate thinning and hypokinesis of the anterior wall consistent with myocardial infarct or hibernation. Cardiac valvular function can be assessed as well. For instance, dynamic images might demonstrate the prolapse of the mitral valve or the incomplete apposition of the aortic valve leaflets, suggesting the presence of aortic regurgitation. In addition to these qualitative assessments of cardiac function, quantitative information can also be obtained. For instance, measurements of the left ventricular volume at end-systole and end-diastole allow the calculation of the stroke volume and ejection fraction. These techniques enable a thorough evaluation of both cardiac anatomy and function.

Cardiac MRI Basics

Nuclear Magnetic Resonance Phenomena

The fundamental physical phenomenon underlying MRI is the fact that certain types of atomic nuclei (including hydrogen, which is abundant in the body in the form of water and fat) have a quantum-mechanical property called *spin* [5–7]. Such nuclei are often informally referred to as "spins." The nuclear spin property leads to the nuclei exhibiting a collective magnetization in the presence of a strong external polarizing magnetic field. This nuclear magnetization is quite weak (the equilibrium magnetization depends on the strength of the field; it is equivalent to a net alignment of the nuclei with the external field of only around one part per million at typical imaging system field strengths), and it is not readily detectable in its equilibrium state, i.e., aligned with the external field.

The nuclear spin property also leads to the nuclei exhibiting an effective angular momentum. This angular momentum combines with the nuclear magnetization to create the possibility of exciting a nuclear resonance condition at a characteristic resonance frequency that is proportional to the magnetic field strength. For the field strengths used in MRI systems, this resonance frequency is in the radiofrequency (RF) range. For example, for a typical imaging field strength of 1.5 T (approximately 30,000 times stronger than Earth's magnetic field), the hydrogen resonance frequency is approximately 64 MHz.

In the phenomenon of nuclear magnetic resonance (NMR), if a suitable short-duration pulse of RF magnetic field oscillating at the resonance frequency is applied to the nuclei, the nuclear magnetization can be induced to rotate away from its equilibrium orientation ("to be excited"). The net rotation angle produced will depend on the strength of the applied oscillating field and its duration. This resonance phenomenon will only be exhibited for a narrow band of frequencies around the central resonance frequency. When the RF magnetic field is turned off, the nuclear magnetization is left at a final net angle called the *flip angle* relative to the external polarizing magnetic field. The component of the nuclear magnetization that is perpendicular to the external polarizing field (*transverse magnetization*) will then rotate around the external field at the resonance frequency; this spinning magnetization will induce a weak but detectable signal in a suitable electrically conducting receiver coil. This signal is the basis of MRI and other applications of NMR [5,6]. Differences in the local tissue magnetization due to different amounts of nuclei (*proton density*) can provide a source of image contrast; for example, the lungs normally have less tissue density than the mediastinal tissues, and appear correspondingly darker. The magnetic resonance signal will not persist indefinitely but decays over time. Typically, the magnetic resonance signal decays exponentially with time, with a characteristic time constant, T2, that depends on the state of the tissue; for example, fluids typically have a larger T2 than solid tissue, and edematous tissue typically has a larger T2 than normal tissue. These differences in the values of T2 provide another potential source of image contrast if the signal detection is delayed to a later time; those regions with T2 values greater than or on the order of signal observation time will tend to appear brighter than regions with lesser values of T2, all other factors being equal (*T2 weighting*). The nuclear magnetization will gradually recover toward its equilibrium state, aligned with the polarizing field (*longitudinal magnetization*). Typically, this recovery is exponential in time with a characteristic time constant, T1, that also depends on the state of the tissue. The T1 value is on the order of or greater than the T2 value. As MRI typically involves the use of repeated excitations, if these excitations are repeated with a repetition time, TR, that is on the order of or smaller than T1, the magnetization will only recover part of its magnetization between consecutive excitations and will appear correspondingly darker in the image. The larger the flip angle, the larger this *T1-weighting* effect will be.

Although the resonance frequency is proportional to the magnetic field experienced by the nucleus, the different screening effects of the electron orbitals can result in different nuclear positions within a molecule having different characteristic resonance frequencies; this effect is known as a *chemical shift*. The chemical shift is a small effect; for example, there is approximately a 3.4 ppm difference between the resonance frequencies of hydrogen nuclei in water and fat. In the presence of different frequencies, the magnetic resonance signal will not decay as a simple exponential function of time, as there will be interference between the signals at different frequencies. The resulting complex signal as a function of time can be used to recover the corresponding distribution of different frequencies in the signal through a mathematical operation, the Fourier transform. The distribution of frequencies due to chemical shift differences can be used for magnetic resonance spectroscopy studies. If there is a wide range of frequencies present, the net observed signal can appear to disappear prematurely due to the resulting interference between them. However, the signal can be induced to transiently reappear at the full strength (limited by the T2 relaxation time) by applying suitable refocusing RF pulses; this reappearance of the signal is known as a *spin echo*, and the time of appearance of the echo is the echo time, TE. If a series of exciting RF pulses is applied at repetition times, TR, on the order of or smaller than the T2 time, the residual transverse magnetization can be refocused by the subsequent excitation pulses, adding to the new transverse magnetization being produced and leading to a condition known as *steady-state free precession*, with an increased signal that depends on the ratio of T2 to T1.

Image contrast depends on a combination of the relative contributions of the different relaxation times of the tissue and the different repetition and echo times and the flip angle used in the imaging. In addition to the T1- and T2-weighting effects described previously, we can create additional T1-weighting effects through the use of an additional RF pulse applied immediately before the signal excitation pulse, so that the recovery from the effects of the pulse at the time of the signal excitation will reflect the local T1 value. For example, such a pulse could have a net flip angle of 90° (saturation recovery, as the starting state of the magnetization is zero, or saturation) or 180° (inversion recovery, as the starting state of the magnetization is inverted). In addition, we can alter the image contrast through the administration of magnetic resonance contrast agents that shorten the tissue relaxation times. As will be discussed further, motion can also affect the magnetic resonance signal.

Imaging Methods

Although the basic principles of the NMR phenomena have been known for over 50 years, their use for imaging was relatively more recent [7]. In part, this delay was because the NMR signal cannot be focused or collimated like other medical imaging signals. The use of localized signal detection coils can provide a limited amount of localization of the signal sources, but this cannot be used for imaging by itself (although it can be useful in speeding up more conventional imaging, as described later). The key to performing MRI is the use of magnetic field *gradients*, supplementary magnetic fields that are computer-controllable and that are designed to increase linearly along some desired direction in space [7]. With the use of gradients, we can couple the position of the signal sources along the direction of the gradient to the corresponding resonance frequency of the signal. The resonance frequency of a source will vary proportionally to the component of its position along the gradient direction and the strength of the gradient. The direction and strength of the gradient can be rapidly and flexibly changed by the MRI system computer during the data acquisition, and can be turned on and off as pulses.

The most straightforward use of gradients in MRI is for the frequency encoding of position by applying the gradient during signal detection. The distribution of the strength of signal sources along the direction of the gradient will be reflected in the resulting distribution of signal frequencies. These source locations can then be separated by performing a Fourier transform on the signal detected as a function of time, to find the corresponding distribution as a function of frequency (similar to its nonimaging use of the Fourier transform to find the distribution of chemical shift frequencies in magnetic resonance spectroscopy). These locations are then mapped to the corresponding distribution as a function of position along the gradient by knowledge of the strength of the applied gradient. By itself, the frequency-encoded signal in the presence of a gradient only provides information about the component of the image positions along the gradient direction, i.e., the projection of the signal sources onto the gradient direction. However, by repeating the signal excitation and detection process with the gradient direction being systematically changed to provide the projection data along different directions in space, we can build a set of radially oriented projection data analogous to that used for x-ray CT imaging. Image reconstruction using this approach, called *projection-reconstruction imaging*, was originally carried out using the same mathematical approaches as x-ray CT.

However, now computational methods are generally used that effectively inter-polate the acquired data set onto an equivalent rectangular grid of samples of the Fourier transform of the image. The image is then reconstructed by the use of Fourier transform processing of this data.

Whereas projection-reconstruction imaging is simpler to understand, most MRI is currently carried out with *phase-encoded imaging*. In phase encoding, a pulse of magnetic field gradient is applied after the excitation but prior to the signal detection. Immediately after the excitation, in the absence of any gradients, the signal sources will all have the same resonance frequency and will be synchronized with the same signal phase. While the pulse is applied, the local resonance frequencies will vary along the direction of the gradient with a resulting accumulation of differences between the phases of the signal from different locations along the gradient. After the gradient is turned off, the frequencies will revert to their initial value, but the signal sources will be left with a difference in their phases that depends on their position and is proportional to the strength and duration of the gradient. If we now acquire the signal data in the presence of a frequency-encoding gradient along another direction, as described previously, the resulting projection data along that direction will be altered compared to the values that would be obtained in the absence of the phase-encoding gradient. In fact, by repeating this process and acquiring a set of such phase-encoded data with a set of different values of the strength of the phase-encoding gradient along the same direction, we can build up a set of samples of the Fourier transform of the image along that direction that can be used to reconstruct the image with corresponding Fourier transform processing. Typically, phase-encoding and frequency-encoding approaches are used jointly in MRI, with signal detections in the presence of a fixed frequency-encoding gradient pulse along one direction being used together with a set of preceding phase-encoding gradient pulses along a perpendicular direction.

As the MRI data are acquired at discrete sampled locations in the Fourier transform of the final image, the number and locations of these samples will determine the final achievable resolution and field of view (FOV) limits of the final image. Specifically, the extent of the data acquired in the Fourier transform domain along a given direction limits the corresponding resolution along that direction in the reconstructed image. To increase the resolution, we must either use stronger gradients or apply them for a longer time. The sparseness of the spacing between the samples in the Fourier transform domain along the phase-encoded direction limits the achievable imaged region FOV along that direction. Any structures located beyond the FOV will appear as if they were "aliased" back into the region, and can be superimposed on the images of structures that are really located in the region being imaged.

We can use magnetic field gradient pulses applied during the excitation pro-cess, together with RF pulses that are designed to have a limited frequency content, to achieve a corresponding spatially limited *selective excitation* of a desired slab or slice to be imaged. As the direction of the slice-selection gradient in space can be freely chosen, as can the frequency content of the RF pulse, we can very flexibly choose the orientation, location, and thickness of the slice. Thus, we can reduce a potentially 3D image reconstruction task to a two-dimensional one, with the imaging gradients applied along the directions in the plane of the slice.

As the repeated excitations and signal detections that are required for acquiring the data used in magnetic resonance image reconstruction take time, and there is a limited signal-to-noise ratio (SNR) of the detected signal, there are trade-offs that must be considered in choosing the imaging parameters. In particular, as only a limited number of data samples can be acquired in a given time period, there will be a trade-off in choosing how to optimize the resolution versus the FOV. Furthermore, as the signal per picture element (pixel) decreases with the decreasing size of the pixel, higher spatial resolution will come at the cost of a decreased SNR.

An obvious difference in imaging the heart compared to other organs is the cyclical contractions it undergoes. As the time required to acquire enough data to reconstruct a high-resolution image can be a large fraction of a cardiac cycle, there would be significant motion blur degrading the image. To avoid this motion blur, we generally use the synchronization of the data acquisition with the cardiac cycle, called *cardiac gating*, and gather the data needed for imaging each phase of the cardiac cycle from a set of relatively small temporal windows (or segments) within each of a series of heart beats. Cardiac gating can be applied in either a prospective or a retrospective manner. In *prospective gating*, the data acquisition is initiated at fixed times after detection of a synchronizing trigger, e.g., derived from detection of the QRS complex in the ECG. In *retrospective gating*, the data are acquired continuously and then interpolated onto equivalent consistent cardiac cycle times as part of the image reconstruction processing. Another potential source of motion blur in cardiac MRI is respiratory motion. To avoid this distortion, we can either keep the imaging times short enough that the patient can suspend respiration during the data acquisition or we can perform an additional gating process, only acquiring data during relatively consistent and motionless phases of the respiratory cycle (generally near end-tidal expiration).

There are two principal potential sources of effects of motion on the magnetic resonance signal due to blood flow or myocardial motion in cardiovascular MRI: "time-of-flight" effects and phase shifts. *Time-of-flight effects* reflect the fact that alterations of the local magnetization (either transverse or longitudinal) will persist for times on the order of the corresponding relaxation times and will move with the underlying blood or tissue; this effect can lead to motion-induced changes in signal intensity. *Phase shift effects* reflect the changing magnetic fields experienced by excited nuclei as they move along magnetic field gradients. Although the signal phase is not displayed in conventional magnetic resonance images, the imaging methods can be modified with suitable additional gradient pulses so that a magnetic resonance image is produced whose phase is directly proportional to the local velocity component along some desired direction in space. Note that due to the limited range of possible phases, the velocity sensitization may need to be adjusted for a given flow condition to avoid aliasing of the apparent velocity.

Imaging Systems

A central component of an MRI system is the imaging magnet itself. This magnet must be both very strong (generally using a superconducting magnet) to boost the magnetization and thus the corresponding achievable SNR, and uniform so that there are minimal pre-existing field gradients [7]. The associated system for generating magnetic field gradients must be both strong and fast-switching (within safety limits for rapidly changing magnetic fields) as well produce gradient fields that are quite linear over the imaging region.

The RF coils (which may or may not be different physical coils for transmitting excitation pulses and receiving the resulting signal) must be designed to be uniform and efficient over the desired response region. The coil can actually be composed of an array of multiple elements. There are safety limits on the amount of RF power that can be deposited in the human body per unit time. The RF receiver electronics must be of high quality, and may need to be multichannel to handle the signals from multiple receiver coils. The whole system is controlled by using a computer or computers to synchronize the RF and gradient pulses for signal excitation, as well as for the image reconstruction and other associated data handling.

Speeding Up Imaging

To get around the imaging speed limitations referred to previously, we need to optimize the system hardware and software performance and tailor the imaging to the individual [7]. This customization includes choosing the smallest FOV dimension we can for orienting the phase-encoded (the "slowest") direction, and optimizing associated trade-offs between spatial and temporal resolution. Acquiring multiple sets of samples of the Fourier transform from each excitation by creating multiple spin echoes, each with a different value of the phase-encoding gradient, is used in echoplanar imaging. Various approaches can be applied to reduce the amount of data that must be acquired, such as using the limited spatial localizing information available from the use of arrays of receiver coils to eliminate the aliasing that would otherwise result from undersampling the data; this is often referred to as *parallel imaging*. In *serial imaging*, similar and other approaches can be used to allow relative undersampling in the time dimension.

Imaging Protocols

In a cardiovascular MRI examination, protocols generally include initial quick localizing images to define the desired region of focus as well as some overall survey images of the general region [7]. Images are then acquired in multiple orientations to define the anatomy and function of different regions. These images can be acquired with different sensitivity to relaxation times to vary the image contrast. Contrast agents are often administered to assess both the early enhancement phases, as a relative measure of perfusion, and the delayed phases, as a sensitive (although not specific) indicator of local processes such as scarring or inflammation. Velocity imaging is often useful to assess flows, e.g., in the great vessels as a means to find the cardiac output.

Image Display and Analysis

A typical cardiovascular examination will generate hundreds or even thousands of individual images; many of these are best viewed as movie frames with a dynamic display. The calculation of functional parameters such as cardiac volume dimensions or velocities requires additional specialized analysis programs.

Summary

In this chapter, we have presented an overview of the basic concepts and principles of cardiac CT imaging and MRI. Knowledge of these fundamental principles is important when selecting the best examination for a particular patient and clinical scenario. Future technological advances will build upon these fundamental principles and address current weaknesses and limitations of each modality. In the chapters that follow, the clinical applications that use current technologies will be discussed.

References

1 Achenbach, S. (2006) Computed tomography coronary angiography. *J Am Coll Cardiol* **48**: 1919–1928.
2 Pannu, H.K., Flohr, T.G., Corl, F.M., Fishman, E.K. (2003) Current concepts in multi-detector row CT evaluation of the coronary arteries: principles, techniques, and anatomy. *Radiographics* **23** Spec No: S111–125.
3 Ferencik, M., Ropers, D., Abbara, S., *et al.* (2007) Diagnostic accuracy of image post processing methods for the detection of coronary artery stenoses by using multidetector CT. *Radiology* **243**: 696–702.
4 Pannu, H.K., Jacobs, J.E., Lai, S., Fishman, E.K. (2006) Coronary CT angiography with 64-MDCT: assessment of vessel visibility. *AJR Am J Roentgenol* **187**: 119–126.
5 MRI Clinics of North America. (1999) *Physics of MR imaging*. Vol. 7. Philadelphia: W.B. Saunders Company.
6 Boxt, L.M. (1999) Cardiac MR imaging: a guide for the beginner. *Radiographics* **19**: 1009–1025; disc. 1026–1008.
7 Lee, V.S. (ed). (2005) *Cardiovascular MRI: Physical Principles to Practical Protocols*. Philadelphia: Lippincott, Williams & Wilkins.

Chapter 2

Clinical Considerations on the Use of Contrast Agents for CT and MRI

Federico E. Mordini and Robert R. Edelman

Contrast Agents for MRI

As discussed in Chapter 1, one of the remarkable aspects of magnetic resonance imaging (MRI) is its ability to generate a contrast between tissues without the use of exogenous agents. As such, standard T1 and T2 weighted sequences provide inherent, "natural" contrast that is the basis of many functional and morphological cardiac exams in clinical practice. MRI contrast agents further alter T1 and T2 signals to depict vascular structures, evaluate tissue content, and assess tissue perfusion. The development of contrast-enhanced sequences has transformed MRI into one of the most powerful modalities in the detection of ischemic heart disease and its sequela.

Basic Properties

Gadolinium produces its effect through paramagnetism, meaning that it has a magnetic moment that is induced by an external magnetic field. Gadolinium has seven unpaired electrons that create this paramagnetic property. The unpaired electrons essentially shorten the T1 relaxation time of the protons in the water molecule. Although primarily a T1 agent, gadolinium produces $T2^*$ effects at high concentrations that decrease the tissue signal. This effect is exploited in neurological MRI but is currently considered undesirable in most cardiovascular applications.

Because gadolinium in its elemental form is toxic to humans, chelates have been developed that abrogate the toxic effects (e.g., DTPA, albumin, DOTA) (Table 2.1). Some common characteristics of gadolinium agents are that they

Novel Techniques for Imaging the Heart, 1st edition. Edited by M. Di Carli and R. Kwong.
© 2008 American Heart Association, ISBN: 9-781-4051-7533-3.

Table 2.1 Commercially Available Gadolinium Contrast Agents in the US [1]

Name of Compound	Trade Name (Company)	Distribution	Elimination	Structure	T1 Relaxivity (1.0 T)	Viscosity (mPa-sec, 20°C)	Osmolality (mOsm/kg)	Concentration (mg/ml)
Gadopentate dimeglumine	Magnevist (Bayer)	Intravascular extacellular	Renal	Linear	$r_1 = 3.4$	4.9	1960	469
Gadodiamide	Omniscan (GE)	Intravascular extacellular	Renal	Linear	$r_1 = 3.9$	2.0	789	287
Gadoteridol	ProHance (Bracco)	Intravascular extacellular	Renal	Cyclic	$r_1 = 3.7$	2.0	630	279
Gadoversetamide	Optimark (Mallinckrodt)	Intravascular extacellular	Renal	Linear	N/A	3.1	1110	331
Gadobenate dimeglumine	Multihance (Bracco)	Intravascular extacellular	Renal Biliary	Linear	$r_1 = 4.6$	5.3 (37°C)	1970	529

Reprinted with permission from Edelman, R. (2004) *Radiology* **232**: 653–668.

distribute rapidly into the intravascular and extravascular spaces, have a short plasma half-life of 20 min, and are eliminated through the kidneys [1]. An exception to this is albumen-bound gadolinium (Phase III trials completed), which initially behaves like an intravascular agent [2,3]. Although safe, commonly used in practice, and well-described in the literature, gadolinium is not FDA-approved for cardiovascular imaging including magnetic resonance angiography (MRA), and its use is an off-label application.

Manganese is the other paramagnetic element approved for use in humans. Its utility in cardiac imaging is being evaluated by clinical trials at the present time. Manganese is chemically similar to calcium and is taken up by cells through voltage-dependent calcium channels. This property is analogous to the uptake of thallium, a potassium analog, and makes manganese promising in the evaluation of ischemic heart disease.

Also in the clinical trial stage are the coated iron particle agents, which are known as *ultrasmall superparamagnetic iron oxides* (USPIO). These shorten T2 relation rates and are primarily intravascular. The application of these agents will likely be in MRA and potentially in plaque imaging, where iron particles are taken up by plaque macrophages.

Myocardial Perfusion Imaging

First-pass contrast enhanced imaging is the most studied method for evaluating myocardial perfusion. Although a purely intravascular contrast agent has theoretical benefits in this application, the commercially available agents have proven practical and accurate. Furthermore, not only is magnetic resonance imaging valuable in the qualitative assessment of perfusion, it is also performs well in the quantitative assessment of myocardial perfusion. Finally, comparisons against angiography, positron emission tomography (PET), and single photon emission computed tomography (SPECT) have been highly favorable in experienced centers [4].

Dosing has been addressed by a multicenter trial that concluded that 0.05 mmol/kg was the optimal dose of gadolinium [5]. However, it has been observed that larger doses of gadolinium in the range of 0.1 to 0.2 mmol/kg provide better myocardial enhancement and image quality. As a technical note, although this larger dosing of contrast is useful for qualitative analysis, quantitation is compromised at high concentrations. Many quantitative approaches have therefore used lower doses such as 0.025 to 0.05 mmol/kg. An alternative strategy that allows qualitative and quantitative assessment is the dual bolus method of perfusion, whereby a very low-dose 0.005 mmol/kg bolus is used to calculate the delivery of contrast and a traditional 0.1 mmol/kg bolus is used for both qualitative analysis and the quantitation of tissue perfusion [6]. Although the optimal injection rate of contrast has not been fully addressed in the literature to date, the delivery of contrast has been cited between 3 and 5 cc/sec. It is generally believed that faster injection rates provide better contrast to noise in visualizing perfusion defects.

Infarct Imaging

The development of *delayed-enhancement imaging* (or delayed hyperenhancement imaging) was a significant step in the field of cardiac MRI. It was initially developed as a means to detect myocardial infarction; however, its use has been extended to the assessment of various cardiomyopathic processes including myocarditis, hypertrophic cardiomyopathy, and infiltrative disease. The high contrast-to-noise and spatial resolution make this technique the gold standard for infarct detection. Furthermore, the prediction of recovery of function and the correlation to adverse clinical outcomes make this technique particularly relevant in today's practice [7,8].

Gadolinium produces its effect by becoming distributed in damaged cells and the engorged extracellular space in the acute setting and in the extracellular space of scar tissue in the chronic setting. In either case, the washout of gadolinium is slower in these areas, resulting in high signal intensity compared to normal myocardium on T1-weighted imaging.

The dosing of gadolinium for infarct imaging has been more consistent in the literature as compared to first-pass perfusion. The original method used 0.2 mmol/kg; however, doses from 0.1 to 0.2 mmol/kg have been described [9–11]. Delay time (time between contrast administration and the commencement of imaging) was originally cited at 5 min so that acquisition occurs between 5 and 30 min post-injection. Early imaging (less than 5 min) leads to overestimation of infarct size, whereas late imaging (greater than 30 min) results in excessive washout of the gadolinium [12]. Lower doses require shorter delay times, which can be exploited as a time-saving technique. Selection of the inversion time (TI, time from radiofrequency excitation to acquisition) is critical to adequate imaging and is initially chosen between 200 and 300 ms. The TI frequently requires adjustment to obtain the appropriate "nulling" of myocardium and the enhancement of infarct. One technique to determine the correct TI is to image the same slice with increasing TI values, e.g., at 200, 225, 250, 275, and 300 ms, which can be performed in one breath-hold on some systems. Once the initial TI is selected, it is commonly necessary to increase the TI by 25 to 50 ms as time progresses to account for contrast loss. Ultimately, it is advisable to be consistent in dosing and in delay time so that the TI is the only variable that requires adjustment.

One of the most helpful techniques in obtaining optimal delayed enhancement imaging is the use of phase-sensitive sequences, which allow adequate imaging even if the TI is suboptimal by 100 ms in either direction [13]. This greater margin of error in selecting the TI value becomes important for inexperienced operators, in cases with atypical enhancement, and for more consistent visualization of myocardial infarction.

Vascular Imaging

The primary application of MRA in cardiology extends to diseases of the aorta, congenital heart disease, and peripheral arterial disease. Each institution has established imaging protocols and each vendor has various strategies for the proper timing of the contrast bolus. In general, the dosages of gadolinium range from 0.1 to 0.3 mmol/kg, and the injection rates are in the 1.5 to 2.0 cc/sec range.

Adverse Effects

Experience with a large number of patients has shown that the commercially available gadolinium chelates are safe and without side effects in the majority (more than 98%) of patients. When side effects do occur, they are usually mild and transient. These include coldness in the arm during the injection, headache, and nausea. More severe reactions (shortness of breath, wheezing, or hypotension) are extremely rare and occur in less than 1% of the population. Nevertheless, gadolinium use during pregnancy is discouraged unless the potential benefit justifies the risk to the fetus. Caution is also advised in sickle cell patients due to the theoretical concern that gadolinium might potentiate sickle cell alignment, although a case of true sickle cell crisis precipitated by gadolinium administration has never been reported.

The use of gadolinium in patients with renal insufficiency has been quelled by reports of nephrogenic systemic fibrosis (NSF), which was first described as nephrogenic fibrosing dermopathy (NFD) in 1997. There is an epidemiologic association between gadolinium and NSF but no causal link has been elucidated. The disease manifests cutaneously as skin swelling or hardening, discoloration, or discomfort that may occur from 2 days to 18 months post-exposure. Joints and muscles can become stiff, leading to debilitation. Multiple organs can become involved, and death may occur. Deposition of collagen is the primary finding in pathological specimens; however, gadolinium has also been found in tissue samples. As of December 2006, there have been 215 cases of NSF reported worldwide. Three of the five approved agents are implicated, but the FDA issued an advisory for all gadolinium products. Patients that have been affected all had severe (GFR < 30 ml/min/1.73 m^2) to end-stage renal disease (GFR < 15 ml/min/1.73 m^2), and either low or high doses were involved. The FDA recommends pursuing alternative imaging methods in patients with moderately and severely impaired renal function and the consideration of prompt dialysis, although it is currently unknown if this is an effective therapy. Contrast clearance rates from hemodialysis average 78, 96, and 99% in successive sessions [14].

FDA recommendations involve patients in acute or chronic renal failure with a GFR of less than 30 ml/min/1.73 m^2, which is a cohort of approximately 700,000 [15]. Another high risk group are those with acute renal dysfunction due to hepatorenal syndrome or perioperative liver transplantation. At this point, there is no general consensus with regard to screening patients, gadolinium dosing, or the implementation of hemodialysis. Institutional guidelines have become common and are aimed at the practical application of FDA recommendations to minimize risk to the patient. One group published the following approach for patients with GFR under 30 ml/min/1.73 m^2 [16]:

1 Consider an alternate imaging modality with the referring physician.

2 Obtain informed consent in writing.

3 Perform nonenhanced sequences that may negate the need for contrast.

4 Use the lowest dose of gadolinium necessary to provide diagnostic information, or consider half the usual dosing.

5 For patients on hemodialysis, perform the first session within 3 hours of contrast administration and a second session within 24 hours of the first, if clinically safe.

6 For patients on peritoneal dialysis, no periods of dry abdomen and performing additional exchanges for 48 hours are recommended. Hemodialysis may be more effective in clearing gadolinium and can be considered as an alternative.

7 Initiating hemodialysis in patients not on chronic dialysis exclusively for removing gadolinium requires further risk/benefit assessment due to the potential complications associated with dialysis.

8 Avoid in pregnancy due to accumulation in amniotic fluid.

9 Avoid gadodiamide due to its association with many NSF cases.

There are a few additional precautions that some centers advocate, such as avoiding contrast in acute renal failure, strongly discouraging contrast in peritoneal dialysis patients, and using a maximum gadolinium dose of 0.1 mmol/kg.

Approaches to patient screening are not established at the current time. Obtaining serum creatinine levels in patients with the following conditions may be reasonable due to the increased risk of renal disease: age 65 or greater, diabetes, hypertension, a personal history of renal disease, a family history of renal disease, on a history of liver transplantation. Calculation of the GFR using the Modification of Diet in Renal Disease (MDRD) formula allows further risk stratification of these patients. Ultimately, it is the responsibility of each institution to determine the best practice for dealing with the issues of screening and renal replacement therapy.

Contrast Agents for CT

Non-contrast computed tomography (CT), with its exquisite sensitivity for calcium, has long established its utility in the detection of coronary artery disease and pericardial abnormalities. However, the development of multidetector computed tomography (MDCT) has made coronary computed tomographic angiography (CTA) a new and compelling endeavor. Because iodinated contrast is necessary for imaging, an understanding of contrast characteristics, dosage, delivery, and side effects is of paramount importance in this technique.

Basic Properties

Iodinated contrast produces its effect through x-ray attenuation. The degree of attenuation is based on the density of iodine, and thus several concentrations of contrast are manufactured to serve the different applications in CT imaging. Properties and nomenclature of some of the available agents are summarized in Table 2.2 [17]. Some basic categories are ionic versus nonionic contrast agents, and high-osmolar versus low-osmolar versus iso-osmolar contrast agents. Compounds are termed *ionic* when they dissociate into a cation (sodium or meglumine) and an anion (carboxylated, iodinated benzene ring). Compounds are termed *nonionic* when they remain as a single molecule and do not dissociate into components. This property accounts for the low osmolality of nonionic agents. The ratio of iodine atoms to total dissolved molecules varies among the osmotic classes: high-osmolar contrast media (HOCM) has a ratio of 1.5, low-osmolar contrast media (LOCM) a ratio of 3, and iso-osmolar contrast media (IOCM) a ratio of 6 [18]. For example, iodixanol (Visipaque^{TM}) has six iodine atoms in its structure and dissolves as a single molecule; it has a ratio of 6:1 and is iso-osmolar. Iopamidol (Isovue®) has three iodine atoms in its structure and dissolves as a single molecule; it has a ratio of 3:1 and is low-osmolar.

Studies involving 64-slice MDCT used high-density contrast ranging from 300 to 400 mgI/ml that was nonionic and either low-osmolar or iso-osmolar. Iodixanol-320 (Visipaque^{TM}) is unique in that it is iso-osmolar and tends to induce moderate and severe sensations of warmth less frequently than low-osmolar media; however, this does not translate into a statistically significant difference in heart rate change compared to LOCM according to the present literature [19]. There is a theoretical benefit to using higher-density media for better contrast enhancement but there is no comparison trial in coronary imaging to verify this potential advantage with regard to improved sensitivity and specificity.

Delivery

There are four basic methods of contrast delivery. The simplest method uses a single injector for a monophasic injection of contrast. This method tends to cause streak artifacts in the right side of the heart from excessive contrast, which may impair the interpretation of the right coronary artery. The second method is the biphasic injection where contrast is chased by saline. This technique is well described in the 64-slice MDCT literature, and has generated impressive sensitivity and specificity results [20–24]. The minor disadvantage of biphasic injection is its poor opacification of the right side of the heart. To circumvent this, a triphasic technique uses a major bolus of contrast followed by a slow injection of contrast, followed by saline (e.g., 60 cc contrast at 5 cc/sec + 20 cc contrast at 3 cc/sec + 40 cc saline). Additionally, there are injectors with

Table 2.2 Commercially Available Iodinated Contrast Agents in the US

Compound	Trade Name (Company)	Ionic vs. Nonionic	Cation Salt	Iodine Concentration (mgI/ml)	Viscocity (cps, 25°C)	Osmolality (mOsm/kg)	Osmotic Class
Diatrizoate	Hypaque Sodium 50 (Amersham)	Ionic	Sodium	300	3.25	1515	HOCM
Iopamidol	Isovue 300 (Bracco)	Nonionic	None	300	8.8 (20°C)	616	LOCM
Iohexol	Omnipaque 300 (Amersham)	Nonionic	None	300	11.8 (20°C)	672	LOCM
Ioversol	Optiray 300 (Mallinckrodt)	Nonionic	None	300	8.2	651	LOCM
Ioxilan	Oxilan 300 (Guerbet)	Nonionic	None	300	9.4 (20°C)	585	LOCM
Iopramide	Ultravist 300 (Bayer)	Nonionic	None	300	9.2	607	LOCM
Ioxaglate	Hexabrix (Mallinckrodt)	Ionic	Meglumine sodium	320	15.7 (20°C)	600*	LOCM
Ioversol	Optiray 320 (Mallinckrodt)	Nonionic	None	320	9.9	702	LOCM
Iodixanol	Visipaque 320 (General Electric)	Nonionic	None	320	26.6	290	IOCM

Iohexol	Optiray 350 (Mallinckrodt)	Nonionic	None	350	14.3	792	LOCM
Ioversol	Omnipaque 350 (Amersham)	Nonionic	None	350	20.4 (20°C)	844	LOCM
Ioxilan	Oxilan 350 (Guerbet)	Nonionic	None	350	16.3 (20°C)	695	LOCM
Diatrizoate	Hypaque 76 (Amersham)	Ionic	Meglumine sodium	370	NA	2016	HOCM
Iopamidol	Isovue 370 (Bracco)	Nonionic	None	370	20.9 (20°C)	796	LOCM
Diatrizoate	MD-76 R (Mallinckrodt)	Ionic	Meglumine sodium	370	16.4	1551	HOCM
Diatrizoate	RenoCal 76 (Bracco)	Ionic	Meglumine sodium	370	15	1870	HOCM
Iopramide	Ultravist 370 (Bayer)	Nonionic	None	370	22 (20°C)	774	LOCM
Iothalamate	Conray 400 (Mallinckrodt)	Ionic	Sodium	400	7	2300*	HOCM

*Approximate value. Reprinted with permission from King, B., Segal, A., Berg, G., et al. (2004) *Am Coll Radiology* 1–68. For latest data see http://www.acr.org/SecondaryMainMenuCategories/quality_safety/contrast_manual.aspx

the ability to administer a mixture of contrast and saline as the second step in a triphasic injection to provide low-level opacification in the right side of the heart. Although most studies document injection rates of 5 cc/sec, this can range from 4 to 6 cc/sec, with the higher injection rates generally reserved for larger patients.

Timing

The timing of acquisition is critical in CTA. Most authors describe the timing bolus method using 10 to 20 cc of contrast and 40 to 50 cc of saline while imaging the proximal aorta at the level of the coronaries. Due to the different kinetics of small versus large boluses, 2 to 4 sec are generally added to the time to peak enhancement of the test run to ensure that the peak enhancement is obtained with the larger volume. The other timing method uses automated bolus tracking, whereby a region of interest is placed in the proximal aorta and acquisition is triggered when 100 to 150 HU is attained.

Dosing

Unlike MRI where contrast dosing is weight-based, the dosing of CT contrast is less defined. Only a limited number of studies have used weight-based dosing. Most 64-slice MDCT studies have cited volumes of 65 to 100 cc of contrast and 40 to 50 cc of saline. A very rational approach is to base bolus volume on scan time, which tends to limit the amount administered. One particular study provided a volume calculation based on scan time, which was

Volume = (scan time + 5 sec) × 5 cc/sec (injection rate)[25].

Special Applications

There are situations where delivery, timing, and dosing must be modified to address the clinical scenario. For example, when coronary artery bypass grafts are imaged, shorter time to acquisition and more contrast are required. The so-called "triple rule-out" protocol (evaluating coronary artery disease, pulmonary embolism, and aortic dissection) requires similar modifications. Pulmonary venography may require earlier timing, although standard coronary protocols are definitely adequate. The assessment of congenital heart disease can require a slower injection rate and more contrast volume, depending on the condition.

Adverse Effects

Total adverse events with intravenously administered iodinated media are estimated between 1% and 3% with nonionic LOCM and between 5% and 12% with ionic HOCM (Table 2.3) [17]. Serious adverse events have a much lower incidence of 1 to 2 per 1000 patients for HOCM and 1 to 2 per 10,000 patients for LOCM. Finally, the risk of death is extremely rare and ranges from 1 to 2 per 100,000 patients.

Table 2.3 Classification of Adverse Contrast Reactions

Severity	Symptoms	Level of Risk	Comments
Mild	Nausea/vomiting Warm sensation Mild urticaria	No treatment required Not life-threatening	Monitor patient for 20 to 30 min.
Moderate	Mild vagal reactions Mild bronchospasm Mild laryngeal edema Symptomatic urticaria	Treatment required Not life-threatening	Monitor patient until resolution.
Severe	Vagal reactions Bronchospasm Laryngeal edema Loss of consciousness Seizures Cardiac arrest	Treatment required Life-threatening	Occur within 20 min of injection. Consider basic life support. Consider advanced cardiac life support.

Reprinted with permission from King, B., Segal, A., Berg, G., *et al.* (2004) *Am Coll Radiology* 1–68. For latest data see http://www.acr.org/SecondaryMainMenu Categories/quality_safety/contrast_manual.aspx

Because LOCM is associated with lower adverse events, it is recommended for high-risk populations: those with previous adverse reaction, asthma, severe allergy history, cardiac dysfunction, and renal dysfunction. Furthermore, pre-medication with steroids and antihistamines is recommended to decrease the overall reaction rate in those with prior reactions; however, it is unclear if this administration decreases the incidence of severe adverse effects. A key concern is to pre-medicate several hours in advance (typically 12 hours prior to contrast administration) as preparation of less than 3 hours is ineffective.

Contrast-Induced Nephropathy

Contrast-induced nephropathy (CIN) is the most clinically relevant side effect of contrast media because of the incidence, morbidity, and mortality. The definition of CIN has varied among studies but is described in many series as an absolute increase of 0.5 mg/dl in creatinine or a relative increase of 25% in creatinine from baseline. The incidence of CIN is difficult to quantify due to dated studies, varied definitions, and mixed populations used in the literature. In patients undergoing percutaneous coronary interventions with serum creatinine less than 2.0, renal impairment has been reported to be less than 2.5% [26]. In patients undergoing contrast CT, cardiac angiography, or peripheral angiography, the incidence of renal impairment has been reported to be 1.1%. Furthermore, the incidence of dialysis is very uncommon in the latter population at less than 0.2%. However, when CIN occurs it is associated with a greater than five-fold increase in death independent of co-morbid conditions [27].

Prevention is aimed at the identification of patients at risk and the application of proven measures. Effective measures include the use of LOCM and hydration, especially before contrast administration. The AHA and ACC endorsed the use of iso-osmolar contrast in chronic kidney disease patients (GFR < 60 ml/min/1.73 m^2 by the MDRD equation) undergoing angiography in the setting of unstable angina or non-ST elevation myocardial infarction (NSTEMI) based on the RECOVER trial and a meta-analysis of randomized trials [28]. Thus, the use of iso-osmolar contrast may be a reasonable option for patients with this degree of renal impairment undergoing CTA. The use of acetylcysteine is controversial but often used due to its low risk. As for the identification of patients at risk, it is recommended that creatinine be measured in the following situations [17]:

- History of any kidney disease
- Family history of kidney failure
- Diabetes
- Multiple myeloma
- Collagen vascular disease (rheumatoid arthritis, lupus, scleroderma)
- Nephrotoxic medications, including NSAIDs

Conclusions

The diverse applications of contrast in myocardial perfusion, infarct imaging, and angiography make MRI unique among cardiac imaging modalities. Side effects from gadolinium are quite limited. However, patients with impaired renal function now require a risk-benefit analysis given the remote possibility of NSF. The administration of iodinated contrast is a necessary component of coronary CTA. Although there is a non-negligible risk of adverse events related to intravenous contrast administration, the benefit of the noninvasive approach provides a distinct advantage over traditional cardiac angiography in selected patient groups.

References

1 Edelman, R. (2004) Contrast-enhanced MR imaging of the heart: overview of the literature. *Radiology* **232**: 653–668.

2 Rapp, J., Wolff, S., Quinn, S., *et al.* (2005) Aortoiliac occlusive disease in patients with known or suspected peripheral vascular disease: safety and efficacy of gadofosveset-enhanced MR angiography—multicenter comparative phase III study. *Radiology* **236**: 71–78.

3 Goyen, M., Edelman, M., Perreault, P., *et al.* (2005) MR angiography of aortoiliac occlusive disease: a phase III study of the safety and effectiveness of the blood-pool contrast agent MS-325. *Radiology* **236**: 825–833.

4 Schwitter, J., Nanz, D., Kneifel, S., *et al.* (2001) Assessment of myocardial perfusion in coronary artery disease by magnetic resonance: a comparison with positron emission tomography and coronary angiography. *Circulation* **103**: 2230–2235.

5 Wolff, S., Schwitter, J., Coulden, R., *et al.* (2004) Myocardial first-pass perfusion magnetic resonance imaging: a multicenter dose-ranging study. *Circulation* **110**: 732–737.

6 Christian, T., Rettmann, D., Aletras, A., *et al.* (2004) Absolute myocardial perfusion in canines measured by using dual-bolus first-pass MR imaging. *Radiology* **232**: 677–684.

7 Kwong, R., Chan, A., Brown, K., *et al.* (2006) Impact of unrecognized myocardial scar detected by cardiac magnetic resonance imaging on event-free survival in patients presenting with signs or symptoms of coronary artery disease. *Circulation* **113**: 2733–2743.

8 Kim, R., Wu, E., Rafael, A., *et al.* (2000) The use of contrast-enhanced magnetic resonance imaging to identify reversible myocardial dysfunction. *NEJM* **343**: 1445–1453.

9 Wu, E., Judd, R.M., Vargas, J.D., *et al.* (2001) Visualisation of presence, location, and transmural extent of healed Q-wave and non-Q-wave myocardial infarction. *Lancet* **357**: 21–28.

10 Simonetti, O., Kim, R., Fieno, D., *et al.* (2001) An improved MR imaging technique for the visualization of myocardial infarction. *Radiology* **218**: 215–223.

11 Ricciardi, M.J., Wu, E., Davidson, C.J., *et al.* (2001) Visualization of discrete microinfarction after percutaneous coronary intervention associated with mild creatine kinase-MB elevation. *Circulation* **103**: 2780–2783.

12 Oshinski, J., Yang, Z., Jones, J., *et al.* (2001) Imaging time after Gd-DTPA injection is critical in using delayed enhancement to determine infarct size accurately with magnetic resonance imaging. *Circulation* **104**: 2838–2842.

13 Kellman, P., Arai, A.E., McVeigh, E.R., Aletras, A.H. (2002) Phase-sensitive inversion recovery for detecting myocardial infarction using gadolinium-delayed hyperenhancement. *Magn Res Med* **47**: 372–383.

14 "Gadolinium-based contrast agents for magnetic resonance imaging scans (marketed as Omniscan, OptiMARK, Magnevist, ProHance, and MultiHance)." FDA Information for Healthcare Professionals, 2006.

15 Levey, A.S., Coresh, J., Balk, E., *et al.* (2003) National Kidney Foundation practice guidelines for chronic kidney disease: evaluation, classification, and stratification. *Ann Intern Med* **139**: 137–147.

16 Kuo, P., Kanal, E., Abu-Alfa, A., Cowper, S. (2007) Gadolinium-based MR contrast agents and nephrogenic systemic fibrosis. *Radiology* **242**: 647–649.

17 King, B., Segal, A., Berg, G., *et al.* (2004) Manual on contrast media, version 5.0. *Am Coll Radiology* 1–68.

18 Katzberg, R. (1997) Urography into the 21st century: new contrast media, renal handling, imaging characteristics, and nephrotoxicity. *Radiology* **204**: 297–312.

19 Bergstra, A., van Dijk, R.B., Brekke, O., *et al.* (2000) Hemodynamic effects of iodixanol and iohexol during ventriculography in patients with compromised left ventricular function. *Catheter Cardiovasc Interv* **50**: 314–321.

20 Leber, A., Knez, A., Von Ziegler, F., *et al.* (2005) Quantification of obstructive and nonobstructive coronary lesions by 64-slice computed tomography. *J Am Coll Cardiol* **46**: 147–154.

21 Mollet, N.R., Cademartiri, F., van Mieghem, C.A., *et al.* (2005) High-resolution spiral computed tomography coronary angiography in patients referred for diagnostic conventional coronary angiography. *Circulation* **112**: 2318–2323.

22 Raff, G.L., Gallagher, M.J., O'Neill, W.W., Goldstein, J.A. (2005) Diagnostic accuracy of noninvasive coronary angiography using 64-slice spiral computed tomography. *J Am Coll Cardiol* **46**: 552–557.

23 Leschka, S., Alkadhi, H., Plass, A., *et al.* (2005) Accuracy of MSCT coronary angiography with 64-slice technology: first experience. *Eur Heart J* **26**: 1482–1487.

24 Ropers, D., Rixe, J., Anders, K., *et al.* (2006) Usefulness of multidetector row spiral computed tomography with 64- × 0.6-mm collimation and 330-ms rotation for the noninvasive detection of significant coronary artery stenoses. *Am J Cardiol* **97**: 343–348.

25 Goldstein, J., Gallagher, M., O'Neill, W., *et al.* (2007) A randomized controlled trial of multi-slice coronary computed tomography for evaluation of acute chest pain. *JACC* **49**: 863–871.

26 Rihal, C., Textor, S., Grill, D., *et al.* (2002) Incidence and prognostic importance of acute renal failure after percutaneous coronary intervention. *Circulation* **105**: 2259–2264.

27 Levy, E., Viscoli, C., Horwitz, R. (1996) The effect of acute renal failure on mortality. *JAMA* **275**: 1489–1494.

28 Anderson, J.L., Adams, C.D., Antman, E.M., *et al.* (2007) ACC/AHA 2007 guidelines for the management of patients with unstable angina/non-ST-elevation myocardial infarction: a report of the American College of Cardiology/American Heart Association Task Force on Practice Guidelines (Writing Committee to Revise the 2002 Guidelines for the Management of Patients with Unstable Angina/Non-ST-Elevation Myocardial Infarction) developed in collaboration with the American College of Emergency Physicians, the Society for Cardiovascular Angiography and Interventions, and the Society of Thoracic Surgeons endorsed by the American Association of Cardiovascular and Pulmonary Rehabilitation and the Society for Academic Emergency Medicine. *J Am Coll Cardiol* **50**: e1–e157.

Chapter 3

Radiation Dose Considerations in Cardiac CT

Mannudeep K. Kalra and Suhny Abbara

Over the past decade, computed tomography (CT) has emerged as an important imaging modality for the noninvasive evaluation of the heart and coronary circulation. Rapid advances in CT have aided this change, particularly with the development of multidetector or multislice technology, and recently of the dual-source or dual x-ray tube technology. However, due to the smaller pitch with greater overlap to facilitate multisegmental reconstruction over multiple cardiac cycles and the need for a higher tube current to obtain a reasonable contrast-to-noise ratio in images, cardiac CT studies are associated with a higher radiation dose compared to uncomplicated diagnostic coronary catheterization as well as a routine CT of the chest. This chapter outlines the physical aspects and risks of ionizing radiation associated with cardiac CT examinations and describes strategies for reducing the radiation dose.

Physical Aspects of Radiation Dose

The terms and units for measurement of radiation are described in Table 3.1. Of these terms, the *absorbed dose* and the *effective dose* are the most important in quantifying radiation exposure and risks with medical radiation-based procedures. They help in comparing relative doses from different examinations performed with the same or different radiation-based imaging techniques such as CT, coronary catheterization, and nuclear medicine examinations. Table 3.2 summarizes the radiation dose to the general population from natural and man-made sources, including radiation based-medical procedures [1–4].

Novel Techniques for Imaging the Heart, 1st edition. Edited by M. Di Carli and R. Kwong.
© 2008 American Heart Association, ISBN: 9-781-4051-7533-3.

Table 3.1 Commonly Used Terms in Radiation with Their Units

Dose Term	Definition	SI Units	ICRU Units
Radioactivity	Transformation of nucleus of an atom with emission of radiation	Becquerel (Bq)	Curie (Ci)
Exposure	Measure of ionization in air	Coulomb/ kilogram (C/kg)	Roentgen (R)
Absorbed dose	Energy deposited by radiation in a standard mass of tissue	Gray (Gy)	Rad
Dose equivalent	Absorbed dose weighted for biological harm of different types of radiation	Sievert (Sv)	Rem
Effective dose	"Manufactured" term representing total equivalent dose weighted for different types of tissues or organs	Sievert (Sv)	Rem

SI = Systeme Internationale
IRCU = International Council for Radiological Units

Measures of CT Radiation Dose

Radiation dose in CT is described using absorbed dose descriptors such as the *CT dose index volume* (CTDI vol) and the *dose length product* (DLP). The CTDI vol represents the average absorbed dose within a single CT slice or section volume, and is expressed in Grays (Gy). The DLP represents the total absorbed dose within the entire scan volume or length of the scan coverage. It is the product of the CTDI vol and scan length in centimeters, and is expressed in Gray-centimeters (Gy-cm).

All vendors display both CTDI vol and DLP on the control console of the scanner [5]. It is important to remember that these dose descriptors are not the actual absorbed dose to patients but represent approximate absorbed dose with selected scan parameters or protocols in reference to a standard-sized body phantom. Both CTDI vol and DLP represent easily available information for comparing the dose between different CT examinations and protocols and for determining a broad estimate of the effective dose. For example, for a broad estimate of the effective dose with cardiac CT, one can multiply the DLP by 0.017.

Table 3.2 Summary of Effective Doses to General Population from Natural and Artificial Sources [1–4]

Sources	Effective Dose (mSv)
Natural background radiation (US)	3
Pilot and air crew with 1000 hours	5
Current U.S. dose limit for most radiation workers	50
NCRP and ICRP recommended dose limit for most radiation workers	20
Hand radiograph	<0.01
Chest radiograph	<0.01
Mammograph	0.3–0.6
Barium enema	3–6
Diagnostic coronary angiogram	5–10
Bone nuclear scan	3–5
Heart scan, ^{99Tcm}Sestamibi (rest/stress)	13–16
Heart scan, ^{201}Thallium (rest/stress)	35–50
Heart scan, ^{13}N-ammonia (rest/stress)	3–5
Heart scan, ^{82}Rubidium (rest/stress)	10–15
Coronary artery calcium MDCT	1–3
Coronary MDCT angiography	5–15
Electron beam CT for coronary calcium	1.0 (men), 1.3 (women)
Electron beam coronary CT angiography	1.5 (men), 2.0 (women)
Chest MDCT	5–7
Abdomen MDCT	5–7
Pelvis MDCT	3–4
Head MDCT	1–2

Risks Associated with CT Radiation Dose

The adverse effects of ionizing radiation have been traditionally classified into deterministic and stochastic effects. The *deterministic effects* are threshold-dependent effects that occur only after the radiation dose exceeds a threshold level. These adverse effects include radiation-induced cataracts, blood count effects, skin erythema and burns, hair loss, sterility, and death from acute exposure. Embryonic and fetal deterministic effects include mental retardation, fetal demise, growth retardation, mental retardation, congenital anomalies, and a low intelligence quotient. For example, skin erythema occurs at a single acute exposure of 2 Gy, which is much greater than the dose associated with cardiac CT (0.005 to 0.012 Gy) as well as that associated with diagnostic and most interventional cardiology procedures (0.28 to 1.03 Gy) [6,7]. Although rare, deterministic effects have been reported with complicated coronary and noncoronary fluoroscopic interventions [8].

When describing radiation risks in the context of diagnostic medical procedures, typically a stochastic risk is implied. The *stochastic effects* of radiation can occur at any dose level (nonthreshold effects) and include mutagenesis and carcinogenesis. According to the Biological Effects of Ionizing Radiation (BEIR 5) report, of these mutagenesis in the offspring of radiated patients has not been demonstrated in humans, although these effects have been demonstrated in plants and animals at high radiation doses [7].

Radiation-induced carcinogenesis is the most important concern with medical diagnostic radiation, including that from CT scanning. A recent 47-year follow-up study of 86,572 Hiroshima and Nagasaki atomic explosion survivors suggest that the risk of solid cancer appears to be linear even in those who received up to 150 mSv, a low level of radiation exposure [9].

The eleventh edition of the Report on Carcinogens from the National Institute of Environmental Health Sciences (NIEHS), a subsidiary of the Department of Health and Human Services, has declared that X-radiation and gamma-radiation are 'known human carcinogens' because human studies show that exposure to these kinds of radiation causes many types of cancer including leukemia and cancers of the thyroid, breast and lung. The risk of developing cancers due to these forms of ionizing radiation depends, at least in part, on the subject's age at the time of exposure. Childhood exposure is linked to an increased risk for leukemia and thyroid cancer. Exposure during reproductive years increases the risk for breast cancer and exposure later in life increases risk for lung cancer. Exposure to X-radiation and gamma radiation has also been linked cancer of the salivary glands, stomach, colon, bladder, ovaries, central nervous system and skin. Of the total worldwide exposure to X-radiation and gamma-radiation, 55 percent is from low-dose medical diagnosis such as bone, chest and dental X-rays, and 43 percent is from natural sources like radon. Other sources, such as industry, scientific research, military weapons testing, nuclear accidents and nuclear power generation, account for about 2 percent.

Strategies for Radiation Dose Reduction with CT

It is important to remember that "no dose" is that lowest dose possible with any medical radiation procedure. Therefore, all cardiac CT studies must be carefully

Table 3.3 Strategies for Reducing Radiation Dose with Cardiac CT [10–16]

Justification for cardiac CT

Limit scan coverage to area of interest only

Prospective ECG triggering
- Coronary artery calcium CT
- Coronary CT angiography (regular and slow heart rate)

ECG-controlled tube current modulation or ECG pulsing
- Lowering heart rate maximizes dose reduction

Low voltage (80–100 kV$_p$)
- Children
- Small adults
- Delayed acquisition (in myocardial delayed enhancement imaging)

Lower tube current
- Children
- Small adults

Non-ECG gated studies
- When not interested in coronary arteries or cardiac function
- Automatic exposure control techniques

Noise reduction filters (available on some scanners, limited evidence)

In-plane shielding for breast (bismuth-based in-beam shield)

Pitch adaptation
- Faster heart rate: higher pitch; faster scan: lower dose

scrutinized and performed when there is a suitable indication. Justification is perhaps the most important part of radiation dose reduction.

Predefined scan protocols based on study indication, patient age, or patient size also help in eliminating guesswork and in reducing radiation dose. In addition, users can adapt several strategies to reduce radiation dose associated with cardiac CT (Tables 3.3 and 3.4) [10–16]. In addition, vendors have also introduced some techniques such as bow-tie or beam-shaping filters and noise-reduction filters to reduce the radiation dose for cardiac CT studies. The former are pre-patient x-ray beam collimators that help in reducing radiation to the thinner portions of the patients' cross-section, whereas the latter are software that helps in "smoothing" noisy images acquired at a lower radiation dose.

Limiting Scan Coverage

As mentioned before, the DLP or the total absorbed dose increases as the scan length or coverage increases. Therefore, users must ensure that the scan length is

Table 3.4 Dose Reduction for Coronary Artery Calcium CT [1,9–15]

Strategy	Study	Effective Dose or Dose Reduction
Prospective ECG triggering	Knez *et al.* [10]	1 mSv
	Morin *et al.* [1]	1 mSv
Low voltage		
• 80 instead of 120 kV$_p$	Thomas *et al.* [11]	57%
• 80 instead of 120 kV$_p$	Jakobs *et al.* [12]	65%
Low tube current		
• 55 instead of 164 mA	Shemesh *et al.* [13]	67%
• Body weight adapted mA	Mahnken *et al.* [14]	24.8% (women),
• Automated attenuation-	Muhlenbruch *et al.* [15]	11.6% (men)
based mA modulation		20.1–31.1%
Breast shields (bismuth-based)	Yilmaz *et al.* [16]	37.12% to breast

limited to the area of interest. When a coronary artery calcium CT is performed before the coronary CT angiography in the same imaging session, the scan start location and end location can be carefully defined. Prior studies have shown that a substantial dose reduction can be achieved by limiting scan coverage to the area of interest [17]. In a large patient, reducing the scan length will also allow the user to increase the tube current in the area of interest so as to obtain better image quality.

Prospective ECG Triggering or ECG-Synchronized CT Acquisition

Most cardiac CT examinations are performed with retrospective electrocardiogram (ECG) gating so that images can be reconstructed at particular time points within the cardiac cycles with less motion. *Prospective ECG triggering* refers to the use of "step-and-shoot" or a non-spiral mode of acquisition of images in only predefined phases of cardiac cycles. In other words, with ECG triggering the x-ray tube emits x-rays only during a predefined portion (phase) of the R–R interval of the cardiac cycle, and is switched off during the remaining duration of the R–R interval. The ECG triggering relies on the average duration of the R–R interval in the prior three cardiac cycles. Therefore, in case of an irregular heart rate or a premature ventricular contraction, the estimation of the appropriate phase within the R–R interval will be inappropriate with ECG triggering, and it will not be possible to reconstruct images in other more appropriate phases. So if 60% of the R–R interval is the predefined phase, image data will be acquired only during that time in the cardiac cycle, and it will not be possible to reconstruct this in any other phase of the cardiac cycle. Several studies have shown that ECG triggering helps reduce radiation dose substantially with coronary artery calcium CT. Typical doses with prospective ECG triggering for coronary artery calcium CT have been reported to be 1 to 2 mSv, which is substantially lower than those associated with coronary CT angiography [1,10].

Most coronary CT angiography examinations are performed in a spiral mode to enable the acquisition of a volume data set while retaining the option of reconstructing images at more than one R–R interval for finding the "best phase" of coronary arteries, as well as for cardiac function analysis with multiphase reconstructions. Some vendors have proposed the successful use of prospective ECG triggering for coronary CT angiography in patients with very low and stable heart rates, which results in a substantial radiation dose savings, although comprehensive data is still awaited at this time. With this technique, it is also important to remember the phase limitation of ECG triggering as stated previously.

ECG Controlled Tube Current Modulation or ECG Pulsing

ECG pulsing is perhaps the most commonly used technique for radiation dose reduction for coronary CT angiography. As stated previously for ECG-gated coronary CT angiography, images are reconstructed at phases within the R–R interval with the least motion for coronary arteries. The ECG pulsing keeps the tube current at the highest level at the user-defined R–R interval and uses a lower tube current for the remaining phase. Typically, at our center ECG pulsing at 65% is performed for all patients with a regular heart rate of less than 65 beats per min. On Siemens multidetector CT (MDCT) scanners, CT scanning is performed at a user-specified full tube current, at a user-defined R–R interval, and is dropped by 80% for the remainder of the cardiac cycle. Other vendors (GE Healthcare and Philips Medical Systems) allow users to control the R–R interval range within which full tube current is desired, as well as the extent of tube current reduction for the remainder of the cardiac cycle. Also on the dual-source CT (Definition®, Siemens Medical Solutions), it is possible to specify these parameters or alternatively pick the system-recommended pulsing windows for full exposure estimated from the patients' heart rate [2]. These parameters allow the user to employ ECG pulsing even in the presence of a higher heart rate (more than 65 beats per minute) with a wider ECG pulsing window (for example, a pulsing window at 35 to 70% of the R–R interval at a heart rate of 80 beats per minute). Conversely, a tighter ECG pulsing window can be applied to save further radiation dose at slower heart rates with the dual-source CT (for example, a pulsing window at 50 to 60% of the R–R interval at a heart rate of 60 beats per minute). Thus, substantial dose savings are obtained in phases that are "less useful" for coronary arteries while maintaining full exposure and quality for the "most appropriate" phases. The extent of dose savings with ECG pulsing depends on the heart rate with greater savings at slower heart rates and vice versa (Figure 3.1). In this respect, the administration of beta-blockers can help in slowing the heart and can enhance the dose savings with ECG pulsing.

(a)

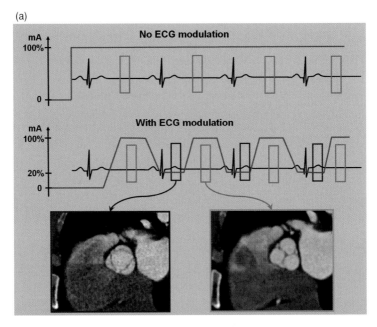

(b)

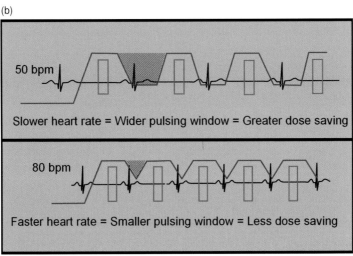

Fig. 3.1 (a) Without ECG pulsing, a constant specified tube current (100%) is used for CT. With ECG pulsing, the current drops during systole to about 20% of the specified current and rises back to 100% during the predefined diastolic reconstruction window. The low current during systole results in more noise (grainy image) compared to the diastolic noise level. (b) At slower heart rates, the duration for which lower current can be used (pulsing window) is wider compared to higher heart rates where there is less dose savings (blue area above the curve), resulting in greater radiation savings at lower heart rates.

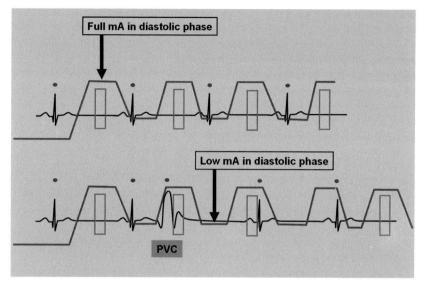

Fig. 3.2 ECG pulsing predicts the diastolic phase for full current based on the R–R interval of three prior cardiac cycles. Thus, a premature ventricular contraction causes an erroneous calculation of the R–R interval, which results in a low tube current in the diastolic phase, resulting in compromised image quality (diastolic images with high noise level).

Like prospective ECG triggering, ECG pulsing must also be avoided for patients with irregular or higher heart rates (Figure 3.2). With ECG pulsing, it may be possible to reconstruct images in other phases, but the images from other phases (that is, in the systolic phase) will have higher noise levels as they were acquired with 80% less x-ray tube output. Another concern with ECG pulsing is that functional multiphase reconstructions of the heart will have more noisy images (acquired at a lower dose) interspersed with less noisy images (acquired at full exposure). However, the data set is usually sufficient for cardiac function and valve evaluation as thicker images are reconstructed. The radiation dose reduction with the use of ECG pulsing is summarized in Table 3.4.

Automatic Pitch Adaptation

For MDCT scanners, the *pitch* is defined as the ratio of table travel per x-ray tube rotation divided by the total width of the active detector rows or the x-ray beam width. A pitch of less than 1.0 implies overlapping scan acquisition, whereas a pitch greater than 1.0 implies nonoverlapping scan acquisition. Generally, a small overlapping pitch (0.20 to 0.35) is selected for a single-source cardiac MDCT, so that images can be reconstructed from one or more cardiac cycles at relatively constant slice positions. A lower pitch implies greater overlap and longer scanning time. Conversely, a wider pitch implies less overlap and faster scanning.

For patients with slower heart rates, a wider pitch would reduce the extent of overlapping scan data due to the larger change in patient position by the time of the next cardiac cycle. This technique can make it difficult to do multisegmental reconstructions. Conversely, at faster heart rates, some scanners including the dual-source CT (Definition®) increase the pitch and thus reduce the radiation dose substantially [2]. Some scanners also adapt the pitch automatically to the heart rate. Recent studies have shown that pitch adaptation to patients' heart rate can result in radiation dose reduction up to 30 to 50%, with higher dose savings at higher heart rates [18]. For dual-source CT, the pitch can be dynamically adapted to a changing heart rate from 0.25 to 0.50.

Shielding

Recent studies suggest that bismuth-based breast shields can help in reducing radiation dose to the breasts by up to 37% without compromising image quality [16]. However, these shields are expensive and disposable to prevent the risk of transferring infections. Some authors have also recommended the displacing of breast tissues from the cardiac region of interest by using tapes to reduce the radiation dose to the breasts and decrease the amount of noise in the cardiac images [2].

Kilovoltage

The use of lower voltage (kV_p) reduces x-ray beam energy and therefore reduces radiation dose (Tables 3.3 and 3.4). Several studies have shown that a low voltage, less than the 120 kV_p used in most centers, can reduce radiation dose substantially without affecting diagnostic information for coronary artery calcium CT as well as for coronary CT angiography, particularly in small adults and children [11,12,15].

Tube Current

There is a linear relationship between radiation dose and tube current. Studies have shown that a lower tube current provides the same accuracy for coronary artery calcium CT as a higher current [13–15]. In general, when possible a lower tube current should be used for children and small adults. When non-ECG gated CT is being acquired for cardiac evaluation, one may use anatomically adapted automatic tube current modulation or adapt the tube current to patient weight to the reduce radiation dose. The anatomically adapted techniques automatically modulate tube current based on patient size, using lower tube currents for smaller patients and higher currents for larger patients.

Noise Based Approach

A recent study has also reported the use of a pre-scan single slice (120 kV_p and 20 mA) at the level of the left ventricle to measure image noise (standard deviation of the mean attenuation value) [2]. In this study, the authors used 80 to 100 kV_p and 700 mA for patients with lower noise (less than 20) on the pre-scan single slice, and 120 to 140 kV_p and 500 to 900 mA for noise equal to or greater than 20 [15].

Conclusions

The benefits to health from diagnostic imaging are well established. However, equally established is the need to minimize the possible deleterious effects from ionizing radiation that may be overprescribed or improperly applied. Several strategies can be adopted to reduce the radiation dose associated with cardiac CT studies. Most importantly, cardiac imagers must prospectively recognize opportunities for radiation dose reduction based on patients' age, size, clinical indication, and desired scan information.

References

1 Morin, R.L., Gerber, T.C., McCollough, C.H. (2003) Radiation dose in computed tomography of the heart. *Circulation* **107**: 917–922.

2 Paul, J.F., Abada, H.T. (2007) Strategies for reduction of radiation dose in cardiac multislice CT. *Eur Radiol* Feb 22; e-pub ahead of print.

3 Hunold, P., Vogt, F.M., Schmermund, A., *et al.* (2003) Radiation exposure during cardiac CT: effective doses at multi-detector row CT and electron-beam CT. *Radiology* **226**: 145–152.

4 Huda, W., Vance, A. (2007) Patient radiation doses from adult and pediatric CT. *AJR* **188**: 540–546.

5 Kalra, M.K., Maher, M.M., Toth, T.L., *et al.* (2004) Strategies for CT radiation dose optimization. *Radiology* **230**: 619–628.

6 Trianni, A., Chizzola, G., Toh, H., *et al.* (2005) Patient skin dosimetry in haemodynamic and electrophysiology interventional cardiology. *Radiat Prot Dosimetry* **117**: 241–246.

7 National Academy of Sciences/National Research Council. (1990) Health effects of exposure to low levels of ionizing radiation. Committee on the Biological Effects of Ionizing Radiation. BEIR V. Washington, DC: National Academy Press.

8 Koenig, T.R., Mettler, F.A., Wagner, L.K. (2001) Skin injuries from fluoroscopically guided procedures: part 2, review of 73 cases and recommendations for minimizing dose delivered to patient. *AJR* **177**: 13–20.

9 Preston, D.L., Shimizu, Y., Pierce, D.A., *et al.* (2003) Studies of mortality of atomic bomb survivors. Report 13: Solid cancer and noncancer disease mortality: 1950–1997. *Radiat Res* **160**: 381–407.

10 Knez, A., Becker, C.R., Becker, A., *et al.* (2002) Determination of coronary calcium with multi-slice spiral computed tomography: a comparative study with electron-beam CT. *Int J Cardiovasc Imaging* **18**: 295–303.

11 Thomas, C.K., Muhlenbruch, G., Wildberger, J.E., *et al.* (2006) Coronary artery calcium scoring with multislice computed tomography: in vitro assessment of a low tube voltage protocol. *Invest Radiol* **41**: 668–673.

12 Jakobs, T.F., Wintersperger, B.J., Herzog, P., *et al.* (2003) Ultra-low-dose coronary artery calcium screening using multislice CT with retrospective ECG gating. *Eur Radiol* **13**: 1923–1930.

13 Shemesh, J., Evron, R., Koren-Morag, N., *et al.* (2005) Coronary artery calcium measurement with multi-detector row CT and low radiation dose: comparison between 55 and 165 mAs. *Radiology* **236**: 810–814.

14 Mahnken, A.H., Wildberger, J.E., Simon, J., *et al.* (2003) Detection of coronary calcifications: feasibility of dose reduction with a body weight-adapted examination protocol. *AJR* **181**: 533–538.

15 Muhlenbruch, G., Hohl, C., Das, M., *et al.* (2007) Evaluation of automated attenuation-based tube current adaptation for coronary calcium scoring in MDCT in a cohort of 262 patients. *Eur Radiol* Feb 17; e-pub ahead of print.

16 Yilmaz, M.H., Yasar, D., Albayram, S., *et al.* (2007) Coronary calcium scoring with MDCT: the radiation dose to the breast and the effectiveness of bismuth breast shield. *Eur J Radiol* **61**: 139–143.

17 Campbell, J., Kalra, M.K., Rizzo, S., *et al.* (2005) Scanning beyond anatomic limits of the thorax in chest CT: findings, radiation dose, and automatic tube current modulation. *AJR* **185**: 1525–1530.

18 Johnson, T.R., Nikolaou, K., Wintersperger, B.J., *et al.* (2006) Dual-source CT cardiac imaging: initial experience. *Eur Radiol* **16**: 1409–1415.

Chapter 4

Safety Considerations of Current and Evolving CMR Techniques and Hardware*

Saman Nazarian, Henry R. Halperin, and David A. Bluemke

Due to unsurpassed soft tissue resolution, lack of ionizing radiation, and multiplanar imaging capability, magnetic resonance imaging (MRI) has become an important tool in the evaluation and treatment of cardiovascular disorders. However, an increasing proportion of patients with cardiovascular disease have higher acuity of disease, diminished organ function, and implanted devices with the potential for interaction with the MRI environment. Familiarity with safety issues is essential for radiologists and cardiologists performing MRI examinations in this population of patients.

The issues related to patient safety are frequently in flux either because of new implanted medical devices that have been developed or new safety concerns, as in the case of gadolinium contrast agents. The final decision to perform MRI is frequently made by considering the potential benefit of MRI relative to its attendant risks. Minimization of risk may additionally involve considerations of alternative methods of diagnostic imaging (e.g., computed tomography or ultrasound) relative to MRI. If multiple MRI scanners are available, the MRI risk may also be lower in low field strength magnets relative to high field units. Because of the wide range of circumstances encountered in the MRI suite, the descriptions that follow should not be construed as recommendations that are appropriate for all patients. The reader is therefore encouraged to consult web

---

* Portions of this chapter are adapted from Nazarian, S., Halperin, H.R., Bluemke, D.A. Safety and monitoring for cardiac magnetic resonance imaging. In: Kwong, R. (ed.), *Cardiovascular Magnetic Resonance Imaging*, Humana Press (in press).

Novel Techniques for Imaging the Heart, 1st edition. Edited by M. Di Carli and R. Kwong.
© 2008 American Heart Association, ISBN: 9-781-4051-7533-3.

sites from device manufacturers, those related to listings of device safety with MRI (e.g., http://www.mrisafety.com), standard handbooks for MRI safety, or the Food and Drug Administration (http://www.fda.gov) for specific information regarding individual devices and MRI contrast agents.

Patient Condition and Monitoring

Patients with cardiovascular disease are often referred for imaging in the setting of brady- and tachyarrhythmias, hypotension, myocardial ischemia, or congestive heart failure. Contrast administration, prolonged supine imaging, and interaction with implantable or temporary devices can lead to changes in the patient's condition during the MRI examination. Appropriate monitoring with continuous electrocardiogram (ECG) telemetry, pulse oximetry, and noninvasive blood pressure measurements, in addition to monitoring of patients symptoms, is essential. To perform an MRI scan with adequate margins of safety, some devices may have to be disabled, and patient monitoring is limited. To increase safety, steps must be taken to replace the disabled function of the device with a well-rehearsed plan for monitoring and treatment.

Given the potential risks listed here, it is essential to conduct a systematic review of the patient's physiological condition, implanted devices, and safety for MRI. At our institution, all patients are asked to review and answer a safety questionnaire (Figure 4.1). Note that these screening forms are unable to capture all information that is potentially relevant to MRI scanning but are intended to screen for possible devices. Specific questions that arise as a result of the screening form are to be followed by verbal questioning of the patient by the MRI technologist or physician. Additional detail regarding many of the points on this screening form are discussed further.

Gadolinium Contrast Agents

Gadolinium contrast agents are frequently used for magnetic resonance angiography (MRA) as well as for imaging the heart for myocardial scar, perfusion, or masses. Safety issues related to gadolinium contrast agents are discussed in detail in Chapter 2.

Potential for Interaction with Implanted Devices

Ferromagnetic materials in a magnetic field are subject to force and torque. The potential for movement of an implanted device in the MRI environment depends upon the magnetic field strength, the ferromagnetic properties of the material, the implant distance from the magnet bore, and the stability of the implant [1].

**THE JOHNS HOPKINS HOSPITAL
DEPARTMENT OF RADIOLOGY AND
RADIOLOGICAL SCIENCE**

MRI Patient Screening

for addressograph plate

This section is to be filled out by the PATIENT/ Patient representative. Please complete the following:

Programmable Shunt/shunt ☐Yes ☐ No		Tracheostomy ☐Yes ☐ No	
Epidural or Swan Ganz catheter ☐Yes ☐ No		Stimulator/Wires ☐Yes ☐ No	
Ear Implant ☐Yes ☐ No		Infusion Pump ☐Yes ☐ No	
Cochlear Implant ☐Yes ☐ No		Penile Prosthesis ☐Yes ☐ No	
Eye Implant ☐Yes ☐ No		IUD ☐Yes ☐ No	
Aneurysm Clips ☐Yes ☐ No		Surgical Clips ☐Yes ☐ No	
Pacemaker/wires ☐Yes ☐ No		Bullets, Pellets, BBs ☐Yes ☐ No	
Internal Defibrillator ☐Yes ☐ No		Medication Patch ☐Yes ☐ No	
Tissue expander ☐Yes ☐ No		Tattoo ☐Yes ☐ No	
Recent Stent Placement ☐Yes ☐ No		Artificial Limb ☐Yes ☐ No	
Blood Vessel Coil ☐Yes ☐ No		Other implanted metal or device _____	
*Kidney disease ☐Yes ☐ No		On dialysis ☐Yes ☐ No	
Liver or kidney transplant ☐Yes ☐ No		*Diabetes ☐Yes ☐ No	

*Age :_____   Weight (lbs):_____   Height :_____

Have you ever been a machinist, welder, or metal worker?   ☐Yes ☐ No

Have you ever had a facial injury from metal and/or metal removed
from your eyes?   ☐Yes ☐ No

Are you pregnant? (Last menstrual period _____)   ☐Yes ☐ No

Allergies? (specify):   _____

Current Medications: _____

Surgeries?   _____

Signature of person completing form: _____   Date: _____

This section is to be filled out by RADIOLOGY STAFF:

Orbit Films?   ☐Yes ☐ No   *Requires GFR?   ☐Yes ☐ No   GFR:_____

Disposition of valuables: ☐ Family member ☐ MRI Locker # _____   ☐ No valuables
                                                Patient/Family has key

Anyone with patient in the MRI room has been cleared for safety requirements?   ☐Yes ☐ No

MRI Technologist name: _____   Date: _____

Fig. 4.1 Sample patient safety questionnaire.

The radiofrequency and pulsed gradient magnetic fields in the MRI environment can induce electrical currents in leads and other ferromagnetic wires within the field. Implant length (versus the radiofrequency wavelength) and conformations such as loops favor the improved transition of energy to the implanted device, thus enhancing the risk of local heating. Repetitive radiofrequency pulses used in some MRI sequences can also lead to implant heating and tissue damage at the device-tissue interface.

Sophisticated electronic implants, such as those in neurostimulators, pacemakers, and implantable cardioverter defibrillators, have the potential for receiving electromagnetic interference in the MRI environment, resulting in programming changes or loss of function.

Cardiovascular Devices with Potential for Interaction with MRI

ECG Leads

Metallic telemetry leads used routinely for patient monitoring can induce artifacts and can heat up in the MRI environment, resulting in skin burns. Specially designed nonferromagnetic ECG leads and filtered monitoring systems have been designed for the MRI environment (e.g., S/5 MRI Monitor, Datex-Ohmeda, Finland). Such systems also offer continuous SpO_2 monitoring, which in our experience is an invaluable tool for monitoring of the cardiac rhythm, especially when the ECG signal — despite filtering — becomes unreadable in the setting of specific MRI pulse sequences.

Sternal Wires

Sternal wires used for closure after thoracotomy procedures are typically made of stainless steel, which is minimally ferromagnetic. Animal studies have suggested the safety of MRI use in this setting [2]. Over the course of 15 years in the authors' large acute care hospital setting, one patient had chest discomfort that was classified as "possibly" related to sternal wires; the MRI in this case was discontinued with the resolution of symptoms and no further complications. However, similar to any other metallic implant, sternal wires typically induce susceptibility artifacts in the immediate area and can limit imaging of the anterior right ventricle [3].

Epicardial Wires

Temporary epicardial pacing wires are routinely cut short at the skin and left in place after cardiac surgery. There are reports of the safe performance of MRI in patients with such retained temporary wires [4,5]. However, permanent epicardial pacing leads and patches placed at cardiac surgery have more ferromagnetic materials and are prone to heating in the MRI environment. Unlike endovascular leads, these devices are not cooled by the blood pool, and in experimental models up to 20°C of heating has been observed [6]. For this reason, at our institution we do not scan patients with permanent epicardial leads and patches. Temporary epicardial wires are removed prior to MRI whenever possible, but retained wires are not considered a contraindication to MRI.

Prosthetic Valves and Annuloplasty Rings

Studies to determine the force required to cause partial or total detachment of a heart valve prosthesis in patients with degenerative valvular disease have found that forces significantly higher than those induced at 4.7 T would be required to pull a suture through the valve annulus tissue [7]. The only prosthetic valves thought to have potential for experiencing enough force and torque to cause clinically concerning problems are the Star-Edwards pre-6000 series prostheses. Deflection measurements at 1.5 T revealed forces similar to peak forces exerted by the beating heart itself, leading to initial recommendations to exclude patients with this device series from MRI procedures. However, later studies revealed lower peak forces exerted even on this prosthetic series [8,9]. Mechanical valves do not appear to be prone to induced lead currents [10].

Although there are no reports of patient injury in the MRI environment due to the presence of a heart valve, there are theoretical concerns about MRI at 1.5 T and higher field strengths [9]. One such theoretical concern is the tendency of a metallic object to develop an opposing magnetic field to that in which it moves through (the Lenz effect). Such a secondary magnetic field may result in a resistive pressure to opening and closing of a disc prosthesis within the valve [11]. Björk-Shiley convex/concave heart valves (Shiley, Irvine, CA) are associated with an increased risk of mechanical failure due to outlet strut fracture. These valves are associated with large susceptibility artifacts under MRI and such artifacts may be increased in size in fractured valves [12].

Edwards *et al.* evaluated multiple heart valve prostheses for MRI-related forces in static fields up to 4.7 T. Most were found to be safe based on current criteria. However, valves made of Elgiloy — a Ni-Co-Cr base paramagnetic engineering material, such as the Carpentier-Edwards Physio® Ring — were found to be prone to rotational forces at such high field strengths [13,14].

Coronary Stents

In vitro studies have shown minimal heating of coronary stents in the MRI environment [15]. Stent dislodgement, even microdislodgement, is of theoretical concern due to the potential for dissection, embolism, and thrombosis. However, most stents are made of materials with little or no ferromagnetic materials such as stainless steel, nitinol (nickel/titanium alloy), or titanium. In vitro and in vivo studies of stent movement have shown minimal movement due to MRI [16,17]. Despite manufacturer recommendations to wait eight weeks after stent placement prior to imaging, no adverse effects have been noted due to MRI even in the acute post-stent period [18,19]. A study of acute MRI after deployment of drug-eluting coronary stents (TAXUS®, Boston Scientific, Natick, MA; and Cypher™, Cordis, New Brunswick, NJ) revealed no acute thrombosis and nine-month adverse events comparable to that expected without MRI [20]. In vitro testing of another drug-eluting stent (Endeavor™ cobalt alloy, Medtronic

Vascular, Santa Rosa, CA) has also been performed, revealing minor magnetic field interactions, heating (+0.5°C), and artifacts [21].

Coils

In vitro tests of nonferromagnetic platinum microcoils have revealed no coil migration and minimal susceptibility artifacts [22]. Three-dimensional time-of-flight MRI has been performed for follow-up of patients with Guglielmi detachable coils within a week post-deployment for treatment of intracranial aneurysms [23]. The substitution of digital subtraction angiography by MRI in this patient population was safe, produced minimal artifacts, and helped identify thromboembolic events associated with balloon-assisted deployment [24,25]. Chronic studies have revealed that time-of-flight MRI is not only safe but might indeed be more sensitive at identifying residual flow in coiled aneurysms than traditional plain radiographs and digital subtraction angiography [26,27]. In a recent case series of diffusion and perfusion MRI in patients with ruptured and unruptured intracranial aneurysms treated by intravascular coiling, no MRI-related complications were reported, and stents and platinum coils added negligible effects on the quality of images [28].

Filters

Initial testing of Greenfield filters for deflection at 1.5 Tesla found large variations in the amount of deflection experienced by each device [29]. However, in vivo studies showed no evidence of migration [29,30]. Although the stainless-steel filters such as Tulip and Bird's Nest filters cause extensive signal voids, the susceptibility artifacts associated with most filters appear to be minimal [31]. Imaging of the tantalum or titanium-alloy filters is associated with such minimal artifact that even intraluminal tilting of the device, post-filter turbulence, and thrombi trapped within the filters can be visualized [32–34].

Septal Defect Closure Devices

An in vitro study to evaluate the safety of 12 different occluders used to treat patients with patent ductus arteriosus, atrial septal defects, and ventricular septal defects in a 1.5-T system was performed by Shellock *et al.* Occluders made of 304 stainless steel were ferromagnetic and displayed deflection forces of 248 to 299 dynes, whereas those made of MP35n were nonferromagnetic. Artifacts were variable depending upon the type and amount of metal used to construct the implant. The authors recommended a waiting period of six weeks post-implant to allow tissue growth and a stronger implant tissue interface prior to MRI [35].

Guidewires, Angiography, and Electrophysiology Catheters

Guidewires are typically made from stainless steel or nitinol and are prone to heating and lead currents in the MRI environment. Angiography and electrophysiology catheters with any form of internal or external conductive wire may be prone to heating or induced lead currents, and are contraindicated in the MRI environment [1].

Swan-Ganz and Thermodilution Catheters

Swan-Ganz and thermodilution catheters contain long wires made of paramagnetic or magnetic materials, and the tip is not fixed. Therefore, they can be prone to movement, heating, and induction of current, and are not safe in the MRI environment [36].

Temporary Pacemakers

Unlike permanent devices, temporary pacemakers typically have unfixed leads and are more prone to movement. Furthermore, the leads are longer and can be more prone to induction of lead currents. Finally, the electronic platform of external temporary pacemakers is less sophisticated and has less filtering compared to modern implantable pacemakers. Temporary pacemakers are generally considered a contraindication to MRI.

Permanent Pacemakers and Implantable Cardioverter Defibrillators

It has been estimated that a patient with a pacemaker or implantable cardioverter defibrillator (ICD) has a 50 to 75% likelihood of having a clinically indicated MRI over the lifetime of their device [37]. The potential for movement of the device, programming changes, asynchronous pacing, activation of tachyarrhythmia therapies, inhibition of demand pacing, and induced lead currents leading to heating and cardiac stimulation have led to concerns from device manufacturers and MRI authorities regarding the performance of MRI procedures in cardiac implantable device recipients [1,38–45].

However, in recent years several case series have reported the safety of MRI in the setting of pacemakers [46–51]. A small case series has also reported neurological MRI in the setting of selected ICD systems [52]. Overall safety has been reported, but acute changes in battery voltage, lead thresholds, and programming can be seen [49,52].

We are currently evaluating a research protocol for MRI with these devices involving device selection based on previous in vitro and in vivo testing, device programming to minimize inappropriate activation or inhibition of brad/tachyarrhythmia therapies, and limitation of the specific absorption rate of MRI sequences (Figure 4.2) [6]. However, it is important to note that due to poor correlation of heating at different specific absorption rates across different scanners, even within the same manufacturer, the specific absorption rates from the authors' results should not be directly applied to other MRI systems [53].

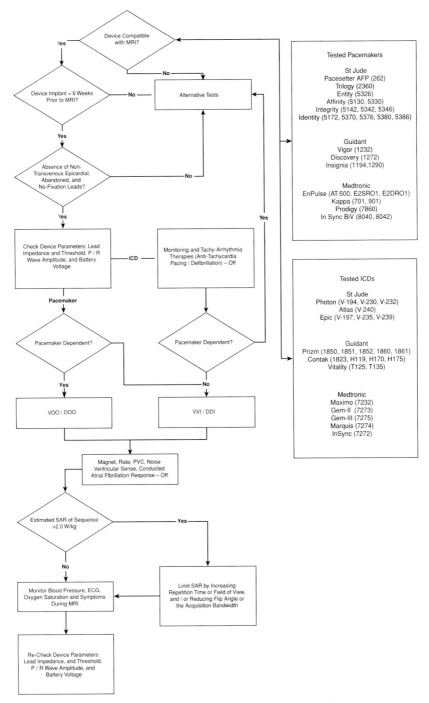

Fig. 4.2 Safety protocol for MRI of patients with permanent pacemakers and implantable defibrillators. Reprinted with permission from Nazarian, S., Roguin, A., Zviman, M.M., *et al.* (2006) *Circulation Sep* 19: **114**(12); 1277–1284.

Intra-aortic Balloon Pumps

Intra-aortic balloon pumps are considered to be a contraindication to MRI. More studies are needed to assess the safety of MRI in the setting of intra-aortic balloon counter-pulsation prior to human studies with MRI.

Ventricular Assist Devices

Ventricular assist devices have a high metal content, complicated circuitry, and in some cases magnetic field dependence for appropriate function. MRI is an absolute contraindication in patients with current ventricular assist devices.

Conclusions

As indications for the referral of patients for cardiovascular MRI evolve, acuity of illness and potential for interaction with implanted devices in those referred will likely increase. Although techniques for safe imaging in the setting of certain devices have been developed, the potential for catastrophic complications exists and dictates a high degree of vigilance for safe imaging. The reader is encouraged to consult web sites that provide more specific information regarding individual devices (e.g., http://www.mrisafety.com) for specific device testing details.

References

1 Prasad, S.K., Pennell, D.J. (2004) Safety of cardiovascular magnetic resonance in patients with cardiovascular implants and devices. *Heart* **90**(11): 1241–1244.

2 Manner, I., Alanen, A., Komu, M., *et al.* (1996) MR imaging in the presence of small circular metallic implants: assessment of thermal injuries. *Acta Radiol* **37**(4): 551–554.

3 Okamura, Y., Yamada, Y., Mochizuki, Y., *et al.* (1997) Evaluation of coronary artery bypass grafts with magnetic resonance imaging. *Nippon Kyobu Geka Gakkai Zasshi* **45**(6): 801–805.

4 Hartnell, G.G., Spence, L., Hughes, L.A., *et al.* (1997) Safety of MR imaging in patients who have retained metallic materials after cardiac surgery. *AJR* **168**(5): 1157–1159.

5 Murphy, K.J., Cohan, R.H., Ellis, J.H. (1999) MR imaging in patients with epicardial pacemaker wires. *AJR* **172**(3): 727–728.

6 Roguin, A., Zviman, M.M., Meininger, G.R., *et al.* (2004) Modern pacemaker and implantable cardioverter/defibrillator systems can be magnetic resonance imaging safe: in vitro and in vivo assessment of safety and function at 1.5 T. *Circulation* **110**(5): 475–482.

7 Edwards, M.B., Draper, E.R., Hand, J.W., *et al.* (2005) Mechanical testing of human cardiac tissue: some implications for MRI safety. *J Cardiovasc Magn Reson* **7**(5): 835–840.

8 Soulen, R.L., Budinger, T.F., Higgins, C.B. (1985) Magnetic resonance imaging of prosthetic heart valves. *Radiology* **154**(3): 705–707.

9 Shellock, F.G. (2002) Magnetic resonance safety update 2002: implants and devices. *J Magn Reson Imaging* **16**(5): 485–496.

10 Shellock, F.G. (2001) Prosthetic heart valves and annuloplasty rings: assessment of magnetic field interactions, heating, and artifacts at 1.5 Tesla. *J Cardiovasc Magn Reson* **3**(4): 317–324.

11 Condon, B., Hadley, D.M. (2000) Potential MR hazard to patients with metallic heart valves: the Lenz effect. *J Magn Reson Imaging* **12**(1): 171–176.

12 van Gorp, M.J., van der Graaf, Y., de Mol, B.A., *et al.* (2004) Bjork-Shiley convexoconcave valves: susceptibility artifacts at brain MR imaging and mechanical valve fractures. *Radiology* **230**(3): 709–714.

13 Ho, J.C., Shellock, F.G. (1999) Magnetic properties of Ni-Co-Cr-base Elgiloy. *J Mater Sci Mater Med* **10**(9): 555–560.

14 Edwards, M.B., Ordidge, R.J., Hand, J.W., *et al.* (2005) Assessment of magnetic field (4.7 T) induced forces on prosthetic heart valves and annuloplasty rings. *J Magn Reson Imaging* **22**(2): 311–317.

15 Strohm, O., Kivelitz, D., Gross, W., *et al.* (1999) Safety of implantable coronary stents during 1H-magnetic resonance imaging at 1.0 and 1.5 T. *J Cardiovasc Magn Reson* **1**(3): 239–245.

16 Scott, N.A., Pettigrew, R.I. (1994) Absence of movement of coronary stents after placement in a magnetic resonance imaging field. *Am J Cardiol* **73**(12): 900–901.

17 Hug, J., Nagel, E., Bornstedt, A., *et al.* (2000) Coronary arterial stents: safety and artifacts during MR imaging. *Radiology* **216**(3): 781–787.

18 Kramer, C.M., Rogers, W.J., Jr., Pakstis, D.L. (2000) Absence of adverse outcomes after magnetic resonance imaging early after stent placement for acute myocardial infarction: a preliminary study. *J Cardiovasc Magn Reson* **2**(4): 257–261.

19 Gerber, T.C., Fasseas, P., Lennon, R.J., *et al.* (2003) Clinical safety of magnetic resonance imaging early after coronary artery stent placement. *J Am Coll Cardiol* **42**(7): 1295–1298.

20 Porto, I., Selvanayagam, J., Ashar, V., *et al.* (2005) Safety of magnetic resonance imaging one to three days after bare metal and drug-eluting stent implantation. *Am J Cardiol* **96**(3): 366–368.

21 Shellock, F.G., Forder, J.R. (2005) Drug eluting coronary stent: in vitro evaluation of magnet resonance safety at 3 Tesla. *J Cardiovasc Magn Reson* **7**(2): 415–419.

22 Marshall, M.W., Teitelbaum, G.P., Kim, H.S., Deveikis, J. (1991) Ferromagnetism and magnetic resonance artifacts of platinum embolization microcoils. *Cardiovasc Intervent Radiol* **14**(3): 163–166.

23 Okahara, M., Kiyosue, H., Hori, Y., *et al.* (2004) Three-dimensional time-of-flight MR angiography for evaluation of intracranial aneurysms after endosaccular packing with Guglielmi detachable coils: comparison with 3D digital subtraction angiography. *Eur Radiol* **14**(7): 1162–1168.

24 Soeda, A., Sakai, N., Sakai, H., *et al.* (2003) Thromboembolic events associated with Guglielmi detachable coil embolization of asymptomatic cerebral aneurysms: evaluation of 66 consecutive cases with use of diffusion-weighted MR imaging. *Am J Neuroradiol* **24**(1): 127–132.

25 Albayram, S., Selcuk, H., Kara, B., *et al.* (2004) Thromboembolic events associated with balloon-assisted coil embolization: evaluation with diffusion-weighted MR imaging. *Am J Neuroradiol* **25**(10): 1768–1777.

26 Cottier, J.P., Bleuzen-Couthon, A., Gallas, S., *et al.* (2003) Follow-up of intracranial aneurysms treated with detachable coils: comparison of plain radiographs, 3D time-of-flight MRA and digital subtraction angiography. *Neuroradiology* **45**(11): 818–824.

27 Yamada, N., Hayashi, K., Murao, K., *et al.* (2004) Time-of-flight MR angiography targeted to coiled intracranial aneurysms is more sensitive to residual flow than is digital subtraction angiography. *Am J Neuroradiol* **25**(7): 1154–1157.

28 Cronqvist, M., Wirestam, R., Ramgren, B., *et al.* (2005) Diffusion and perfusion MRI in patients with ruptured and unruptured intracranial aneurysms treated by endovascular coiling: complications, procedural results, MR findings and clinical outcome. *Neuroradiology* **47**(11): 855–873.

29 Williamson, M.R., McCowan, T.C., Walker, C.W., Ferris, E.J. (1988) Effect of a 1.5-Tesla magnetic field on Greenfield filters in vitro and in dogs. *Angiology* **39**(12): 1022–1024.

30 Liebman, C.E., Messersmith, R.N., Levin, D.N., Lu, C.T. (1988) MR imaging of inferior vena caval filters: safety and artifacts. *AJR* **150**(5): 1174–1176.

31 Honda, M., Obuchi, M., Sugimoto, H. (2003) Artifacts of vena cava filters ex vivo on MR angiography. *Magn Reson Med Sci* **2**(2): 71–77.

32 Teitelbaum, G.P., Ortega, H.V., Vinitski, S., *et al.* (1988) Low-artifact intravascular devices: MR imaging evaluation. *Radiology* **168**(3): 713–719.

33 Teitelbaum, G.P., Ortega, H.V., Vinitski, S., *et al.* (1990) Optimization of gradient-echo imaging parameters for intracaval filters and trapped thromboemboli. *Radiology* **174**(3 Pt 2): 1013–1019.

34 Grassi, C.J., Matsumoto, A.H., Teitelbaum, G.P. (1992) Vena caval occlusion after Simon nitinol filter placement: identification with MR imaging in patients with malignancy. *J Vasc Interv Radiol* **3**(3): 535–539.

35 Shellock, F.G., Morisoli, S.M. (1994) Ex vivo evaluation of ferromagnetism and artifacts of cardiac occluders exposed to a 1.5-T MR system. *J Magn Reson Imaging* **4**(2): 213–215.

36 Ahmed, S., Shellock, F.G. (2001) Magnetic resonance imaging safety: implications for cardiovascular patients. *J Cardiovasc Magn Reson* **3**(3): 171–182.

37 Kalin, R., Stanton, M.S. (2005) Current clinical issues for MRI scanning of pacemaker and defibrillator patients. *Pacing Clin Electrophysiol* **28**(4): 326–328.

38 Shellock, F.G., Tkach, J.A., Ruggieri, P.M., Masaryk, T.J. (2003) Cardiac pacemakers, ICDs, and loop recorder: evaluation of translational attraction using conventional ("long-bore") and "short-bore" 1.5- and 3.0-Tesla MR systems. *J Cardiovasc Magn Reson* **5**(2): 387–397.

39 Erlebacher, J.A., Cahill, P.T., Pannizzo, F., Knowles, R.J. (1986) Effect of magnetic resonance imaging on DDD pacemakers. *Am J Cardiol* **57**(6): 437–440.

40 Hayes, D.L., Holmes, D.R., Jr., Gray, J.E. (1987) Effect of 1.5-tesla nuclear magnetic resonance imaging scanner on implanted permanent pacemakers. *J Am Coll Cardiol* **10**(4): 782–786.

41 Smith, J.M. (2005) Industry viewpoint: Guidant: pacemakers, ICDs, and MRI. *Pacing Clin Electrophysiol* **28**(4): 264.

42 Stanton, M.S. (2005) Industry viewpoint: Medtronic: pacemakers, ICDs, and MRI. *Pacing Clin Electrophysiol* **28**(4): 265.

43 Levine, P.A. (2005) Industry viewpoint: St. Jude Medical: pacemakers, ICDs and MRI. *Pacing Clin Electrophysiol* **28**(4): 266–267.

44 Shellock, F.G., Crues, J.V. (2004) MR procedures: biologic effects, safety, and patient care. *Radiology* **232**(3): 635–652.

45 Faris, O.P., Shein, M.J. (2005) Government viewpoint: U.S. Food & Drug Administration: pacemakers, ICDs and MRI. *Pacing Clin Electrophysiol* **28**(4): 268–269.

46 Gimbel, J.R., Johnson, D., Levine, P.A., Wilkoff, B.L. (1996) Safe performance of magnetic resonance imaging on five patients with permanent cardiac pacemakers. *Pacing Clin Electrophysiol* **19**(6): 913–919.

47 Sommer, T., Vahlhaus, C., Lauck, G., *et al.* (2000) MR imaging and cardiac pacemakers: in-vitro evaluation and in-vivo studies in 51 patients at 0.5 T. *Radiology* **215**(3): 869–879.

48 Vahlhaus, C., Sommer, T., Lewalter, T., *et al.* (2001) Interference with cardiac pacemakers by magnetic resonance imaging: are there irreversible changes at 0.5 Tesla? *Pacing Clin Electrophysiol* **24**(4 Pt 1): 489–495.

49 Martin, E.T., Coman, J.A., Shellock, F.G., *et al.* (2004) Magnetic resonance imaging and cardiac pacemaker safety at 1.5 Tesla. *J Am Coll Cardiol* **43**(7): 1315–1324.

50 Del Ojo, J.L., Moya, F., Villalba, J., *et al.* (2005) Is magnetic resonance imaging safe in cardiac pacemaker recipients? *Pacing Clin Electrophysiol* **28**(4): 274–278.

51 Shellock, F.G., Fieno, D.S., Thomson, L.J., *et al.* (2006) Cardiac pacemaker: in vitro assessment at 1.5 T. *Am Heart J* **151**(2): 436–443.

52 Gimbel, J.R., Kanal, E., Schwartz, K.M., Wilkoff, B.L. (2005) Outcome of magnetic resonance imaging (MRI) in selected patients with implantable cardioverter defibrillators (ICDs). *Pacing Clin Electrophysiol* **28**(4): 270–273.

53 Nazarian, S., Roguin, A., Zviman, M.M., *et al.* (2006) Clinical utility and safety of a protocol for noncardiac and cardiac magnetic resonance imaging of patients with permanent pacemakers and implantable-cardioverter defibrillators at 1.5 Tesla. *Circulation* **114**(12): 1277–1284.

PART II

Clinical Applications of CT and CMR Imaging

Chapter 5

Evaluating the Symptomatic Patient with Suspected CAD

Bernhard L. Gerber

In addition to evaluating asymptomatic patients for cardiovascular risks, cardiologists are also often confronted to evaluate symptomatic patients for suspected coronary artery disease (CAD). The question of whether an individual patient does or does not have CAD may arise in different clinical settings. Most commonly, CAD is suspected in patients complaining of stable exercise-induced chest pain. However, evaluation for CAD is even more important in patients with acute chest pain presenting to the emergency room. It is also important in patients prior to cardiac valve surgery and in patients undergoing high-risk noncardiac surgery.

Presently, the reference standard for diagnosis of CAD remains cardiac catheterization and coronary angiography. However, the invasive nature and associated risks and costs of this test limit its use to patients with a high suspicion of CAD. Therefore, symptomatic patients are generally investigated first using noninvasive tests for detection of myocardial ischemia, such as exercise electrocardiogram (ECG), nuclear scintigraphy, or stress echocardiography. Newer imaging techniques such as multidetector computed tomography (MDCT) and cardiac magnetic resonance (CMR) are very promising alternatives for the noninvasive evaluation of patients with suspected CAD as they can noninvasively image the coronary arteries and directly reveal the presence of atherosclerosis. In addition, CMR offers the ability to detect myocardial ischemia either as perfusion abnormalities during a vasodilatation stress test or as wall motion abnormalities during the infusion of dobutamine. Both CMR and MDCT can also demonstrate the consequences of CAD, such as regional wall motion abnormalities or myocardial necrosis.

Novel Techniques for Imaging the Heart, 1st edition. Edited by M. Di Carli and R. Kwong.
© 2008 American Heart Association, ISBN: 9-781-4051-7533-3.

Evaluation of Patients with Stable Chest Pain

Stable exercise-induced angina pectoris in the setting of chronic CAD is associated with a relatively good prognosis and a fairly low overall risk of mortality or myocardial infarction (MI) [1]. However, there are clear individual variations of risk. Therefore, it is important to identify high-risk patients (e.g., multivessel disease), particularly if they present with significant left ventricular dysfunction or heart failure. In such high-risk patients, their clinical outcomes can be improved by revascularization therapy. By contrast, revascularization does not affect survival in other lower-risk patients with stable chest pain, but it is more efficient than medical treatment in alleviating symptoms.

Current guidelines suggest a stepwise approach for the assessment of patients with stable chest pain. Symptomatic patients with a high probability of CAD should be directly referred for cardiac catheterization. In patients with an intermediate probability, noninvasive stress tests are proposed to exclude chest pain from noncardiac causes from CAD. Both MDCT and CMR have been well studied in this setting of patients with stable chest pain.

Coronary Calcification on Unenhanced EBCT or MDCT

Because coronary calcium is absent in normal coronary arteries but commonly present in the advanced stages of atherosclerosis, it has been hypothesized that the identification of coronary calcification on unenhanced electron beam computed tomography (EBCT) or MDCT might be helpful for revealing obstructive CAD in patients with chest pain. As discussed in more detail in Chapter 16, this approach appears to work in at-risk, screening populations [2,3]. However, because noncalcified plaques can also be obstructive, it may not be as reliable in patients with chest pain as a low calcium score or its absence may not be able to exclude noncalcified, albeit significant, CAD [4]. In addition, the specificity for excluding obstructive coronary stenosis in patients with a high calcium score is low (45 to 66%). This result is due to the fact that coronary calcification may already be present in nonobstructive coronary plaques.

Contrast-Enhanced MDCT

MDCT offers the unique ability to directly and noninvasively visualize the presence of coronary atherosclerosis. With the latest generation of 64-slice MDCT systems, it is possible to image the entire coronary tree, including small branch vessels, with excellent image quality. An overall success rate of more than 95% and a high diagnostic accuracy for the identification of CAD compared to invasive coronary angiography on a per-patient basis has been reported (Table 5.1). In the populations studied with a high prevalence of CAD, the test is especially interesting because of its high negative predictive value. Indeed, a normal coronary MDCT scan reliably excludes the probability of significant CAD,

Table 5.1 Diagnostic Accuracies of 64/40-Slice CT for the Detection of CAD on a Per-Patient Basis in Patients with Chronic Chest Pain

CT	Patients	Prevalence of CAD	Sensitivity	Specificity	PPV	NPV	Accuracy
Leber [53]	45	56%	88%	100%	100%	87%	93%
Raff [5]	70	57%	95%	90%	93%	93%	93%
Leschka [54]	67	70%	100%	100%	100%	100%	100%
Mollet [55]	52	73%	100%	93%	97%	100%	98%
Pugliese [56]	35	71%	100%	90%	96%	100%	97%
Muhlenbruch [57]	51	88%	98%	50%	94%	75%	92%
Ehara [58]	67	90%	98%	86%	98%	86%	97%
Schuijf [59]	60	52%	94%	97%	97%	93%	95%
Watkins [60]	85	53%	98%	93%	94%	97%	95%
Ghostine [61]	66	44%	97%	95%	93%	97%	95%
Scheffel [62]	30	50%	93%	100%	100%	94%	97%
Shapiro [63]	32	84%	96%	100%	100%	83%	97%
All	660	65%	97%	94%	97%	94%	96%

and could thus avoid invasive coronary angiography or other noninvasive tests (Figure 5.1). However, the relatively limited spatial resolution (compared to invasive coronary angiography) prevents MDCT from providing exact, quantitative measures of stenosis severity, especially in the presence of extensive coronary calcification, where MDCT can overestimate the severity of coronary

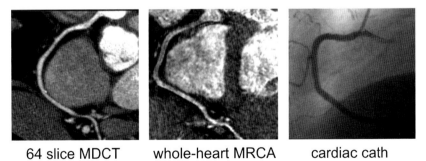

64 slice MDCT   whole-heart MRCA   cardiac cath

Fig. 5.1 An example of direct coronary imaging of a normal coronary artery by MDCT, whole-heart MRCA, and its comparison to coronary angiography.

stenosis [5]. Therefore, many studies have excluded severely calcified vessels from their analysis. Another major limitation is that because of the need of retrospective ECG gating, MDCT is limited to image patients with irregular heart rhythms, such as those with atrial fibrillation or premature heart beats.

Magnetic Resonance Coronary Angiography

Similar to MDCT, direct magnetic resonance coronary angiography (MRCA) has also been proposed for the detection of CAD in patients with chest pain. Chapter 14 includes a detailed discussion of the relative merits of CT and magnetic resonance imaging (MRI) for evaluating the coronary arteries. Currently, the best image quality is obtained using three-dimensional steady-state free precession (SSFP) bright blood pulse sequences and free-breathing respirator navigator gating [6]. Most recently, it was proposed to perform whole-heart imaging — i.e., the acquisition of one large stack of axial images — which, similar to MDCT, can be reformatted to follow the complex course or the coronary arteries [7]. This technique obviated the need for the localization of individual coronary arteries and substantially accelerated and simplified image acquisition. Despite these technical improvements, MRCA still remains technically more challenging to perform than MDCT. Compared to MDCT, relatively fewer studies have evaluated the diagnostic accuracy of MRCA in patients with chest pain (Table 5.2). Although the success rate and diagnostic accuracy of MRCA has certainly improved over time, it remains lower than that of MDCT. In 2001, a large multicenter trial using an older gradient echo imaging technique with individual localization of coronary arteries reported that only 83% of proximal and mid-coronary segments were interpretable, and that sensitivity for detection of CAD on a per-patient basis was high (93%) but specificity was very low (43%) [8]. Currently, using the most recent whole-heart MRCA technique, 83% to 94% of all coronary segments including side branches and small vessels were reported interpretable, whereas sensitivity and specificity on a segmental basis were 78 to 82% and 91 to 96%, respectively [9,10]. On a per-patient basis, a pooled analysis of seven studies involving a total of 483 patients showed an average sensitivity for MRCA of 84% and a specificity of 73% (Table 5.3). The advantage of MRCA over MDCT is that the technique does not use ionizing radiation or injection of a contrast agent to image the coronary arteries, as contrast is obtained from spontaneous difference in T2/T1 times. Currently, the major limitation of MRCA remains the low signal-to-noise ratio and lower spatial resolution than MDCT. Another important limitation of MRCA is the long acquisition time (20 min) and high failure rates (15 to 20%) due to navigator drift. It is hoped that 3-T systems, newer cardiac coils with greater numbers of elements, parallel imaging techniques, as well as intravascular contrast agents may allow a step-up in signal-to-noise ratio, spatial resolution, and acquisition speed.

Table 5.2 Diagnostic Accuracies of MRCA for the Detection of CAD on a Per-Patient Basis in Patients with Chronic Chest Pain

Source	Technique	Patients	Prevalence of CAD	Sensitivity	Specificity	PPV	NPV	Accuracy
Kim [64]	Gradient echo-localized	103	58%	93%	42%	69%	82%	72%
Bogaert [65]	Localized SSFP	19	32%	85/92%	83/50%	72/75%	92/80%	84/79%
Dewey [66]	Localized SSFP	108	56%	69%	74%	78%	65%	71%
Kefer [32]	Localized SSFP	52	65%	88%	50%	77%	69%	75%
Sakuma [67]	Whole-heart SSFP	20	60%	83%	75%	83%	75%	80%
Sakuma [68]	Whole-heart SSFP	113	45%	82%	90%	88%	86%	87%
Pouleur [51]	Whole-heart SSFP	68	22%	100%	81%	60%	100%	85%
All	—	483	49%	84%	73%	75%	82%	78%

Table 5.3 Diagnostic Accuracy of Dobutamine Stress CMR for the Detection of CAD on a Per-Patient Basis in Patients with Chronic Chest Pain

Source	Technique	Patients	Prevalence of CAD	Sensitivity	Specificity	PPV	NPV	Accuracy
Nagel [11]	GRE	172	63%	86%	86%	91%	78%	86%
Hundley [12]	GRE	41	73%	83%	83%	97%	45%	83%
Schalla [69]	EPI/Realtime	22	73%	81/88%	83%	93%	63/71%	82/86%
Paetsh [30]	SSFP	79	67%	89%	81%	90%	78%	86%
Jahnke [70]	KTBLAST-SSFP	40	70%	89%	83%	93%	77%	88%
All		354	67%	87%	84%	92%	75%	86%

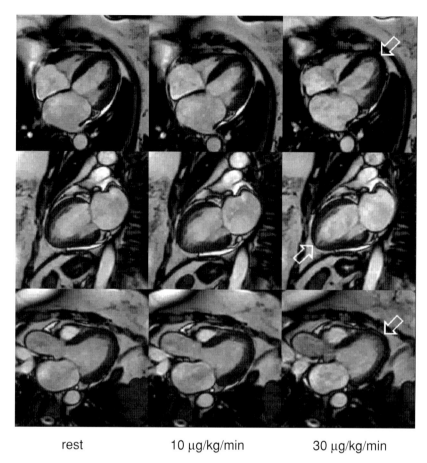

| rest | 10 μg/kg/min | 30 μg/kg/min |

Fig. 5.2 An example of dobutamine stress magnetic resonance in a patient with stenosis of the mid-LAD, showing ischemia in the apical and anterior region at high-dose infusion (arrow). See video clip 1 ⊙.

Dobutamine Stress CMR

Similar to stress echocardiography, high-dose dobutamine stress magnetic resonance can detect CAD by demonstrating inducible wall motion abnormalities in myocardial territories subtended by significant epicardial stenoses (Figure 5.2). The major advantage of dobutamine CMR over dobutamine echocardiography is better image quality and a sharper definition of endocardial borders against blood pool. Consequently, dobutamine CMR appears to have a higher diagnostic accuracy than dobutamine echocardiography for the detection of CAD, especially in patients with a poor acoustic window [11,12]. The overall diagnostic accuracy of dobutamine CMR for the detection of CAD in symptomatic patients

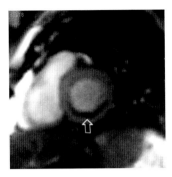

Fig. 5.3 An example of dipyridamole perfusion magnetic resonance showing an inferior perfusion defect (arrow) in a patient with stenosis of the right coronary artery. See video clip 2 ⟨👁⟩. Courtesy of Jerome Garot, Hopital Mondor, Paris, France.

on a per-patient basis was found to be high (Table 5.3). Several studies have shown that dobutamine stress CMR can also predict prognosis in patients with chest pain [12–15]. Indeed, patients with a negative dobutamine stress test have an excellent prognosis, with a very low rate of cardiovascular events. A limitation of high-dose dobutamine stress CMR is that it bears the potential risk of severe side effects, such as hypotension, and severe ventricular arrhythmias, in the inhospitable environment of the magnetic resonance scanner; therefore, it requires the availability of trained personnel and resuscitation facilities. Fortunately, severe complications only occur very infrequently. Indeed, in a series of 1000 consecutive dobutamine magnetic resonance studies, only seven severe nonlethal complications were observed. All of them resolved after stopping the infusion of the drug [16,17].

Myocardial Perfusion CMR

Similar to nuclear imaging, perfusion CMR allows the detection of suspected CAD in patients with chest pain by demonstrating perfusion defects during maximal coronary vasodilation induced by the infusion of either dipyridamole or adenosine (Figure 5.3). Several single-center studies and two multicenter studies have reported high diagnostic accuracy (Table 5.4) of stress perfusion CMR imaging for the detection of CAD in patients with chest pain [18,19]. The advantage of perfusion CMR over single photon emission computed tomography (SPECT) is its clearly greater spatial resolution, allowing the detection of subendocardial defects that can be missed by SPECT [20]. The major limitation of perfusion CMR is the common presence of so-called "dark-rim" artifacts, which may cause false positive readings. Some authors have proposed adding a delayed enhancement in a stepwise interpretation algorithm to avoid false positive readings [21]. Accordingly, fixed perfusion defects without delayed enhancement are interpreted as artifacts, whereas the presence of

Table 5.4 Diagnostic Accuracy of Perfusion Magnetic Resonance for the Detection of CAD on a Per-Patient Basis in Patients with Chronic Chest Pain

Author	Remarks	Patients	Prevalence of CAD	Sensitivity	Specificity	PPV	NPV	Accuracy
Schwitter [71]	Semiquantitative analysis (up-slope)	57	65%	86%	85%	91%	77%	86%
Nagel [72]	Semiquantitative analysis (up-slope)	84	51%	88%	90%	90%	88%	89%
Ishida [20]	Visual analysis	104	74%	90%	85%	95%	74%	88%
Wolff [19]	Visual analysis, low-dose group	26	54%	93%	75%	81%	90%	85%
Giang [18]	Semiquantitative analysis (up-slope) Groups 2 and 3	44	64%	93%	75%	87%	86%	86%
Paetsh [30]	Visual analysis	79	67%	91%	62%	83%	76%	81%
Plein [73]	Semiquantitative analysis (up-slope)	92	64%	88%	82%	90%	79%	86%
Sakuma [29]	Visual analysis	40	53%	81%	68%	74%	76%	75%
Klem [21]	Visual analysis of perfusion and late images	92	40%	89%	87%	83%	92%	88%
All		618	60%	89%	81%	87%	83%	86%

delayed enhancement identifies true perfusion abnormalities related to MI. In one study, specificity (87% versus 58%) and overall diagnostic accuracy (88% versus 68%) was significantly improved when delayed enhancement was employed in this way to identify artifacts [21]. A current point of debate is whether perfusion CMR exams should be analyzed only visually or using semiquantitative indices such as regional signal up-slope. Absolute quantification has also been proposed but currently remains too tedious for general clinical practice. Perfusion CMR commonly engenders mild side effects such as flushing, mild chest discomfort, or headaches. Severe side effects such as angina pectoris, MI, auricular-ventricular conduction blocks, bronchospasm, and cerebral hypoperfusion are fortunately rare (less than 1%) and usually self-limiting after stopping infusion of the drug. Similar to dobutamine stress magnetic resonance, perfusion CMR however requires careful monitoring of patients and the availability of resuscitation equipment.

Additional Parameters of Importance in Patients with Chest Pain: Resting Function and Myocardial Necrosis

The assessment of resting contractile function and the detection of myocardial necrosis provides additional important information in patients with suspected CAD [22]. Indeed, the prognosis in patients with CAD is largely predicted by impaired resting left ventricular function. Both CMR cine imaging and, more recently, MDCT can accurately measure left ventricular volumes and ejection fractions [23]. Given the important prognostic value of left ventricular function and cavity size in patients with CAD, these parameters should be systematically assessed in all patients with suspected CAD that undergo MDCT, MRCA, perfusion, or stress CMR. The detection of myocardial necrosis is also important in the setting of chronic CAD. Kwong *et al.* demonstrated in 195 patients with symptoms of suspected CAD that the previously unrecognized presence of myocardial necrosis was the single strongest predictor of major cardiovascular events and mortality [24]. Infarct characterization has also recently been demonstrated to be feasible using MDCT, but prognostic information of infarct detection by MDCT has not yet been reported [25,26].

Relative Accuracy of Noninvasive Approaches to the Diagnosis of CAD

Figure 5.4 compares the accuracy of different noninvasive tests for diagnosing obstructive CAD. This comparison suggests that perfusion and dobutamine CMR have similar high diagnostic sensitivity and specificity, which is slightly greater than that reported for stress SPECT and ECG stress testing but similar to stress positron emission tomography (PET) perfusion imaging [27,28]. MDCT appears to have the greatest sensitivity and specificity of all tests. In contrast, MRCA appears to be more limited than either MDCT, stress perfusion, or dobutamine stress CMR. Of course, such comparison of pooled data is limited by the inclusion of patient populations with different clinical characteristics and

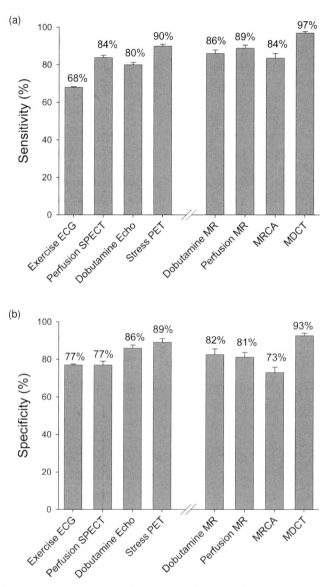

Fig. 5.4 A comparison of the (a) sensitivities and (b) specificities of tests on a per-patient basis. The diagnostic accuracy for exercise ECG, nuclear scintigraphy, stress echocardiography, and stress PET were derived from Schinkel *et al.*, Di Carli and Hachamovitch, and Gianrossi *et al.*, respectively [27,28,52].

different inclusion and exclusion criteria. So far, there are only a few head-to-head comparisons between tests in the same patient population, and no study has compared all tests against each other. For example, one study reported a greater diagnostic accuracy for dobutamine CMR than for dobutamine echocardiography [11]. In another study, perfusion CMR was found to have a greater diagnostic accuracy than stress SPECT for the detection of significant CAD [20]. However, in another smaller study the diagnostic accuracy for perfusion CMR and for ^{201}Tl SPECT was similar [29]. In direct comparison, dobutamine stress CMR was superior to adenosine stress cine CMR [30]. Also, the diagnostic accuracy and specificity of dobutamine stress CMR appeared greater than that of perfusion CMR. Finally, four different studies compared the diagnostic accuracies of MRCA and MDCT. In the first study, comparing 4-slice MDCT to MRCA, MDCT had greater sensitivity, whereas MRCA had greater specificity and overall diagnostic accuracy [31]. In another study comparing 16-slice MDCT to MRCA with individually localized coronaries, and restricting comparisons to patients that successfully completed both tests, there was no statistically significant difference in sensitivity, specificity, or diagnostic accuracy between these tests [32]. In another study, 16-slice MDCT had greater sensitivity (82% versus 54%, $p < 0.001$) for detecting clinically significant stenosis because of the greater failure rate of MRCA [33]. However, the specificity of MDCT and MRCA was similar (90% versus 87%, $p = NS$). In the most recent comparison of 64-slice MDCT and whole-heart MRCA, MDCT allowed the identification of more diseased segments (97%) than MRCA (73%) [34]. If noninterpretable segments were excluded, MRCA and MDCT had similar sensitivity, specificity, and diagnostic accuracy for the detection of CAD. However, if noninterpretable segments were considered in the analysis, MRCA had lower sensitivity (71% versus 92%, $p < 0.001$), lower specificity (68% versus 92%, $p < 0.001$), and lower diagnostic accuracy (68% versus 92%, $p < 0.001$) for the detection of coronary stenosis than MDCT.

Selecting a Testing Strategy for Patients with Suspected CAD

Current guidelines suggest a stepwise approach for the assessment of patients with stable chest pain based on Bayesian analysis of pre-test probability of disease. Indeed, the clinical value of any test will be greatest in patients with an intermediate likelihood of disease [35]. Patients whose clinical presentation suggests a very high (e.g., typical chest pain and an unambiguously positive stress test) or very low (young patients with nonanginal chest pain) probability of CAD will benefit very little from even the most powerful test. The new imaging techniques MDCT and CMR compete with well-established techniques for the detection of CAD, such as exercise ECG, nuclear cardiology, and stress echocardiography. The relative clinical utility of anatomic and functional tests is discussed in more detailed in Chapter 10. It is possible that stress ECG, stress SPECT, or stress echocardiography may remain a first line of investigation for

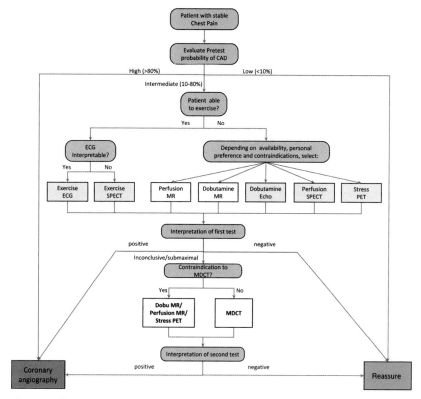

Fig. 5.5 A flow diagram illustrating the potential place perfusion and dobutamine stress CMR and MDCT (yellow) could occupy in a stepwise approach for the assessment of patients with stable chest pain suspected to result from CAD. Perfusion and stress magnetic resonance could be used in patients unable to exercise as an alternative to dobutamine echocardiography, perfusion SPECT, and stress PET. The tests could also be used as second-line tests when first-line stress tests are inconclusive. This algorithm is not a validated guideline but a personal recommendation of the author.

the majority of patients with an intermediate to high likelihood of CAD (Figure 5.5). MDCT, CMR, or PET/CT could be useful alternatives in patients unable to exercise, or those with equivocal findings on exercise stress tests with or without imaging. In such patients, perfusion and stress CMR, PET/CT, or MDCT can substitute for stress echocardiography or pharmacological SPECT imaging.

In view of the fact that MDCT appears to have the highest diagnostic accuracy on a per-patient basis, and that this test is more available than CMR, less costly, and faster to perform than any CMR study, it would be straightforward to propose MDCT for the detection of CAD in every patient. However, MDCT has significant disadvantages, which consist of high radiation exposure (10 to 15 mSv, or

Table 5.5 Major Contraindications to Tests

Test	Relative	Contraindication
MDCT		Renal insufficiency Allergy to iodated contrast Arrhythmias (atrial fibrillation) Pregnancy
All CMR techniques		Pacemaker/AICD implantation Claustrophobia Unsafe metal objects in brain/eye Neurostimulators/insulin pumps
MRCA		None
Adenosine/dipyridamole stress perfusion		Asthma/COPD AV block Carotid stenosis Pregnancy
Stress dobutamine		Obstructive cardiomyopathy Severe aortic/mitral stenosis Pregnancy

three times more than conventional coronary angiography) and a potential toxicity of iodinated contrast agents. Another major limitation of contrast-enhanced MDCT is that the test is a purely anatomical investigation of coronary stenosis severity, with a limited positive predictive value compared to either an anatomic gold standard (invasive angiography) or a test of ischemia [28]. Finally, MDCT has a poor performance record in patients with extensive coronary calcification. Thus, the choice of test should be individually targeted. It should not only depend on diagnostic performance but also on local availability, costs, specific preferences, contraindications (Table 5.5), and potential side effects in individual patients. For example, in view of the potential risk of radiation-induced cancer, MDCT would probably not be the best choice in young patients (under 45 years of age). Similarly, in patients with multiple coronary risk factors (old patients, diabetics) where coronary calcifications are very likely, MDCT would also not be an optimal choice. In such patients, as well as in patients that have contraindications to MDCT, perfusion or dobutamine magnetic resonance, or PET/CT might be better choices.

The cost-effectiveness of different strategies should also be considered. To date, a single study compared the cost-effectiveness of calcium scoring, contrast-enhanced MDCT, stress CMR, exercise ECG, stress echocardiography, and direct coronary angiography for the diagnosis of CAD in patients with chest pain [36]. The study concluded that cost-effectiveness depends on the pre-test likelihood of the probability of disease. For patients with a 10 to 50% pre-test likelihood of CAD, MDCT was the most cost-effective approach. At a pre-test likelihood of 60%, MDCT and coronary angiography were equally effective, whereas invasive cardiac catheterization was most cost-effective when the pre-test likelihood was greater than 70%. CMR was not found to be cost-effective for any pre-test likelihood. However, the conclusions are limited by being based on assumptions and statistical modeling from diagnostic accuracies published in the literature and not on actual outcome data. Indeed, there are only a few studies to date that have published prognostic information for the detection of ischemia by stress and perfusion magnetic resonance, and no prognostic data have yet been published for MRCA or MDCT [12–15].

Evaluation of Patients with Acute Chest Pain in the Emergency Department

The evaluation of patients with acute chest pain is more complex and differs significantly from that of patients with stable chest pain. Patients with suspected acute coronary syndrome (ACS) have significantly higher risks than patients with stable CAD. The initial diagnostic workup and risk stratification of these patients is well-defined and requires the assessment of clinical history, resting ECG, and the analysis of cardiac biomarkers, such as troponin I. If these tests are positive, they allow patients to be rapidly diagnosed with ST-elevation MI, non-ST elevation MI, or unstable angina. However, many patients presenting to the emergency department with acute chest pain have normal or nondiagnostic ECGs and negative biomarkers. This group of patients clearly represents a cohort with a lower clinical risk where noninvasive tests may be of benefit to define a management strategy. Current guidelines suggest repeat ECG and biomarker assessment followed by a negative stress test, often with imaging, to allow discharge. However, this current management requires patients to stay in the emergency room for prolonged times, and it is responsible for the higher costs. Consequently, noninvasive imaging techniques allowing a rapid and potentially more accurate diagnosis of patients with acute chest pain may be of great benefit by allowing faster management decisions and potentially reduced costs. Recent studies suggest a potential value for both MDCT and CMR in this setting.

Contrast-Enhanced MDCT

The potential use of MDCT in the early triage of patients presenting to the emergency room with acute chest pain has been evaluated by several studies. Negative predictive values ranging between 87% and 100% and positive predictive values ranging between 38 and 95% for the detection of ACS by MDCT were reported [37–40]. In one small, nonrandomized study, 64-slice MDCT showed better sensitivity than SPECT (86% versus 71%) and comparable specificity (92% versus 90%) for the detection of ACS [39]. Finally, a recent pilot study randomized 197 patients to MDCT versus a standard of care that included stress SPECT [41]. The strategy employing MDCT appeared equally effective to stress SPECT to identify patients without ACS with a very low six-month risk (88% versus 91%, respectively). However, the number of patients undergoing cardiac catheterization in the MDCT group (12%) with a 67% true positive rate was slightly greater than that in the group undergoing the standard care (7%) with only a 14% true positive rate. The main advantage of the MDCT strategy over the standard care was a significantly shorter time to diagnosis (median 3.4 hours versus 15 hours, respectively, $p < 0.001$), reduced costs ($1586 versus $1872, $p < 0.001$), and a trend to reduced cardiovascular re-evaluation (2% versus 7%, $p = 0.10$) during follow-up. Larger prospective studies are currently under way to evaluate the efficacy of MDCT in patients with acute chest pain.

Perfusion/Late-Enhancement CMR

The potential use of CMR in patients with acute chest pain was addressed in two studies. In a first study evaluating the diagnostic performance of regional function, resting perfusion, and late-enhancement MRI in patients presenting with chest pain to the emergency room, this test had an 84% sensitivity and an 85% specificity for detecting ACS [42]. In a subsequent study from the same group, the combination of adenosine perfusion and late-enhancement CMR had a 100% sensitivity and a 93% specificity for predicting significant CAD, defined as coronary artery stenosis greater than 50% on angiography, abnormal correlative stress test, new MI, or death in patients with acute chest pain [43].

Selecting a Testing Strategy for Patients with Acute Chest Pain

Given the low number of studies and the absence of direct comparison of techniques, it remains unclear whether and how MDCT or CMR should be used for assessing patients with acute chest pain. MDCT is quicker to perform and usually more available in off-hours than CMR. In addition, MDCT has the potential advantage of uncovering other etiologies for acute chest pain, such as pericardial or pulmonary effusion, pulmonary embolism, or aortic dissection. Nevertheless, MDCT has significant limitations in patients with suspected ACS. It requires the injection of iodinated contrast media, which can add to the contrast media that patients may receive during subsequent cardiac catheterization procedures. This media could potentially increase the risk of renal failure in patients. Another major disadvantage is that plaques in unstable ACS tend to be more rich in lipids, less calcified, and less stenotic, and could be more difficult to identify in patients with chronic chest pain. Alternatively, many patients without ACS may also have plaques on MDCT. For example, in the study by Hoffmann *et al.* 63 out of 107 patients with acute chest pain had plaques; however, only 14 of these had ACS [40]. Overdetection of plaque by MDCT might result in unnecessary hospital admissions, coronary angiography, or revascularization procedures. Given that MDCT appears to have a high negative predictive value, it seems plausible that MDCT might allow the early discharge of patients with normal coronary angiograms. Alternatively, given the inability to determine the physiological significance of stenosis and the inability to identify culprit lesions in ACS, patients in which MDCT identifies CAD will likely need further stress testing, and perfusion or dobutamine stress CMR could play a potential role as a secondary test [41]. More research is needed to warrant the use of either MDCT or CMR in the setting of acute chest pain. Also, these novel tests must prove their benefit over established techniques for the evaluation of low-risk patients with chest pain, such as nuclear imaging or stress echocardiography.

Evaluation for CAD in Symptomatic Patients with Valve Disease Prior to Surgery

As discussed in greater detail in Chapter 12, the evaluation of CAD is also important in patients undergoing surgery for valvular disease. Indeed, in patients having both valve and coronary disease, combined valve and coronary artery bypass graft surgery reduces the rate of perioperative and late morbidity and mortality, as compared to valve surgery alone [44,45]. Because of the poor predictive value of chest pain and noninvasive stress tests in patients with valvular heart disease, the current guidelines recommend performing preoperative coronary angiograms in almost every patient scheduled to undergo valve surgery, i.e., in male patients older than 35 years, in postmenopausal women, and in premenopausal women older than 35 years with significant coronary risk factors [46].

Several studies have investigated the ability of MDCT to detect CAD in such patients with valve disease, and have reported high sensitivity and negative predictive values ranging between 92% and 100% on a per-patient basis [47–51]. They suggest that MDCT might serve as a gatekeeper by filtering out patients with completely normal coronary MDCTs, referring only those patients to invasive coronary angiography in whom MDCT is frankly abnormal, doubtful, or nondiagnostic. Such a strategy might avoid performing systematic coronary angiography in all patients with valve disease, and might substantially reduce the cost of preoperative investigation in such patients. However, a larger clinical experience will be needed to warrant such use of MDCT to avoid missing patients with significant CAD prior to valve surgery.

Conclusions

The large amount of data and the encouraging results support a potential role for both MDCT and perfusion and dobutamine CMR for the evaluation of patients with chronic stable chest pain. The available evidence suggests that MRCA still lacks stability and therefore does not yet seem ready for widespread clinical use in such patients. These new imaging techniques are competing with existing noninvasive tests and, similar to those tests, should be used in a staged Bayesian approach based on clinical estimates of risk. The choice of noninvasive test in the individual patient should depend on diagnostic performance, individual advantages, and contraindications of tests.

Given the low number of studies and the greater risk of misdiagnosis, neither MDCT nor CMR are sufficiently validated for the diagnosis of CAD in patients with chest paint presenting to the emergency room. However, the encouraging initial results suggest that these techniques could play an important role in this setting in the near future. MDCT also shows promise for the preoperative screening of CAD in symptomatic patients with valve disease, as it might avoid systematic coronary angiography in these patients.

References

1 Fox, K., Garcia, M.A., Ardissino, D., et al. (2006) Guidelines on the management of stable angina pectoris: executive summary: the Task Force on the Management of Stable Angina Pectoris of the European Society of Cardiology. Eur Heart J 27(11): 1341–1381.

2 Rumberger, J.A., Sheedy, P.F., III, Breen, J.F., Schwartz, R.S. (1995) Coronary calcium, as determined by electron beam computed tomography, and coronary disease on arteriogram: effect of patient's sex on diagnosis. Circulation 91(5): 1363–1367.

3 Budoff, M.J., Georgiou, D., Brody, A., et al. (1996) Ultrafast computed tomography as a diagnostic modality in the detection of coronary artery disease: a multicenter study. Circulation 93(5): 898–904.

4 Rubinshtein, R., Gaspar, T., Halon, D.A., et al. (2007) Prevalence and extent of obstructive coronary artery disease in patients with zero or low calcium score undergoing 64-slice cardiac multidetector computed tomography for evaluation of a chest pain syndrome. Am J Cardiol 99(4): 472–475.

5 Raff, G.L., Gallagher, M.J., O'Neill, W.W., Goldstein, J.A. (2005) Diagnostic accuracy of noninvasive coronary angiography using 64-slice spiral computed tomography. J Am Coll Cardiol 46(3): 552–557.

6 Stuber, M., Botnar, R.M., Danias, P.G., et al. (1999) Double-oblique free-breathing high resolution three-dimensional coronary magnetic resonance angiography. J Am Coll Cardiol 34(2): 524–531.

7 Weber, O.M., Martin, A.J., Higgins, C.B. (2003) Whole-heart steady-state free precession coronary artery magnetic resonance angiography. Magn Reson Med 50(6): 1223–1228.

8 Kim, W.Y., Danias, P.G., Stuber, M., et al. (2001) Coronary magnetic resonance angiography for the detection of coronary stenoses. N Engl J Med 345(26): 1863–1869.

9 Sakuma, H., Ichikawa, Y., Suzawa, N., et al. (2005) Assessment of coronary arteries with total study time of less than 30 minutes by using whole-heart coronary MR angiography. Radiology 237(1): 316–321.

10 Jahnke, C., Paetsch, I., Nehrke, K., *et al.* (2005) Rapid and complete coronary arterial tree visualization with magnetic resonance imaging: feasibility and diagnostic performance. *Eur Heart J* **26**(21): 2313–2319.

11 Nagel, E., Lehmkuhl, H.B., Bocksch, W., *et al.* (1999) Noninvasive diagnosis of ischemia-induced wall motion abnormalities with the use of high-dose dobutamine stress MRI: comparison with dobutamine stress echocardiography. *Circulation* **99**(6): 763–770.

12 Hundley, W.G., Hamilton, C.A., Thomas, M.S., *et al.* (1999) Utility of fast cine magnetic resonance imaging and display for the detection of myocardial ischemia in patients not well suited for second harmonic stress echocardiography. *Circulation* **100**(16): 1697–1702.

13 Kuijpers, D., Ho, K.Y., van Dijkman, P.R., *et al.* (2003) Dobutamine cardiovascular magnetic resonance for the detection of myocardial ischemia with the use of myocardial tagging. *Circulation* **107**(12): 1592–1597.

14 Kuijpers, D., van Dijkman, P.R., Janssen, C.H., *et al.* (2004) Dobutamine stress MRI. Part II: risk stratification with dobutamine cardiovascular magnetic resonance in patients suspected of myocardial ischemia. *Eur Radiol.* Ref Type: E-pub.

15 Jahnke, C., Nagel, E., Gebker, R., *et al.* (2007) Prognostic value of cardiac magnetic resonance stress tests: adenosine stress perfusion and dobutamine stress wall motion imaging. *Circulation* **115**(13): 1769–1776.

16 Kuijpers, D., Janssen, C.H., van Dijkman, P.R., Oudkerk, M. (2004) Dobutamine stress MRI. Part I: safety and feasibility of dobutamine cardiovascular magnetic resonance in patients suspected of myocardial ischemia. *Eur Radiol.* Ref Type: E-pub.

17 Wahl, A., Paetsch, I., Gollesch, A., *et al.* (2004) Safety and feasibility of high-dose dobutamine-atropine stress cardiovascular magnetic resonance for diagnosis of myocardial ischaemia: experience in 1000 consecutive cases. *Eur Heart J* **25**(14): 1230–1236.

18 Giang, T.H., Nanz, D., Coulden, R., *et al.* (2004) Detection of coronary artery disease by magnetic resonance myocardial perfusion imaging with various contrast medium doses: first European multi-centre experience. *Eur Heart J* **25**(18): 1657–1665.

19 Wolff, S.D., Schwitter, J., Coulden, R., *et al.* (2004) Myocardial first-pass perfusion magnetic resonance imaging: a multicenter dose-ranging study. *Circulation* **110**(6): 732–737.

20 Ishida, N., Sakuma, H., Motoyasu, M., *et al.* (2003) Noninfarcted myocardium: correlation between dynamic first-pass contrast-enhanced myocardial MR imaging and quantitative coronary angiography. *Radiology* **229**(1): 209–216.

21 Klem, I., Heitner, J.F., Shah, D.J., *et al.* (2006) Improved detection of coronary artery disease by stress perfusion cardiovascular magnetic resonance with the use of delayed enhancement infarction imaging. *J Am Coll Cardiol* **47**(8): 1630–1638.

22 Fox, K., Garcia, M.A., Ardissino, D., *et al.* (2006) Guidelines on the management of stable angina pectoris: executive summary: the Task Force on the Management of Stable Angina Pectoris of the European Society of Cardiology. *Eur Heart J* **27**(11): 1341–1381.

23 Juergens, K.U., Fischbach, R. (2005) Left ventricular function studied with MDCT. *Eur Radiol* **16**(2): 342–357.

24 Kwong, R.Y., Chan, A.K., Brown, K.A., *et al.* (2006) Impact of unrecognized myocardial scar detected by cardiac magnetic resonance imaging on event-free survival in patients

presenting with signs or symptoms of coronary artery disease. *Circulation* **113**(23): 2733–2743.

25 Mahnken, A.H., Koos, R., Katoh, M., *et al*. (2005) Assessment of myocardial viability in reperfused acute myocardial infarction using 16-slice computed tomography in comparison to magnetic resonance imaging. *J Am Coll Cardiol* **45**(12): 2042–2047.

26 Gerber, B.L., Belge, B., Legros, G.J., *et al*. (2006) Characterization of acute and chronic myocardial infarcts by multidetector computed tomography: comparison with contrast-enhanced magnetic resonance. *Circulation* **113**(6): 823–833.

27 Schinkel, A.F., Bax, J.J., Geleijnse, M.L., *et al*. (2003) Noninvasive evaluation of ischaemic heart disease: myocardial perfusion imaging or stress echocardiography? *Eur Heart J* **24**(9): 789–800.

28 Di Carli, M.F., Hachamovitch, R. (2007) New technology for noninvasive evaluation of coronary artery disease. *Circulation* **115**(11): 1464–1480.

29 Sakuma, H., Suzawa, N., Ichikawa, Y., *et al*. (2005) Diagnostic accuracy of stress first-pass contrast-enhanced myocardial perfusion MRI compared with stress myocardial perfusion scintigraphy. *AJR* **185**(1): 95–102.

30 Paetsch, I., Jahnke, C., Wahl, A., *et al*. (2004) Comparison of dobutamine stress magnetic resonance, adenosine stress magnetic resonance, and adenosine stress magnetic resonance perfusion. *Circulation* **110**(7): 835–842.

31 Gerber, B.L., Coche, E., Pasquet, A., *et al*. (2005) Coronary artery stenosis: direct comparison of four-section multi-detector row CT and 3D Navigator MR imaging for detection—initial results. *Radiology* **234**(1): 98–108.

32 Kefer, J., Coche, E., Pasquet, A., *et al*. (2005) Head to head comparison of multislice coronary CT and 3D Navigator MRI for the detection of coronary artery stenosis. *J Am Coll Cardiol* **46**(1): 92–100.

33 Dewey, M., Teige, F., Schnapauff, D., *et al*. (2006) Noninvasive detection of coronary artery stenoses with multislice computed tomography or magnetic resonance imaging. *Ann Intern Med* **145**(6): 407–415.

34 Pouleur, A., le Polain de Waroux, J., Kefer, J., *et al*. (2007) Comparison of whole-heart coronary MR vs. multidetector CT angiography for detection of coronary artery stenosis. *Eur Heart J*. Ref Type: Abstract.

35 Fox, K., Garcia, M.A., Ardissino, D., *et al*. (2006) Guidelines on the management of stable angina pectoris: executive summary: the Task Force on the Management of Stable Angina Pectoris of the European Society of Cardiology. *Eur Heart J* **27**(11): 1341–1381.

36 Dewey, M., Hamm, B. (2006) Cost effectiveness of coronary angiography and calcium scoring using CT and stress MRI for diagnosis of coronary artery disease. *Eur Radiol*. Ref Type: E-pub.

37 Rubinshtein, R., Halon, D.A., Gaspar, T., *et al*. (2007) Usefulness of 64-slice cardiac computed tomographic angiography for diagnosing acute coronary syndromes and predicting clinical outcome in emergency department patients with chest pain of uncertain origin. *Circulation* **115**(13): 1762–1768.

38 Sato, Y., Matsumoto, N., Ichikawa, M., *et al*. (2005) Efficacy of multislice computed tomography for the detection of acute coronary syndrome in the emergency department. *Circ J* **69**(9): 1047–1051.

39 Gallagher, M.J., Ross, M.A., Raff, G.L., *et al.* (2007) The diagnostic accuracy of 64-slice computed tomography coronary angiography compared with stress nuclear imaging in emergency department low-risk chest pain patients. *Ann Emerg Med* **49**(2): 125–136.

40 Hoffmann, U., Nagurney, J.T., Moselewski, F., *et al.* (2006) Coronary multidetector computed tomography in the assessment of patients with acute chest pain. *Circulation* **114**(21): 2251–2260.

41 Goldstein, J.A., Gallagher, M.J., O'Neill, W.W., *et al.* (2007) A randomized controlled trial of multi-slice coronary computed tomography for evaluation of acute chest pain. *J Am Coll Cardiol* **49**(8): 863–871.

42 Kwong, R.Y., Schussheim, A.E., Rekhraj, S., *et al.* (2003) Detecting acute coronary syndrome in the emergency department with cardiac magnetic resonance imaging. *Circulation* **107**(4): 531–537.

43 Ingkanisorn, W.P., Kwong, R.Y., Bohme, N.S., *et al.* (2006) Prognosis of negative adenosine stress magnetic resonance in patients presenting to an emergency department with chest pain. *J Am Coll Cardiol* **47**(7): 1427–1432.

44 Czer, L.S., Gray, R.J., Stewart, M.E., *et al.* (1988) Reduction in sudden late death by concomitant revascularization with aortic valve replacement. *J Thorac Cardiovasc Surg* **95**(3): 390–401.

45 Czer, L.S., Gray, R.J., DeRobertis, M.A., *et al.* (1984) Mitral valve replacement: impact of coronary artery disease and determinants of prognosis after revascularization. *Circulation* **70**(3 Pt 2): I198–I207.

46 Bonow, R.O., de la Carabello, B., Jr., Edmunds, L.H., Jr., *et al.* (1998) Guidelines for the management of patients with valvular heart disease: executive summary: a report of the American College of Cardiology/American Heart Association Task Force on Practice Guidelines (Committee on Management of Patients with Valvular Heart Disease). *Circulation* **98**(18): 1949–1984.

47 Gilard, M., Cornily, J.C., Pennec, P.Y., *et al.* (2006) Accuracy of multislice computed tomography in the preoperative assessment of coronary disease in patients with aortic valve stenosis. *J Am Coll Cardiol* **47**(10): 2020–2024.

48 Reant, P., Brunot, S., Lafitte, S., *et al.* (2006) Predictive value of noninvasive coronary angiography with multidetector computed tomography to detect significant coronary stenosis before valve surgery. *Am J Cardiol* **97**(10): 1506–1510.

49 Manghat, N.E., Morgan-Hughes, G.J., Broadley, A.J., *et al.* (2006) 16-detector row computed tomographic coronary angiography in patients undergoing evaluation for aortic valve replacement: comparison with catheter angiography. *Clin Radiol* **61**(9): 749–757.

50 Meijboom, W.B., Mollet, N.R., van Mieghem, C.A., *et al.* (2006) Pre-operative computed tomography coronary angiography to detect significant coronary artery disease in patients referred for cardiac valve surgery. *J Am Coll Cardiol* **48**(8): 1658–1665.

51 Pouleur, A., le Polain de Waroux, J., Kefer, J., *et al.* Usefulness of 40-slice multidetector row computed tomography to detect coronary disease in patients prior to cardiac valve surgery. *Eur Radiol* (in press).

52 Gianrossi, R., Detrano, R., Mulvihill, D., *et al.* (1989) Exercise-induced ST depression in the diagnosis of coronary artery disease: a meta-analysis. *Circulation* **80**(1): 87–98.

53 Leber, A.W., Knez, A., von Ziegler, F., *et al.* (2005) Quantification of obstructive and nonobstructive coronary lesions by 64-slice computed tomography: a comparative

study with quantitative coronary angiography and intravascular ultrasound. *J Am Coll Cardiol* **46**(1): 147–154.

54 Leschka, S., Alkadhi, H., Plass, A., *et al.* (2005) Accuracy of MSCT coronary angiography with 64-slice technology: first experience. *Eur Heart J* **26**(15): 1482–1487.

55 Mollet, N.R., Cademartiri, F., van Mieghem, C.A., *et al.* (2005) High-resolution spiral computed tomography coronary angiography in patients referred for diagnostic conventional coronary angiography. *Circulation* **112**(15): 2318–2323.

56 Pugliese, F., Mollet, N.R., Runza, G., *et al.* (2006) Diagnostic accuracy of non-invasive 64-slice CT coronary angiography in patients with stable angina pectoris. *Eur Radiol* **16**(3): 575–582.

57 Muhlenbruch, G., Seyfarth, T., Soo, C.S., *et al.* (2007) Diagnostic value of 64-slice multidetector row cardiac CTA in symptomatic patients. *Eur Radiol* **17**(3): 603–609.

58 Ehara, M., Surmely, J.F., Kawai, M., *et al.* (2006) Diagnostic accuracy of 64-slice computed tomography for detecting angiographically significant coronary artery stenosis in an unselected consecutive patient population: comparison with conventional invasive angiography. *Circ J* **70**(5): 564–571.

59 Schuijf, J.D., Pundziute, G., Jukema, J.W., *et al.* (2006) Diagnostic accuracy of 64-slice multislice computed tomography in the noninvasive evaluation of significant coronary artery disease. *Am J Cardiol* **98**(2): 145–148.

60 Watkins, M.W., Hesse, B., Green, C.E., *et al.* (2007) Detection of coronary artery stenosis using 40-channel computed tomography with multi-segment reconstruction. *Am J Cardiol* **99**(2): 175–181.

61 Ghostine, S., Caussin, C., Daoud, B., *et al.* (2006) Non-invasive detection of coronary artery disease in patients with left bundle branch block using 64-slice computed tomography. *J Am Coll Cardiol* **48**(10): 1929–1934.

62 Scheffel, H., Alkadhi, H., Plass, A., *et al.* (2006) Accuracy of dual-source CT coronary angiography: first experience in a high pre-test probability population without heart rate control. *Eur Radiol* **16**(12): 2739–2747.

63 Shapiro, M.D., Butler, J., Rieber, J., *et al.* (2007) Analytic approaches to establish the diagnostic accuracy of coronary computed tomography angiography as a tool for clinical decision making. *Am J Cardiol* **99**(8): 1122–1127.

64 Kim, W.Y., Danias, P.G., Stuber, M., *et al.* (2001) Coronary magnetic resonance angiography for the detection of coronary stenoses. *N Engl J Med* **345**(26): 1863–1869.

65 Bogaert, J., Kuzo, R., Dymarkowski, S., *et al.* (2003) Coronary artery imaging with real-time navigator three-dimensional turbo-field-echo MR coronary angiography: initial experience. *Radiology* **226**(3): 707–716.

66 Dewey, M., Teige, F., Schnapauff, D., *et al.* (2006) Noninvasive detection of coronary artery stenoses with multislice computed tomography or magnetic resonance imaging. *Ann Intern Med* **145**(6): 407–415.

67 Sakuma, H., Ichikawa, Y., Suzawa, N., *et al.* (2005) Assessment of coronary arteries with total study time of less than 30 minutes by using whole-heart coronary MR angiography. *Radiology* **237**(1): 316–321.

68 Sakuma, H., Ichikawa, Y., Chino, S., *et al.* (2006) Detection of coronary artery stenosis with whole-heart coronary magnetic resonance angiography. *J Am Coll Cardiol* **48**(10): 1946–1950.

69 Schalla, S., Klein, C., Paetsch, I., *et al.* (2002) Real-time MR image acquisition during high-dose dobutamine hydrochloride stress for detecting left ventricular wall-motion abnormalities in patients with coronary arterial disease. *Radiology* **224**(3): 845–851.

70 Jahnke, C., Paetsch, I., Gebker, R., *et al.* (2006) Accelerated 4D dobutamine stress MR imaging with k-t BLAST: feasibility and diagnostic performance. *Radiology* **241**(3): 718–728.

71 Schwitter, J., Nanz, D., Kneifel, S., *et al.* (2001) Assessment of myocardial perfusion in coronary artery disease by magnetic resonance: a comparison with positron emission tomography and coronary angiography. *Circulation* **103**(18): 2230–2235.

72 Nagel, E., Klein, C., Paetsch, I., *et al.* (2003) Magnetic resonance perfusion measurements for the noninvasive detection of coronary artery disease. *Circulation* **108**(4): 432–437.

73 Plein, S., Radjenovic, A., Ridgway, J.P., *et al.* (2005) Coronary artery disease: myocardial perfusion MR imaging with sensitivity encoding versus conventional angiography. *Radiology* **235**(2): 423–430.

Chapter 6

Evaluation of Atherosclerotic Plaques with CT and MRI

Ilan Gottlieb and João A.C. Lima

Clinical assessment based on risk factors and the physical examination of atherosclerosis is inexpensive, effective, and should be performed routinely. However, it is likely not sufficient, as underscored by one trial in which 75% of the patients being admitted for acute coronary syndromes did not fulfill the most current clinical indications for statin therapy [1]. The atherosclerotic process in humans is extremely heterogeneous and multifactorial; thus, it is very difficult to find a one-size-fits-all clinical stratification algorithm. The fact that over 200 risk factors have been described in the literature associated with coronary artery disease (CAD) underscores this heterogeneity [2]. This result leads to the conclusion that some form of more precise phenotypic diagnosis of subclinical CAD is desirable. Both computed tomography (CT) and magnetic resonance imaging (MRI) are powerful tools for the detection and quantification of atherosclerosis, and are also being intensively evaluated for the purposes of morphological characterization and monitoring of the atherosclerotic plaque.

Multidetector Computed Tomography

Coronary Calcium Score

The *coronary calcium score* (CCS) provides an overall estimate of the total plaque burden in the coronary arterial system [3]. The magnitude of coronary artery calcification is related to most coronary risk factors including total cholesterol, LDL cholesterol, blood pressure, cigarette smoking, and a family history of CAD [4]. More importantly, the CCS predicts the development of adverse clinical events, independent of the Framingham Risk Score [5–7]. Greenland *et al.*

Novel Techniques for Imaging the Heart, 1st edition. Edited by M. Di Carli and R. Kwong.
© 2008 American Heart Association, ISBN: 9-781-4051-7533-3.

suggested that in asymptomatic individuals with an intermediate risk of coronary risk by Framingham criteria, CCS could be useful to reclassify the patients with initial intermediate clinical risk into an appropriately low (CCS = 0) or high (CCS > 300) risk for adverse events [6]. Although the evidence from prospective studies demonstrating the predictive power of coronary calcification to detect cardiovascular events in asymptomatic individuals is compelling, there is no direct evidence that such screening will lead to reduced morbidity and mortality caused by CAD (as discussed in more detail in Chapter 15) [4]. Patients deemed at intermediate risk for cardiovascular events are the best suited to undergo CCS, whereas patients at low and high clinical risk are less likely to benefit from it due to the fact that CCS will probably not change clinical management [5].

CCS measurements are relatively low-risk as the test does not require the use of iodinated contrast agents and the radiation exposure from it is limited to 1.0 to 2.0 mSv. The main intrinsic clinical limitation of the test is the fact that coronary calcification represents only one of the components of atherosclerotic plaques that can develop late in the natural history of atherosclerosis [8]. Therefore, the amount of calcium accumulated in any given coronary arterial segment reflects not only the magnitude of plaque burden but also the period of time during which plaques were exposed to the factors that underlie calcification. Although the potential contributions of inflammatory, hormonal, metabolic, and physical factors thought to underlie coronary calcification are still incompletely understood, the process is believed to represent a natural biological response to arterial wall injury, which would be activated for the purposes of achieving increased arterial wall stiffness to theoretically make the plaque less vulnerable to rupture or undue deformation caused by mechanical or biological stresses [8,9].

The high density of calcium results in marked x-ray attenuation. Most laboratories use an attenuation coefficient value greater than or equal to 130 Hounsfield units (HU) to define calcification with CT. This threshold represents approximately two standard deviations of the attenuation of blood, and correlates well with histomorphometric measurements of calcified plaque [3]. Both multidetector (MDCT) and electron beam (EBCT) computed tomography can be employed for coronary artery calcium (CAC) detection and quantification [10]. Interstudy reproducibility of calcium measurements, a factor that critically influences the interpretation of changes in CAC scores detected over a period of time, has been a matter of concern, especially for low scores. With newer scanners and optimized methodology, the variability can be reduced to below 10% [11].

Three methods for calcium scoring are currently used, and reference ranges for each approach have been reported [12]. The *Agatston score* is obtained by the summation of areas of the calcified lesions multiplied by a scaling factor derived from the peak attenuation in each plaque (factor of 1 for attenuation between 130 to 200 HU, 2 for attenuation between 200 to 300 HU, 3 for attenuation between 300 to 400 HU, and 4 for attenuation greater than 400 HU) [13]. This score can be subsequently normalized for different imaging parameters such as slice thickness or reconstruction increment [14]. The Agatston score has been the most common method used in clinical and epidemiological investigations. A second approach is the *volumetric method*, which measures the volume of the calcified voxels and performs a continuous isotropic interpolation to avoid the nonlinearity attenuation of the Agatston scaling factors [15]. A third approach is the *quantification of calcium mass*, combining volumetric calculations with density information derived from the mean attenuation of the lesion [14]. Reproducibility is worst for the Agatston method, intermediate for the volumetric approach, and best for the mass score [14]. Interestingly, all three methods appear to stratify cardiovascular risk similarly [12].

Because nonstenotic and noncalcified plaques can rupture and lead to infarction or sudden death, a calcium score of zero does not assure protection. This scenario can be especially true in young individuals in whom those high-risk plaques may not have accumulated enough calcium to cross the threshold of brightness (130 HU), currently used by the Agtaston method to be considered positive [16,17]. Although relatively rare among asymptomatic individuals, such cases have been well documented [17,18]. Finally, given the intrinsic variability associated with measuring individual calcium scores, the method is currently not suitable for the individual assessment of disease progression or plaque regression induced by therapy or lifestyle modifications [19,20]. However, in large populations atherosclerosis progression can be quantified by using large samples to compensate for its variability.

CT Coronary Angiography

Since the development of invasive coronary angiography (ICA), studies had demonstrated that when considering individual lesions, the likelihood of plaque destabilization is greater for severe obstructive lesions [21,22]. Indeed, using data from the Coronary Artery Surgery Study (CASS) program, Alderman *et al.* demonstrated that during a five-year follow-up only less than or equal to 2.3% of segments with luminal narrowings (less than or equal to 49%) resulted in coronary occlusion, whereas occlusion occurred in 10 to 24% of lesions with narrowings (greater than or equal to 50%). In addition, the location of coronary stenoses is also an important predictor of future coronary events, with lesions in the proximal vessels associated with worse prognosis [23]. Although the location and degree of coronary stenosis has been shown to predict cardiovascular events in population-based analyses, it is now clear that the degree of stenosis is not the only factor influencing plaque erosion or rupture [23–25]. Such plaque vulnerability appears to be also associated with other plaque characteristics, such as a large lipidic necrotic core, positive remodeling, a thin fibrous cap, and intraplaque neovascularization and hemorrhage [24,26,27]. Consequently, the noninvasive detection and characterization of plaques would seem to be a reasonable target for improving risk assessment and management strategies.

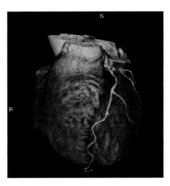

Fig. 6.1 Volume-rendered (3D) data set of the heart with contrast acquired with 64-detector MDCT scanner showing the left anterior descending artery.

Until a few years ago, all noninvasive tests available for the detection of CAD relied on atherosclerotic plaque lumen impingement. ICA is a projection image generated by the attenuation to x-rays created by the iodinated contrast material inside the coronary lumen, whereas stress imaging techniques detect myocardial perfusion or contractile abnormalities resulting from flow-limiting stenoses in epicardial coronary arteries. However, these techniques are not designed to identify or adequately quantify the extent of atherosclerosis.

This limitation can potentially be overcome by MDCT coronary angiography owing to its ability to image coronary atherosclerotic plaques three-dimensionally (Figure 6.1), allowing for the accurate quantification of plaque volumes as compared to intravascular ultrasound, detection, and quantification of positive remodeling, and plaque attenuation (as a potential surrogate for plaque composition) [28–35]. In addition, by tagging contrast molecules with macrophage scavenger receptor ligands, MDCT shows promise to detect macrophage infiltration within plaques as a measure of inflammation [36]. Figure 6.2a is an example of an MDCT angiography of the left anterior descending artery with a severe proximal stenosis. Note the anatomical detail, the visualization of the entire plaque structure, and the positive remodeling associated with this lesion. Also note that the plaque extends proximally into the left main with minimal luminal impingement, which would probably not be seen by ICA. MDCT can also provide valuable complementary information such as the assessment of global and regional left ventricular function, myocardial perfusion, and scar detection by delayed enhancement techniques [37–39].

As discussed in Chapter 1, MDCT uses back projection techniques to acquire volumetric image data sets of the heart, freezing the heart's motion to generate a coronary anatomy with exquisite isotropic spatial resolution as high as 0.4 mm. The performance profile of MDCT angiography with machines equipped with 16 detectors for the detection of obstructive lesions has been reasonably

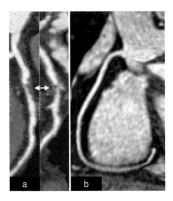

Fig. 6.2 Examples of two different noninvasive coronary angiography techniques.
(a) On the left is an example of two orthogonal views of an MDCT angiography of the
left anterior descending artery with a severe proximal stenosis (arrow). Note the
anatomical detail, the visualization of the entire plaque structure, and the positive
remodeling associated with this lesion. Also note that the plaque extends proximally
into the left main with minimal luminal impingement, which would probably not be
seen by ICA. (b) In MRI 3D angiography of the entire heart showing the right coronary,
no lesions are seen.

well-established in the literature [40]. Although some of the earliest studies reported very high values for both sensitivity and specificity for 16-slice
MDCT angiography, it soon became obvious that whereas specificity estimates
appeared to hold, those for sensitivity had wide limits of confidence associated
with the type of population being examined, the techniques employed, the type
of analytic comparisons made against the invasive coronary angiography gold
standard, small sample size, and the rigor of control for other analytic biases
[40]. The Core64 Trial has been extremely valuable in overcoming such biases
and demonstrating the excellent diagnostic performance for the detection of
greater than or equal to 50% stenosis with an area under the ROC curve of 0.92
($p < 0.001$) [41]. Additionally, the recent development of a dual-source MDCT
scanner has significantly improved temporal resolution, enabling the scanning
of patients at higher heart rates possibly without the use of beta-blockers. Results
from small single center studies are encouraging [42,43].

Although more studies are needed to determine the number of detectors that
will provide a reliable diagnostic profile, there is consensus that a greater number
of detectors and thus greater coverage per gantry rotation has been fundamental
in enabling this technology to image the coronaries and that these factors yield
improved images if all other variables are kept constant. The decreased number of "unevaluable" coronary segments with more than 16 detector scanners
confirms this impression (Figure 6.3) [40]. Moreover, it is important to note that
analyses by segment, by vessel, and by patient yield different results and have

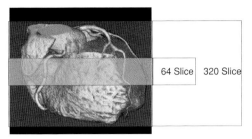

64 Slice   320 Slice

Fig. 6.3 Schematic coverage of the heart by 64- and 320-detector scanners. With the latter, no helical acquisition is necessary.

different meanings relative to the interpretation of these comparisons against invasive angiography [40]. In summary, results from studies performed so far indicate that whereas coronary MDCT angiography has room to evolve and improve relative to ICA, its specificity is great enough to indicate that the test can certainly be used as a tool to exclude the presence of significant coronary stenoses.

Magnetic Resonance Imaging

Atherosclerosis Imaging of Peripheral Arteries

MRI is a noninvasive imaging modality that does not expose the patient to ionizing radiation or iodinated contrast material. Importantly, its ability to characterize soft-tissue structures is far superior to CT, and it has the potential to revolutionize our ability to detect and characterize atherosclerotic plaques. MRI consists of several techniques that can be performed separately or in various combinations during a patient examination. It provides high-resolution images of vascular structures with good reproducibility and accuracy [44–50]. MRI can detect small changes in plaque size with low variability, allowing for smaller sample sizes and shorter follow-up in clinical trials evaluating atherosclerosis progression [51–54].

Quantification of Plaque Dimensions

Accurate quantification of vessel wall dimensions depends on the ability to discern the inner and outer boundaries of the vessel wall. Using techniques to suppress the blood-flow signal (e.g., double inversion recovery combined with fast spin echo) enhances the conspicuity of the vessel wall and its components against the backdrop of a hypointense lumen [55–59]. Several semiautomatic image-processing tools have been proposed for vessel boundary detection [60,61]. In general, three-dimensional measurements are preferred in continuous rather than categorical form to draw conclusions about the regression/progression of plaques in longitudinal studies. Because atherosclerosis is

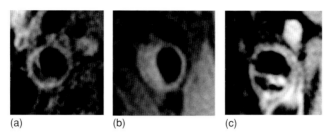

(a)   (b)   (c)

Fig. 6.4 MRI T1W black blood post-contrast acquisitions of three different carotid artery plaque morphologies. (a) A large lipid core can be visualized, in contrast with (b) a predominantly fibrous plaque and (c) a complex plaque, where calcification, intraplaque hemorrhage, and lipid and fibrous tissue can be seen.

generally not a uniform process, an accurate and reproducible determination of vessel wall dimensions is extremely important to draw valid conclusions longitudinally. Arterial wall dimension assessment using MRI has been found to be highly reproducible in arteries such as the carotids and the aorta [52,62,63].

Plaque Morphology

The quest for the vulnerable plaque has been ongoing since the moment it was demonstrated from pathological specimens of patients who died from cardiovascular causes that plaque rupture (and less frequently fissure) was the underlying mechanism for the lethal thrombotic event. Furthermore, plaque rupture seemed to be associated with certain plaque characteristics such as a large lipidic necrotic core, a thin fibrous cap, and intraplaque neovascularization and hemorrhage — and that stenosis severity was not the most important determinant phenomenon [24–27,64]. This pattern of plaque destabilization seems to be generalizable to other vascular beds with larger vessels, like the carotid and ileo-femoral systems, which are better suited to MRI imaging due to their larger diameter and relative lack of motion [65,66]. In medium-sized and large vessels, MRI can accurately differentiate plaque components such as the lipid core, fibrous cap, intraplaque hemorrhage, calcified nodules, and fibrous tissue with a good correlation with pathology [44–47,67]. Figure 6.4 demonstrates examples of three different carotid plaques with discernible differences in their composition. Nonetheless, whether measuring and monitoring these different plaque components will provide more useful information above and beyond plaque burden is still to be defined.

There is substantial evidence to suggest that plaque inflammation also plays an important role in plaque destabilization [24,65]. Recently, a micelle with gadodiamide (an MRI contrast agent) that is able to selectively bind to the macrophage scavenger receptor was developed [68–70]. With macrophage migration, this contrast-enhanced micelle would be carried with it and trapped inside the plaque, generating a bright signal on T1-weighted images. Higher inflammatory activity leads to more macrophage migration and to higher signal intensities in the MRI images. This concept was demonstrated in a recent animal model, where these micelles were injected into mice with atherosclerosis. The authors were able to demonstrate that after 24 hours, the aorta from mice that received the gadodiamide micelle had higher signal intensity than those from mice who received gadodiamide alone [71].

Imaging of the Coronary Arteries

As discussed in more detailed in Chapter 15, the growth of MRI for coronary imaging has been hampered by the following technical limitations: cardiac motion due to contraction/relaxation; diaphragmatic/chest wall motion due to respiration; small caliber of the coronary vessels; tortuosity of the coronaries; and signal from surrounding epicardial fat. To account for intrinsic cardiac motion, electrocardiogram (ECG) gating is absolutely necessary. However, under the influence of a strong static magnetic field, the so-called magnetohydrodynamic effect is enhanced and an artifactual voltage overlaid to the T-wave of the ECG results, leading to the faulty detection of the R-wave detection algorithm and resulting in serious artifacts on coronary magnetic resonance images. To counter that, various gating techniques such as fiber optic gating have been employed to provide a clean ECG signal when the patient is inside the MRI scanner. Most recently, the vector ECG approach (which analyzes the ECG vector in three-dimensional space and separates the true T-wave from the artifactual T-wave) has been used with highly reliable results [72]. Coronary artery motion occurs in a triphasic pattern during the cardiac cycle. Hence, mid-diastolic diastasis has been identified as the preferred time for image acquisition because this "rest period" also coincides with the interval of rapid coronary filling [73]. Thus, to minimize blurring and ensure complete "freezing" of the coronary vessels, a careful selection of the acquisition window is important. Ongoing technical improvement leading to automatic detection of this rest period should further reduce residual coronary motion and improve the image quality of coronary MRI.

Traditionally, MRI is dependent upon the patient's cooperation in breath-holds, which might have to be sustained for up to 20 sec or more. However, breath-holding strategies have several limitations. Some patients may have difficulty sustaining adequate breath-holds, particularly when the duration exceeds a few seconds. Additionally, it has been shown that during a sustained breath-hold there is cranial diaphragmatic drift, which can reach as much as 1 cm in some cases [74]. Among serial breath-holds, the diaphragmatic and cardiac positions frequently vary by up to 1 cm, resulting in registration errors [75]. Misregistration results in apparent gaps between the segments of the visualized coronary arteries, which could be misinterpreted as signal voids from coronary stenoses. Finally, the use of signal enhancement techniques, such as signal averaging or fold-over suppression, is significantly restricted by the duration of the applicable breath-hold duration. Using breath-holding techniques, the spatial resolution of the images is also governed by the patient's ability to hold their breath. Thus, although breath-hold strategies are often successful with motivated volunteers, its applicability to a broad range of patients with cardiovascular disease is limited.

Several approaches have been developed to minimize the effect of respiratory motion. These include free breathing using multiple averages, chest wall bellows, or more recently magnetic resonance "navigators" that consist of continuous tracking of the diaphragmatic position by highly localized imaging (the navigator is positioned at any interface that accurately depicts respiratory motion, such as the dome of the right hemidiaphragm) [73,76]. Advanced magnetic resonance pulse sequences have been developed that can suppress the surrounding epicardial fat and the myocardium, thus enabling the visualization of the coronary arteries with or without contrast enhancement [77]. Finally, to improve the in-plane spatial resolution in imaging the coronary arteries, newer cardiac phase-array coils with enhanced numbers of receiver elements have been developed that support an improved signal-to-noise ratio (SNR) [73].

With these technical developments, three-dimensional cardiac data sets of the heart can be acquired and coronary angiography becomes not only feasible but also reasonably accurate, although limited spatial resolution with MRI still makes MDCT the preferred method for noninvasive coronary angiography at the present time [78–80]. Figure 6.2 compares two average-image quality coronary angiographies, one by MRI (b) and another by MDCT (a); note that the latter yields finer details due to the higher spatial resolution.

Coronary Vessel Wall Imaging

To successfully image the coronary artery vessel wall and the atherosclerotic changes associated with it, a high contrast between the coronary lumen blood pool and the surrounding coronary vessel wall is mandatory. The first successful implementations of coronary vessel wall imaging in humans included the use of a dual-inversion fast spin echo sequence. Using this method, single slices of the coronary artery vessel wall could be acquired during a prolonged breath-hold period, and the relative thickening of the coronary arterial vessel wall was successfully demonstrated in selected cases [59]. Subsequently, to remove the limitations associated with breath-holding, this technique was refined by the use of navigators for free-breathing data acquisition [81]. More recently, the free-breathing navigator approach was combined with three-dimensional spiral imaging in conjunction with a "local inversion" technique [82]. Using this method, a high-quality image can be obtained due to the high SNR associated with three-dimensional imaging on the one hand and the signal-efficient spiral readout on the other. This method enables a larger anatomic coverage, and the reconstructed slices are much thinner than those used in the earlier two-dimensional approaches. Therefore, it is now possible to visualize long, contiguous sections of the coronary arterial wall. Additionally, the spiral approach permits data acquisition in a short acquisition window of only 50 ms, with more effective suppression of artifacts caused by intrinsic myocardial motion or beat-to-beat variability. The disadvantages of this technique include the prolonged scanning time of approximately 12 min during free breathing (image acquisition during every other R–R interval).

Conclusions

The technical developments in CT and MRI are rapidly advancing our ability to quantify and characterize atherosclerotic plaques. These developments allow for early disease diagnosis and have the potential to improve the management of this important public health problem. CT angiography is already used in clinical cardiology practice, and technical advances continue to improve image quality while decreasing radiation dose. MRI angiography of medium and large arteries has been shown to be accurate, reproducible, and fast, allowing for the morphologic depiction of the atherosclerotic plaque. Although MRI coronary angiography development has also progressed at a fast pace, the challenges are greater for MRI and new developments are necessary to enhance spatial resolution, acquisition speed, and image quality. The fact that MRI does not entail ionizing radiation or iodinated contrast material makes it ideal for the noninvasive coronary evaluation of asymptomatic individuals in the future.

Acknowledgments

We gratefully thank Ms. Kathi Lensch for her invaluable secretarial assistance.

References

1 Akosah, K.O., Schaper, A., Cogbill, C., Schoenfeld, P. (2003) Preventing myocardial infarction in the young adult in the first place: how do the National Cholesterol Education Panel III guidelines perform? *J Am Coll Cardiol* **41**: 1475–1479.

2 Naghavi, M., Falk, E., Hecht, H.S., *et al.* (2006) From vulnerable plaque to vulnerable patient—part III: executive summary of the Screening for Heart Attack Prevention and Education (SHAPE) Task Force report. *Am J Cardiol* **98**: 2H–15H.

3 Rumberger, J.A., Simons, D.B., Fitzpatrick, L.A., *et al.* (1995) Coronary artery calcium area by electron-beam computed tomography and coronary atherosclerotic plaque area: a histopathologic correlative study. *Circulation* **92**: 2157–2162.

4 Budoff, M.J., Achenbach, S., Blumenthal, R.S., *et al.* (2006) Assessment of coronary artery disease by cardiac computed tomography: a scientific statement from the American Heart Association Committee on Cardiovascular Imaging and Intervention,

Council on Cardiovascular Radiology and Intervention, and Committee on Cardiac Imaging, Council on Clinical Cardiology. *Circulation* **114**: 1761–1791.

5 Greenland, P., Bonow, R.O., Brundage, B.H., *et al.* (2007) ACCF/AHA 2007 clinical expert consensus document on coronary artery calcium scoring by computed tomography in global cardiovascular risk assessment and in evaluation of patients with chest pain: a report of the American College of Cardiology Foundation Clinical Expert Consensus Task Force (ACCF/AHA Writing Committee to Update the 2000 Expert Consensus Document on Electron Beam Computed Tomography) developed in collaboration with the Society of Atherosclerosis Imaging and Prevention and the Society of Cardiovascular Computed Tomography. *J Am Coll Cardiol* **49**: 378–402.

6 Greenland, P., LaBree, L., Azen, S.P., *et al.* (2004) Coronary artery calcium score combined with Framingham score for risk prediction in asymptomatic individuals. *JAMA* **291**: 210–215.

7 Shaw, L.J., Raggi, P., Schisterman, E., *et al.* (2003) Prognostic value of cardiac risk factors and coronary artery calcium screening for all-cause mortality. *Radiology* **228**: 826–833.

8 Wexler, L., Brundage, B., Crouse, J., *et al.* (1996) Coronary artery calcification: pathophysiology, epidemiology, imaging methods, and clinical implications: a statement for health professionals from the American Heart Association. Writing Group. *Circulation* **94**: 1175–1192.

9 O'Rourke, R.A., Brundage, B.H., Froelicher, V.F., *et al.* (2000) American College of Cardiology/American Heart Association Expert Consensus Document on electron-beam computed tomography for the diagnosis and prognosis of coronary artery disease. *J Am Coll Cardiol* **36**: 326–340.

10 Horiguchi, J., Yamamoto, H., Akiyama, Y., *et al.* (2004) Coronary artery calcium scoring using 16-MDCT and a retrospective ECG-gating reconstruction algorithm. *AJR* **183**: 103–108.

11 Kopp, A.F., Ohnesorge, B., Becker, C., *et al.* (2002) Reproducibility and accuracy of coronary calcium measurements with multi-detector row versus electron-beam CT. *Radiology* **225**: 113–119.

12 Rumberger, J.A., Kaufman, L. (2003) A Rosetta stone for coronary calcium risk stratification: Agatston, volume, and mass scores in 11,490 individuals. *AJR* **181**: 743–748.

13 Agatston, A.S., Janowitz, W.R., Hildner, F.J., *et al.* (1990) Quantification of coronary artery calcium using ultrafast computed tomography. *J Am Coll Cardiol* **15**: 827–832.

14 Ohnesorge, B., Flohr, T., Fischbach, R., *et al.* (2002) Reproducibility of coronary calcium quantification in repeat examinations with retrospectively ECG-gated multisection spiral CT. *Eur Radiol* **12**: 1532–1540.

15 Callister, T.Q., Cooil, B., Raya, S.P., *et al.* (1998) Coronary artery disease: improved reproducibility of calcium scoring with an electron-beam CT volumetric method. *Radiology* **208**: 807–814.

16 Hausleiter, J., Meyer, T., Hadamitzky, M., *et al.* (2006) Prevalence of noncalcified coronary plaques by 64-slice computed tomography in patients with an intermediate risk for significant coronary artery disease. *J Am Coll Cardiol* **48**: 312–318.

17 Haberl, R., Becker A., Leber, A., *et al.* (2001) Correlation of coronary calcification and angiographically documented stenoses in patients with suspected coronary artery disease: results of 1,764 patients. *J Am Coll Cardiol* **37**: 451–457.

18 Raggi, P., Callister, T.Q., Cooil, B., *et al.* (2000) Identification of patients at increased risk of first unheralded acute myocardial infarction by electron-beam computed tomography. *Circulation* **101**: 850–855.

19 Achenbach, S., Ropers, D., Mohlenkamp, S., *et al.* (2001) Variability of repeated coronary artery calcium measurements by electron beam tomography. *Am J Cardiol* **87**: 210–213, A218.

20 Lu, B., Zhuang, N., Mao, S.S., *et al.* (2002) EKG-triggered CT data acquisition to reduce variability in coronary arterial calcium score. *Radiology* **224**: 838–844.

21 Giroud, D., Li, J.M., Urban, P., *et al.* (1992) Relation of the site of acute myocardial infarction to the most severe coronary arterial stenosis at prior angiography. *Am J Cardiol* **69**: 729–732.

22 Alderman, E.L., Corley, S.D., Fisher, L.D., *et al.* (1993) Five-year angiographic follow-up of factors associated with progression of coronary artery disease in the Coronary Artery Surgery Study (CASS). CASS Participating Investigators and Staff. *J Am Coll Cardiol* **22**: 1141–1154.

23 Ellis, S., Alderman, E., Cain, K., *et al.* (1988) Prediction of risk of anterior myocardial infarction by lesion severity and measurement method of stenoses in the left anterior descending coronary distribution: a CASS Registry Study. *J Am Coll Cardiol* **11**: 908–916.

24 Virmani, R., Burke, A.P., Farb, A., Kolodgie, F.D. (2006) Pathology of the vulnerable plaque. *J Am Coll Cardiol* **47**: C13–18.

25 Naghavi, M., Libby, P., Falk, E., *et al.* (2003) From vulnerable plaque to vulnerable patient: a call for new definitions and risk assessment strategies: part I. *Circulation* **108**: 1664–1672.

26 Schmermund, A., Schwartz, R.S., Adamzik, M., *et al.* (2001) Coronary atherosclerosis in unheralded sudden coronary death under age 50: histo-pathologic comparison with 'healthy' subjects dying out of hospital. *Atherosclerosis* **155**: 499–508.

27 Kragel, A.H., Reddy, S.G., Wittes, J.T., Roberts, W.C. (1989) Morphometric analysis of the composition of atherosclerotic plaques in the four major epicardial coronary arteries in acute myocardial infarction and in sudden coronary death. *Circulation* **80**: 1747–1756.

28 Leber, A.W., Becker, A., Knez, A., *et al.* (2006) Accuracy of 64-slice computed tomography to classify and quantify plaque volumes in the proximal coronary system: a comparative study using intravascular ultrasound. *J Am Coll Cardiol* **47**: 672–677.

29 Achenbach, S., Ropers, D., Hoffmann, U., *et al.* (2004) Assessment of coronary remodeling in stenotic and nonstenotic coronary atherosclerotic lesions by multidetector spiral computed tomography. *J Am Coll Cardiol* **43**: 842–847.

30 Imazeki, T., Sato, Y., Inoue, F., *et al.* (2004) Evaluation of coronary artery remodeling in patients with acute coronary syndrome and stable angina by multislice computed tomography. *Circ J* **68**: 1045–1050.

31 Nikolaou, K., Becker, C.R., Muders, M., *et al.* (2004) Multidetector-row computed tomography and magnetic resonance imaging of atherosclerotic lesions in human ex vivo coronary arteries. *Atherosclerosis* **174**: 243–252.

32 Yamagishi, M., Terashima, M., Awano, K., *et al.* (2000) Morphology of vulnerable coronary plaque: insights from follow-up of patients examined by intravascular ultrasound before an acute coronary syndrome. *J Am Coll Cardiol* **35**: 106–111.

33 Cademartiri, F., Mollet, N.R., Runza, G., *et al.* (2005) Influence of intracoronary attenuation on coronary plaque measurements using multislice computed tomography: observations in an ex vivo model of coronary computed tomography angiography. *Eur Radiol* **15**: 1426–1431.

34 Cordeiro, M.A., Lima, J.A. (2006) Atherosclerotic plaque characterization by multidetector row computed tomography angiography. *J Am Coll Cardiol* **47**: C40–47.

35 Motoyama, S., Kondo, T., Sarai, M., *et al.* (2007) Multislice computed tomographic characteristics of coronary lesions in acute coronary syndromes. *J Am Coll Cardiol* **50**: 319–326.

36 Hyafil, F., Cornily, J.C., Feig, J.E., *et al.* (2007) Noninvasive detection of macrophages using a nanoparticulate contrast agent for computed tomography. *Nat Med* **13**: 636–641.

37 Juergens, K.U., Fischbach, R. (2006) Left ventricular function studied with MDCT. *Eur Radiol* **16**: 342–357.

38 George, R.T., Silva, C., Cordeiro, M.A., *et al.* (2006) Multidetector computed tomography myocardial perfusion imaging during adenosine stress. *J Am Coll Cardiol* **48**: 153–160.

39 Lardo, A.C., Cordeiro, M.A., Silva, C., *et al.* (2006) Contrast-enhanced multidetector computed tomography viability imaging after myocardial infarction: characterization of myocyte death, microvascular obstruction, and chronic scar. *Circulation* **113**: 394–404.

40 Hamon, M., Biondi-Zoccai, G.G., Malagutti, P., *et al.* (2006) Diagnostic performance of multislice spiral computed tomography of coronary arteries as compared with conventional invasive coronary angiography: a meta-analysis. *J Am Coll Cardiol* **48**: 1896–1910.

41 Miller, J.M., Rochitte, C.E., Dewey, M., *et al.* (2007) Coronary artery evaluation using 64-row multidetector computed tomography angiography (CORE-64): results of a multicenter, international trial to assess diagnostic accuracy compared with conventional coronary angiography. *Circulation* **116**: 2630.

42 Lell, M.M., Panknin, C., Saleh, R., *et al.* (2007) Evaluation of coronary stents and stenoses at different heart rates with dual source spiral CT (DSCT). *Invest Radiol* **42**: 536–541.

43 Weustink, A.C., Meijboom, W.B., Mollet, N.R., *et al.* (2007) Reliable high-speed coronary computed tomography in symptomatic patients. *J Am Coll Cardiol* **50**: 786–794.

44 Chu, B., Hatsukami, T.S., Polissar, N.L., *et al.* (2004) Determination of carotid artery atherosclerotic lesion type and distribution in hypercholesterolemic patients with moderate carotid stenosis using noninvasive magnetic resonance imaging. *Stroke* **35**: 2444–2448.

45 Chu, B., Kampschulte, A., Ferguson, M.S., *et al.* (2004) Hemorrhage in the atherosclerotic carotid plaque: a high-resolution MRI study. *Stroke* **35**: 1079–1084.

46 Desai, M.Y., Lima, J.A. (2006) Imaging of atherosclerosis using magnetic resonance: state of the art and future directions. *Curr Atheroscler Rep* **8**: 131–139.

47 Fayad, Z.A., Fuster, V. (2001) The human high-risk plaque and its detection by magnetic resonance imaging. *Am J Cardiol* **88**: 42E–45E.

48 Larose, E., Yeghiazarians, Y., Libby, P., *et al.* (2005) Characterization of human atherosclerotic plaques by intravascular magnetic resonance imaging. *Circulation* **112**: 2324–2331.

49 Lima, J.A., Desai, M.Y., Steen, H., *et al.* (2004) Statin-induced cholesterol lowering and plaque regression after 6 months of magnetic resonance imaging-monitored therapy. *Circulation* **110**: 2336–2341.

50 Yuan, C., Mitsumori, L.M., Ferguson, M.S., *et al.* (2001) In vivo accuracy of multispectral magnetic resonance imaging for identifying lipid-rich necrotic cores and intraplaque hemorrhage in advanced human carotid plaques. *Circulation* **104**: 2051–2056.

51 Corti, R., Fuster, V., Fayad, Z.A., *et al.* (2005) Effects of aggressive versus conventional lipid-lowering therapy by simvastatin on human atherosclerotic lesions: a prospective, randomized, double-blind trial with high-resolution magnetic resonance imaging. *J Am Coll Cardiol* **46**: 106–112.

52 Gottlieb, I., Agarwal, S., Sandeep, G., *et al.* Aortic plaque regression as determined by magnetic resonance imaging with high and low dose statin therapy. *J Cardiovasc Med* (in press).

53 Gottlieb, I., Xavier, S.S., Lima, J.A. (2007) Atherosclerosis monitoring in the elderly using magnetic resonance imaging: is the extra step needed? *Am J Geriatr Cardiol* **16**: 363–368.

54 Saam, T., Kerwin, W.S., Chu, B., *et al.* (2005) Sample size calculation for clinical trials using magnetic resonance imaging for the quantitative assessment of carotid atherosclerosis. *J Cardiovasc Magn Reson* **7**: 799–808.

55 Edelman, R.R., Chien, D., Kim, D. (1991) Fast selective black blood MR imaging. *Radiology* **181**: 655–660.

56 Chan, S.K., Jaffer, F.A., Botnar, R.M., *et al.* (2001) Scan reproducibility of magnetic resonance imaging assessment of aortic atherosclerosis burden. *J Cardiovasc Magn Reson* **3**: 331–338.

57 Fayad, Z.A., Fuster, V., Fallon, J.T., *et al.* (2000) Noninvasive in vivo human coronary artery lumen and wall imaging using black-blood magnetic resonance imaging. *Circulation* **102**: 506–510.

58 Fayad, Z.A., Nahar, T., Fallon, J.T., *et al.* (2000) In vivo magnetic resonance evaluation of atherosclerotic plaques in the human thoracic aorta: a comparison with transesophageal echocardiography. *Circulation* **101**: 2503–2509.

59 Yuan, C., Mitsumori, L.M., Beach, K.W., Maravilla, K.R. (2001) Carotid atherosclerotic plaque: noninvasive MR characterization and identification of vulnerable lesions. *Radiology* **221**: 285–299.

60 Ladak, H.M., Thomas, J.B., Mitchell, J.R., *et al.* (2001) A semi-automatic technique for measurement of arterial wall from black blood MRI. *Med Phys* **28**: 1098–1107.

61 Yuan, C., Lin, E., Millard, J., Hwang, J.N. (1999) Closed contour edge detection of blood vessel lumen and outer wall boundaries in black-blood MR images. *Magn Reson Imaging* **17**: 257–266.

62 Desai, M.Y., Rodriguez, A., Wasserman, B.A., *et al.* (2005) Association of cholesterol subfractions and carotid lipid core measured by MRI. *Arterioscler Thromb Vasc Biol* **25**: e110–111.

63 Zhang, S., Hatsukami, T.S., Polissar, N.L., *et al.* (2001) Comparison of carotid vessel wall area measurements using three different contrast-weighted black blood MR imaging techniques. *Magn Reson Imaging* **19**: 795–802.

64 Davies, M.J., Thomas, A. (1984) Thrombosis and acute coronary-artery lesions in sudden cardiac ischemic death. *N Engl J Med* **310**: 1137–1140.

65 Libby, P. (2003) Vascular biology of atherosclerosis: overview and state of the art. *Am J Cardiol* **91**: 3A–6A.

66 Mohler, E.R., III. (2007) Therapy insight: peripheral arterial disease and diabetes—from pathogenesis to treatment guidelines. *Nat Clin Pract Cardiovasc Med* **4**: 151–162.

67 Yuan, C., Zhang, S.X., Polissar, N.L., *et al.* (2002) Identification of fibrous cap rupture with magnetic resonance imaging is highly associated with recent transient ischemic attack or stroke. *Circulation* **105**: 181–185.

68 Lipinski, M.J., Amirbekian, V., Frias, J.C., *et al.* (2006) MRI to detect atherosclerosis with gadolinium-containing immunomicelles targeting the macrophage scavenger receptor. *Magn Reson Med* **56**: 601–610.

69 Lipinski, M.J., Frias, J.C., Fayad, Z.A. (2006) Advances in detection and characterization of atherosclerosis using contrast agents targeting the macrophage. *J Nucl Cardiol* **13**: 699–709.

70 Sirol, M., Fuster, V., Fayad, Z.A. (2006) Plaque imaging and characterization using magnetic resonance imaging: towards molecular assessment. *Curr Mol Med* **6**: 541–548.

71 Amirbekian, V., Lipinski, M.J., Briley-Saebo, K.C., *et al.* (2007) Detecting and assessing macrophages in vivo to evaluate atherosclerosis noninvasively using molecular MRI. *Proc Natl Acad Sci USA* **104**: 961–966.

72 Fischer, R.W., Botnar, R.M., Nehrke, K., *et al.* (2006) Analysis of residual coronary artery motion for breath hold and navigator approaches using real-time coronary MRI. *Magn Reson Med* **55**: 612–618.

73 Manning, W.J., Nezafat, R., Appelbaum, E., *et al.* (2007) Coronary magnetic resonance imaging. *Magn Reson Imaging Clin N Am* **15**: 609–637, vii.

74 Danias, P.G., Stuber, M., Botnar, R.M., *et al.* (1998) Navigator assessment of breath-hold duration: impact of supplemental oxygen and hyperventilation. *AJR* **171**: 395–397.

75 Wang, Y., Grimm, R.C., Rossman, P.J., *et al.* (1995) 3D coronary MR angiography in multiple breath-holds using a respiratory feedback monitor. *Magn Reson Med* **34**: 11–16.

76 Stuber, M., Botnar, R.M., Danias, P.G., *et al.* (1999) Submillimeter three-dimensional coronary MR angiography with real-time navigator correction: comparison of navigator locations. *Radiology* **212**: 579–587.

77 Li, D., Paschal, C.B., Haacke, E.M., Adler, L.P. (1993) Coronary arteries: three-dimensional MR imaging with fat saturation and magnetization transfer contrast. *Radiology* **187**: 401–406.

78 Liu, X., Zhao, X., Huang, J., *et al.* (2007) Comparison of 3D free-breathing coronary MR angiography and 64-MDCT angiography for detection of coronary stenosis in patients with high calcium scores. *AJR* **189**: 1326–1332.

79 Maintz, D., Ozgun, M., Hoffmeier, A., *et al.* (2007) Whole-heart coronary magnetic resonance angiography: value for the detection of coronary artery stenoses in comparison to multislice computed tomography angiography. *Acta Radiol* **48**: 967–973.

80 Sakuma, H., Ichikawa, Y., Chino, S., *et al.* (2006) Detection of coronary artery stenosis with whole-heart coronary magnetic resonance angiography. *J Am Coll Cardiol* **48**: 1946–1950.

81 Botnar, R.M., Stuber, M., Kissinger, K.V., *et al.* (2000) Noninvasive coronary vessel wall and plaque imaging with magnetic resonance imaging. *Circulation* **102**: 2582–2587.

82 Botnar, R.M., Kim, W.Y., Bornert, P., *et al.* (2001) 3D coronary vessel wall imaging utilizing a local inversion technique with spiral image acquisition. *Magn Reson Med* **46**: 848–854.

Chapter 7

Evaluating Chest Pain in Patients with Known CAD

Amit R. Patel and Christopher M. Kramer

Chest pain occurring in a patient with known coronary artery disease (CAD) is often related to the underlying coronary atherosclerosis. Perhaps the most challenging aspect of evaluating a patient with known CAD presenting with recurrent chest pain is determining whether the symptom is a manifestation of an acute coronary syndrome (ACS). The astute clinician can often diagnose an ACS with a thorough history, physical examination, electrocardiogram, and cardiac biomarkers. Despite its usefulness, the electrocardiogram is an imperfect tool for the detection of ACS as it can be normal in up to 17% of cases [1]. Similarly, elevations of CK-MB and troponin might not occur for several hours following the onset of an ACS, and the absence of an elevation does not exclude an ACS [2]. The evaluation and management of these patients is often difficult because other important etiologies such as aortic dissection and pulmonary embolism must also be considered. If a careful history and physical exam lead the clinician to believe that CAD is the cause, several questions must then be answered: Does the patient have an ACS? What is the patient's prognosis? What is the ischemic burden? An additional complexity in evaluating patients with known CAD includes the possibility that the patient may also have prior percutaneous coronary interventions (PCI) or coronary artery bypass grafting (CABG). This chapter will review the role of cardiac magnetic resonance (CMR) and cardiac computed tomography (CT) for the evaluation of chest pain in patients with known CAD.

Novel Techniques for Imaging the Heart, 1st edition. Edited by M. Di Carli and R. Kwong.
© 2008 American Heart Association, ISBN: 9-781-4051-7533-3.

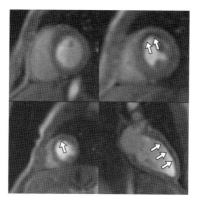

Fig. 7.1 Still frames from a resting first-pass perfusion CMR study in a patient with an ACS are shown. The hypoperfused segments in the anterior wall in multiple views are demarcated with arrows.

Physiologic Approach to Chest Pain in Patients with Known CAD (CMR)

Chest pain resulting from CAD generally reflects an inadequate delivery of blood to jeopardized myocardium. This reduced tissue perfusion can be detected using several imaging modalities. In the acute setting, resting radionuclide injections have been proposed and validated to identify high-risk patients with abnormal myocardial perfusion at rest, and especially to exclude the possibility of an ACS [3–5]. However, radionuclide techniques are limited in their ability to differentiate resting myocardial perfusion defects caused by acute myocardial ischemia from those related to old myocardial infarction [6]. Kwong *et al.* used CMR to evaluate 161 patients who presented with chest pain to an emergency department [7]. These authors performed CMR at rest including regional function, first-pass gadolinium-enhanced myocardial perfusion, and late enhancement to image the spectrum of potential abnormalities in ACS (Figure 7.1). The presence of any abnormality during a resting study had a sensitivity and specificity of 84 and 85% for detecting ACS. In the presence of a myocardial infarction, perfusion is markedly reduced, appearing as hypoenhancement on first-pass imaging. The presence of first-pass hypoperfusion at rest in the setting of a recent infarction is associated with a low likelihood of contractile recovery for that segment of myocardium [8]. The rate of increase in signal intensity in the myocardium has likewise shown to be predictive of recovery of regional function with worse recovery in segments with greater delay to contrast arrival [9].

In the setting of acute and stable coronary syndromes in patients with known CAD, adenosine stress testing can be safely performed and offers additional information regarding the magnitude of myocardium at risk [10]. Although older imaging techniques are commonly used for stress testing, echocardiography is limited by the quality of available acoustic windows and SPECT is often limited by attenuation artifacts, poor spatial resolution, and the use of ionizing radiation. Stress CMR is an attractive alternative as it has excellent spatial and temporal resolution, thereby making it a particularly useful tool for evaluating myocardial ischemia. In 135 patients with acute chest pain, Ingkanisorn *et al.* showed that the presence of an adenosine-induced perfusion abnormality on stress CMR had 100% sensitivity and 93% specificity for predicting the future diagnosis of CAD, myocardial infarction, or death [11]. Importantly, the absence of a perfusion defect was associated with a favorable outcome at one year.

The diagnostic performance of adenosine CMR was further improved in another study by using an interpretation algorithm incorporating late gadolinium enhancement (LGE). The combination of perfusion and LGE imaging had a sensitivity and specificity of 89 and 87% for the diagnosis of CAD [12]. Alternatively, Hundley *et al.* used dobutamine cine CMR to provoke ischemia in 153 patients with inadequate transthoracic echocardiographic windows [13]. Stenoses greater than 50% were safely detected with a sensitivity and specificity of 83% each. Furthermore, the 103 patients without inducible wall motion abnormalities had a 97% event-free survival. Jahnke *et al.* examined 513 patients with adenosine CMR and dobutamine CMR. The absence of ischemia was associated with a three-year event-free survival of 99.2% even though half of the population had known CAD, indicating a high disease prevalence. However, 16.5% of those with any evidence of ischemia experienced cardiovascular events during the ensuing three years [14].

Patients with a large ischemic burden often do better with revascularization than with medical therapy alone. The extent of perfusion abnormalities can be visually assessed as well as quantified. CMR can also be used to measure myocardial perfusion reserve and even absolute myocardial blood flow during both hyperemic and resting conditions [15,16]. In addition to determining patient prognosis, measuring the extent of ischemia may also be useful in determining a patient's response to either medical or mechanical therapy [17]. Preliminary data from our laboratory suggests that measuring perfusion reserve may be more accurate than qualitative assessment for the detection of coronary artery stenoses greater than 70%. Although there are clearly some benefits to the quantitative assessment of CAD, it is unclear at this point whether such a technique is preferred over the simpler qualitative evaluation. Multicenter studies are still needed to better understand the role of each of these methods. Few doubt that stress testing will identify a larger number of patients with hemodynamically significant CAD when compared to resting imaging alone, but it may not be specific enough to identify only patients suffering from ACS. The importance of differentiating unstable coronary disease from stable coronary disease is clearly relevant for implementing an appropriate treatment plan.

Anatomic Approach to Chest Pain in Patients with Known CAD (CT)

During the last few years, significant advances have enabled the noninvasive evaluation of coronary artery anatomy. This evolution can largely be attributed to several important improvements in CT equipment. Increases in the number of detector rows, gantry rotation speed, and number of x-ray sources have led to the improved spatial and temporal resolution needed to image rapidly moving coronary arteries. Although several investigators have demonstrated that the newest generation of CT scanners has a superb diagnostic accuracy, there are still some important limitations to the technology [18–20]. Poor heart rate control, arrhythmia, and coronary artery calcium considerably decrease the specificity and positive predictive value of coronary CT angiography (CTA), at least with 16-row detector scanners [21]. Additionally, CTA can currently only achieve a moderate accuracy of measuring percent stenosis and plaque areas compared to intravascular coronary ultrasound [22].

Despite the inclusion of many patients with CAD in these studies, it is unclear what the diagnostic accuracy of CTA is when evaluating only patients with known CAD. One small study using 16-detector row CT did suggest that CTA overestimated the degree of stenosis and was only moderately correlated with quantitative coronary angiography in patients with ACS [23]. Ropers *et al.* evaluated the native coronary arteries in 50 patients with prior coronary artery bypass grafting. Nine percent of the coronary artery segments were unevaluable, and in the evaluable segments the sensitivity and specificity were 86 and 76%, respectively [24]. A meta-analysis published by Di Carli *et al.* reviewing the diagnostic accuracy of CTA suggested that on a per-segment basis, the sensitivity, specificity, positive predictive value, and negative predictive value were 83, 92, 67, and 97%, respectively [25].

From a clinical viewpoint, the problem of using CTA to make a diagnosis and guide management in the setting of acute chest pain in patients with known CAD is that although highly sensitive for identifying coronary plaque (old and new) and the potential ability to delineate the presence of severe stenosis (Figure 7.2), this approach does not provide information regarding the magnitude of stress-induced ischemia that is required to make decisions regarding revascularization [26]. Indeed, several groups have documented the relationship between the anatomic and physiologic approaches to imaging coronary disease. For example, in a patient population with an intermediate likelihood of having coronary disease, Schuijf *et al.* showed that inducible ischemia was present in 39% of patients with "non-obstructive" CAD and in only 50% of those with "obstructive" CAD [27]. Although some of the discrepancy is likely related to false positive

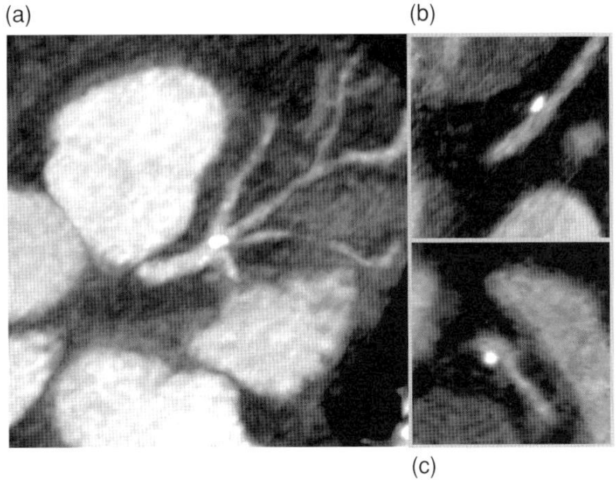

(a)   (b)

(c)

Fig. 7.2 These CT images depict a trifurcating left main coronary artery with a calcified plaque. (a) A maximum intensity projection (MIP) of the left main and its branches. (b,c) Multiplanar reformations (MPR) revealing the plaque to be nonobstructive.

CTA images, the notion that the degree of stenosis is not the only determinant of tissue perfusion is also confirmed. In fact, some have advocated the use of hybrid imaging of function and anatomy using SPECT/CT, PET/CT, or CMR [25,28].

Special Considerations in Patients with Prior Revascularization

Evaluation of Patients with Prior Coronary Artery Bypass Grafting

Surgical revascularization is a common and effective therapy for CAD. However, 25% of coronary artery bypass grafts are occluded within five years [29]. Patients with prior CABG can be safely imaged using either CTA or CMR. In general, bypass grafts are easier targets than native coronary arteries for anatomic imaging due to their relatively larger size and less susceptibility to motion. Using a 16-detector row CT scanner, Schlosser *et al.* demonstrated the patency of all the grafts was reliably determined with a sensitivity and specificity of 96 and 95%, respectively. The majority of false positives were related to metallic surgical clips, poor opacification, or the exaggerated motion that occurs in the right coronary artery. The major limitation of the technique was apparent at the distal anastomosis: 26% of these segments were unevaluable [30].

With 64-detector row CT scanners, both arterial and saphenous vein grafts are readily visualized (Figure 7.3). Meyer evaluated 418 bypass grafts in 138 consecutive patients. CTA had a sensitivity, specificity, positive predictive value, and negative predictive value of 97, 97, 93, and 99%, respectively, for the detection of significant graft disease. Importantly, no difference was noted in the diagnostic

(a)   (b)

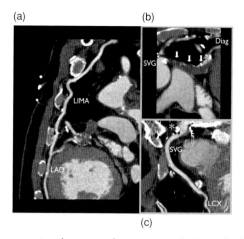

(c)

Fig. 7.3 These coronary artery bypass grafts were imaged using a dual-source CT scanner. (a) A left internal mammary artery (LIMA) graft anastomosed to the left anterior descending artery (LAD). The graft, the distal anastomosis, and runoff vessel are unobstructed. (b) A thrombosed saphenous vein graft (SVG) anastomosed to a diagonal branch of the LAD. (c) A patent and unobstructed SVG anastomosed to a marginal branch of the left circumflex artery (LCX). The asterisk demarcates a surgical clip and its associated beam-hardening artifact.

accuracy between arterial and venous grafts. The diagnostic performance deteriorated in the face of arrhythmia and heart rates greater than 65 beats per minute. In this study population, the radiation dose (18 mSv) was twice as high as x-ray angiography but the contrast dose was significantly less. Of note, the native coronary arteries and the distal anastomoses were not assessed due to their small size, extensive disease, severe calcification, and clip artifacts [31]. Ropers *et al.* addressed this limitation by evaluating bypass grafts, distal anastomoses, and distal runoff vessels. All 138 grafts studied were accurately classified as patent or occluded, and all the significant stenoses in the grafts and the anastomoses were correctly identified with CTA. The sensitivity and specificity of detecting a graft stenosis were 100 and 94%, respectively, and the majority of false positive lesions were located at the distal anastomosis [24]. Despite the high degree of accuracy to detect occlusions and stenoses within venous and arterial grafts, CTA has limited value in the evaluation of the patient with recurrent chest pain after CABG because this also requires an assessment of the native coronary arteries, which tend to be more challenging because they are usually very small and heavily calcified [26].

When CMR is used, the evaluation of the grafts and native circulation is typically based on function and blood flow rather than direct anatomic visualization of the lumen. Over two decades ago, Aurigemma *et al.* demonstrated that contiguous gradient recalled echo (GRE) images in an axial plane could be used to confirm graft patency with a sensitivity and specificity of 88 and 100%, respectively. Unfortunately, stenoses could not be detected because no difference in signal intensity exists between widely patent and severely stenosed grafts [32]. More recently, Gajlee *et al.* combined the assessment of graft patency with the physiologic measurement of graft flow using velocity encoded imaging (VENC). Although 15% of grafts could not be evaluated, patency of the remainder grafts was detected with a sensitivity and specificity of 98 and 88%, respectively. This technique also demonstrated that vein grafts have a unique balanced biphasic forward flow with individual peaks in systole and diastole rather than the typical monophasic diastolic flow seen in native coronary arteries. Additionally, the volume of flow was related to the amount of myocardial territory supplied [33]. Langerak combined VENC imaging with vasodilator stress testing to detect flow-limiting stenoses in coronary artery bypass grafts or recipient vessels (Figure 7.4). Sixty-nine patients with 166 grafts were evaluated, and adequate images could be obtained in 80% of grafts. VENC images of the proximal portion of the grafts were obtained before and during adenosine infusion to estimate the "graft blood flow reserve" or, in actuality, the velocity reserve. The receiver operator characteristics curve had an area of 0.89 for the detection of stenoses greater than or equal to 70%. The failure to increase graft blood flow velocity reserve more than 1.43-fold over resting conditions had a sensitivity and specificity of 91 and 78%, respectively, for the detection of significant CAD [34].

A three-dimensional anatomic evaluation of coronary artery bypass grafts is also possible using CMR. In a study by Langerak *et al.*, 56 grafts were examined with high-resolution gated magnetic resonance angiography (MRA). Eleven percent of grafts were still unevaluable. The receiver operator characteristics curve had an area of 0.81 for the detection of stenoses greater than or equal to 70% and an optimal sensitivity and specificity of 73 and 84%, respectively [35]. Although preliminary data are encouraging, larger multicenter studies are clearly needed. Stress perfusion CMR may be another approach to evaluating bypass grafts, but most stress MRI studies have excluded patients who have had a prior CABG procedure.

Evaluation of Patients with Prior Stenting

Although stents were not reliably visualized using 4-, 8-, or 16-detector row cardiac CT, the insight gained from these earlier-generation CT scanners has been important. Certain stent characteristics such as stent diameter, cell morphology, strut thickness, and stent material influence the diagnostic ability of detecting in-stent restenosis. Important artifacts such as blooming result from the metal used in the stent and are exaggerated by motion and the presence of calcium. The blooming artifact causes the struts to appear thickened, resulting in the artificial narrowing of the stent lumen. Additionally, volume averaging of the "thickened" struts and stent lumen result in falsely increased attenuation.

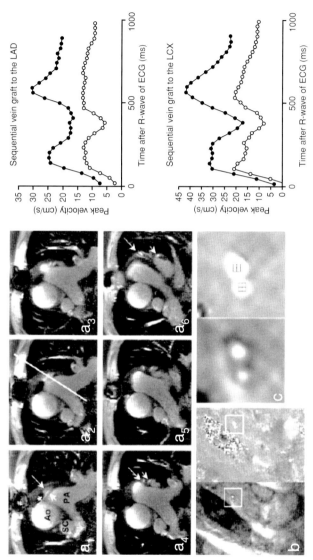

Fig. 7.4 (a) CMR images of vein grafts to the LCX (small arrow) and LAD (large arrow) are shown. (b,c) Phase- and velocity-encoded images of a vein graft during adenosine infusion. The measured velocities during stress and resting conditions are shown in graph form. Courtesy of Langerak *et al.*, with permission [34].

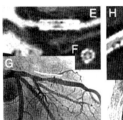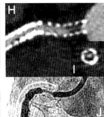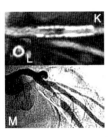

Fig. 7.5 CT images of several stents and the corresponding x-ray angiograms (XA) are shown. The white line is drawn on the XA to show the stent location. Courtesy of Ehara *et al.*, with permission [39].

Although interpretation is difficult in the presence of these artifacts, the careful selection of reconstruction algorithms is helpful. The use of a dedicated sharp convolution kernel significantly increases the amount of stent lumen that can be visualized and substantially minimizes the artificially increased attenuation. These image characteristics improve the diagnostic performance of CTA and clearly outweigh the increased noise that results from the use of the sharp convolution kernel [36,37].

As a result of the excellent spatial and temporal resolution offered by the latest-generation CT scanners, the lumen of some larger stents can now be reliably visualized (Figure 7.5). In fact, Van Mieghem recently used CTA to serially follow patients who had been treated with a left main stent. Most were drug-eluting and had a diameter larger than 3 mm prior to balloon dilatation. In image sets reconstructed with a sharper convolution kernel, the extent of neointimal hyperplasia (when greater than 1 mm) and the absolute stent diameter correlated strongly with measurements derived from intravascular ultrasound. In this ideal stent size and location, only 4 of 74 stents were unevaluable, and the sensitivity and specificity for detecting significant in-stent restenoses were 100 and 91%, respectively. Most importantly, the negative predictive value was 100% [38]. Ehara evaluated the diagnostic performance of 64-detector row CT in the remainder of the coronary tree. Eighty-one patients were imaged after stent implantation. The majority were bare metal stents and larger than 3 mm in diameter. The number of stents with open cell morphology was similar to those with closed cell morphology, as was the number with thick (greater than or equal to 0.005 in.) and thin (less than or equal to 0.005 in.) struts. Using a sharper convolution kernel, the presence of in-stent restenosis was detected with a sensitivity of 92%, specificity of 93%, PPV of 77%, and NPV of 98%. Still, 12% of patients could not be adequately imaged. In fact, 20% of stents with a diameter less than 3.5 mm were uninterpretable, compared to only 6% of stents with a diameter greater than 3.5 mm. Although the sample size was small, stents with thicker struts were more difficult to evaluate. No obvious difference in diagnostic ability was seen between closed cell and open cell stent morphology [39].

In 182 patients with previously implanted stents with a diameter greater than or equal to 2.5 mm, Cadamartiri confirmed the extremely high negative predictive value (99%) and limited positive predictive value (63%) of coronary CT for the diagnosis of in-stent restenosis. Once again, the images were reconstructed using a sharper convolution kernel. Additionally, the images were evaluated using a wider than typical window (1500 HU) centered at 300 HU. In this cohort, 11.2% had in-stent restenosis, 7.3% of stents could not be interpreted, and 10 of these 14 noninterpretable stents had a diameter of less than or equal to 3.0 mm [40]. Collectively, it is apparent that the latest-generation CT scanners can reliably exclude the presence of significant in-stent restenosis in larger stents (typically greater than 3 mm). Unfortunately, restenosis occurs more often in stents with smaller diameters.

The evaluation of stents using CMR remains challenging. Although initial safety concerns about imaging coronary stents early after implantation have been alleviated in several studies, susceptibility artifacts continue to be a major obstacle [41–45]. The artifacts result from local magnetic field inhomogeneities, eddy currents, and radiofrequency shielding of the metallic stent material. The artifacts are related to the size and ferromagnetic properties of the stent, and the resultant signal loss typically extends less than 1 cm beyond the stent and is least pronounced during fast spin echo imaging. Stents made from polyethylene, tantalum, or nitinol seem to produce fewer artifacts than stainless steel stents. Other factors that influence the extent of artifact present include the arrangement of the stent filaments, the echo time, and the relationship of the stent to the frequency encoding gradient and B_0 field [46,47]. In its current state, CMR is not a useful modality for directly visualizing luminal changes within coronary stents. MRI-friendly stent prototypes are currently being developed, but continued attention to the MRI characteristics of future stents will be necessary [48].

Assessment of Prognosis

Perhaps the most important issue in the evaluation of patients with known CAD is the determination of prognosis. Currently, there is limited data on the incremental prognostic value of CTA for risk stratification or for predicting therapeutic benefit. Alternatively, ejection fraction is extremely important as documented in the imaging literature. Patients with an ejection fraction less than 45% have a poorer prognosis regardless of the degree of ischemia that is present when compared to those patients with a preserved left ventricular ejection fraction (LVEF) [49]. CMR provides highly reproducible and accurate measures of left ventricular size and function, and it is considered the gold standard against which other imaging modalities are compared. Gated CTA has also been shown to be a useful tool for determining LVEF, but its use for this purpose alone is limited by exposure to ionizing radiation and iodinated contrast dye [50].

For many patients with ischemic cardiomyopathy, revascularization is not a sufficient treatment. Many of these patients require an implantable cardioverter-defibrillator (ICD) to prevent sudden cardiac death. Although ejection fraction is currently used to identify patients that might benefit from such therapy, it is obvious that other measures of risk are also needed. Kwong *et al.* studied 195 patients with a high clinical suspicion of CAD but no prior known myocardial infarction. LGE was present in 23% and resulted in a greater than seven-fold increase in major adverse cardiac events regardless of the extent of LGE. After 40 months of follow-up, only approximately 25% of patients with LGE had an event-free survival compared to more than 80% of those without LGE [51]. Some investigators have also suggested that the presence of peri-infarct ischemia is an important substrate for ventricular tachycardia. Yan *et al.* demonstrated that the extent of peri-infarct zone as defined by LGE imaging was an independent predictor of post-myocardial infarction mortality [52]. Similarly, Schmidt demonstrated that the mechanism for the increased mortality was related to the arrhythmogenesis of excessive tissue heterogeneity [53].

Conclusions

Both CTA and CMR are emerging techniques that are rapidly being accepted by the cardiology community. The greatest strength of CTA lies in its ability to exclude the presence of obstructive CAD as a cause of chest pain (high NPV). This result would suggest that it might not be an ideal first-line test for evaluating patients with known CAD, in whom we may require to know the magnitude of jeopardized myocardium in addition to the anatomic burden of disease. In the setting of prior CABG, CTA can provide a highly accurate assessment of graft patency. However, concomitant reliable evaluation of distal anastomosis and native coronary arteries remain challenging.

Alternatively, CMR's ability to provide comprehensive physiologic assessments regarding myocardial perfusion and ischemia, left ventricular function, and viability is appealing for the clinical evaluation of patients with known CAD. However, the majority of the current evidence supporting a role for CTA and CMR is based on small, often single-center studies. Larger multicenter trials are needed to determine the diagnostic performance of many of these techniques and whether they improve patient care and outcomes.

References

1 Rouan, G.W., Lee, T.H., Cook, E.F., *et al.* (1989) Clinical characteristics and outcome of acute myocardial infarction in patients with initially normal or nonspecific electrocardiograms (a report from the Multicenter Chest Pain Study). *Am J Cardiol* **64**(18): 1087–1092.

2 Hamm, C.W., Goldmann, B.U., Heeschen, C., *et al.* (1997) Emergency room triage of patients with acute chest pain by means of rapid testing for cardiac troponin T or troponin I. *N Engl J Med* **337**(23): 1648–1653.

3 Wackers, F.J., Sokole, E.B., Samson, G., *et al.* (1976) Value and limitations of thallium-201 scintigraphy in the acute phase of myocardial infarction. *N Engl J Med* **295**(1): 1–5.

4 Wackers, F.J., Lie, K.I., Liem, K.L., *et al.* (1978) Thallium-201 scintigraphy in unstable angina pectoris. *Circulation* **57**(4): 738–742.

5 Kapetanopoulos, A., Heller, G.V., Selker, H.P., *et al.* (2004) Acute resting myocardial perfusion imaging in patients with diabetes mellitus: results from the Emergency Room Assessment of Sestamibi for Evaluation of Chest Pain (ERASE Chest Pain) trial. *J Nucl Cardiol* **11**(5): 570–577.

6 Kjoller, E., Nielsen, S.L., Carlsen, J., *et al.* (1995) Impact of immediate and delayed myocardial scintigraphy on therapeutic decisions in suspected acute myocardial infarction. *Eur Heart J* **16**(7): 909–913.

7 Kwong, R.Y., Schussheim, A.E., Rekhraj, S., *et al.* (2003) Detecting acute coronary syndrome in the emergency department with cardiac magnetic resonance imaging. *Circulation* **107**(4): 531–537.

8 Rogers, W.J., Jr., Kramer, C.M., Geskin, G., *et al.* (1999) Early contrast-enhanced MRI predicts late functional recovery after reperfused myocardial infarction. *Circulation* **99**(6): 744–750.

9 Taylor, A.J., Al-Saadi, N., Abdel-Aty, H., *et al.* (2004) Detection of acutely impaired microvascular reperfusion after infarct angioplasty with magnetic resonance imaging. *Circulation* **109**(17): 2080–2085.

10 Mahmarian, J.J., Shaw, L.J., Filipchuk, N.G., *et al.* (2006) A multinational study to establish the value of early adenosine technetium-99m sestamibi myocardial perfusion imaging in identifying a low-risk group for early hospital discharge after acute myocardial infarction. *J Am Coll Cardiol* **48**(12): 2448–2457.

11 Ingkanisorn, W.P., Kwong, R.Y., Bohme, N.S., *et al.* (2006) Prognosis of negative adenosine stress magnetic resonance in patients presenting to an emergency department with chest pain. *J Am Coll Cardiol* **47**(7): 1427–1432.

12 Klem, I., Heitner, J.F., Shah, D.J., *et al.* (2006) Improved detection of coronary artery disease by stress perfusion cardiovascular magnetic resonance with the use of delayed enhancement infarction imaging. *J Am Coll Cardiol* **47**(8): 1630–1638.

13 Hundley, W.G., Hamilton, C.A., Thomas, M.S., *et al.* (1999) Utility of fast cine magnetic resonance imaging and display for the detection of myocardial ischemia in patients not well suited for second harmonic stress echocardiography. *Circulation* **100**(16): 1697–1702.

14 Jahnke, C., Nagel, E., Gebker, R., *et al.* (2007) Prognostic value of cardiac magnetic resonance stress tests: adenosine stress perfusion and dobutamine stress wall motion imaging. *Circulation* **115**(13): 1769–1776.

15 Al Saadi, N., Nagel, E., Gross, M., *et al.* (2000) Noninvasive detection of myocardial ischemia from perfusion reserve based on cardiovascular magnetic resonance. *Circulation* **101**(12): 1379–1383.

16 Christian, T.F., Rettmann, D.W., Aletras, A.H., *et al.* (2004) Absolute myocardial perfusion in canines measured by using dual-bolus first-pass MR imaging 1. *Radiology* **232**(3): 677–684.

17 Al Saadi, N., Nagel, E., Gross, M., *et al.* (2000) Improvement of myocardial perfusion reserve early after coronary intervention: assessment with cardiac magnetic resonance imaging. *J Am Coll Cardiol* **36**(5): 1557–1564.

18 Mollet, N.R., Cademartiri, F., van Mieghem, C.A., *et al.* (2005) High-resolution spiral computed tomography coronary angiography in patients referred for diagnostic conventional coronary angiography. *Circulation* **112**(15): 2318–2323.

19 Raff, G.L., Gallagher, M.J., O'Neill, W.W., Goldstein, J.A. (2005) Diagnostic accuracy of noninvasive coronary angiography using 64-slice spiral computed tomography. *J Am Coll Cardiol* **46**(3): 552–557.

20 Leschka, S., Alkadhi, H., Plass, A., *et al.* (2005) Accuracy of MSCT coronary angiography with 64-slice technology: first experience. *Eur Heart J* **26**(15): 1482–1487.

21 Garcia, M.J., Lessick, J., Hoffmann, M.H. (2006) Accuracy of 16-row multidetector computed tomography for the assessment of coronary artery stenosis. *JAMA* **296**(4): 403–411.

22 Leber, A.W., Knez, A., von Ziegler, F., *et al.* (2005) Quantification of obstructive and nonobstructive coronary lesions by 64-slice computed tomography: a comparative study with quantitative coronary angiography and intravascular ultrasound. *J Am Coll Cardiol* **46**(1): 147–154.

23 Dragu, R., Rispler, S., Ghersin, E., *et al.* (2006) Contrast enhanced multi-detector computed tomography coronary angiography versus conventional invasive quantitative coronary angiography in acute coronary syndrome patients—correlation and bias. *Acute Cardiac Care* **8**(2): 99–104.

24 Ropers, D., Pohle, F.K., Kuettner, A., *et al.* (2006) Diagnostic accuracy of noninvasive coronary angiography in patients after bypass surgery using 64-slice spiral computed tomography with 330-ms gantry rotation. *Circulation* **114**(22): 2334–2341.

25 Di Carli, M.F., Hachamovitch, R. (2007) New technology for noninvasive evaluation of coronary artery disease. *Circulation* **115**(11): 1464–1480.

26 Anderson, J.L., Adams, C.D., Antman, E.M., *et al.* (2007) ACC/AHA 2007 guidelines for the management of patients with unstable angina/non ST-elevation myocardial infarction: A report of the American College of Cardiology/American Heart Association Task Force on Practice Guidelines (writing committee to revise the 2002 guidelines for the management of patients with unstable angina/non ST-elevation myocardial infarction) developed in collaboration with the American College of Emergency Physicians, the Society for Cardiovascular Angiography and Interventions, and the Society of Thoracic Surgeons endorsed by the American Association of Cardiovascular and Pulmonary Rehabilitation and the Society for Academic Emergency Medicine. *J Am Coll Cardiol* 2007.02.013. Ref Type: E-pub.

27 Schuijf, J.D., Wijns, W., Jukema, J.W., *et al.* (2006) Relationship between noninvasive coronary angiography with multi-slice computed tomography and myocardial perfusion imaging. *J Am Coll Cardiol* **48**(12): 2508–2514.

28 Rispler, S., Keidar, Z., Ghersin, E., *et al.* (2007) Integrated single-photon emission computed tomography and computed tomography coronary angiography for the assessment of hemodynamically significant coronary artery lesions. *J Am Coll Cardiol* **49**(10): 1059–1067.

29 Fitzgibbon, G.M., Kafka, H.P., Leach, A.J., *et al.* (1996) Coronary bypass graft fate and patient outcome: angiographic follow-up of 5,065 grafts related to survival

and reoperation in 1,388 patients during 25 years. *J Am Coll Cardiol* **28**(3): 616–626.

30 Schlosser, T., Konorza, T., Hunold, P., *et al.* (2004) Noninvasive visualization of coronary artery bypass grafts using 16-detector row computed tomography. *J Am Coll Cardiol* **44**(6): 1224–1229.

31 Meyer, T.S., Martinoff, S., Hadamitzky, M., *et al.* (2007) Improved noninvasive assessment of coronary artery bypass grafts with 64-slice computed tomographic angiography in an unselected patient population. *J Am Coll Cardiol* **49**(9): 946–950.

32 Aurigemma, G.P., Reichek, N., Axel, L., *et al.* (1989) Noninvasive determination of coronary artery bypass graft patency by cine magnetic resonance imaging. *Circulation* **80**(6): 1595–1602.

33 Galjee, M.A., van Rossum, A.C., Doesburg, T., *et al.* (1996) Value of magnetic resonance imaging in assessing patency and function of coronary artery bypass grafts: an angiographically controlled study. *Circulation* **93**(4): 660–666.

34 Langerak, S.E., Vliegen, H.W., Jukema, J.W., *et al.* (2003) Value of magnetic resonance imaging for the noninvasive detection of stenosis in coronary artery bypass grafts and recipient coronary arteries. *Circulation* **107**(11): 1502–1508.

35 Langerak, S.E., Vliegen, H.W., de Roos, A., *et al.* (2002) Detection of vein graft disease using high-resolution magnetic resonance angiography. *Circulation* **105**(3): 328–333.

36 Maintz, D., Seifarth, H., Flohr, T., *et al.* (2003) Improved coronary artery stent visualization and in-stent stenosis detection using 16-slice computed-tomography and dedicated image reconstruction technique. *Inv Rad* **38**(12): 790–795.

37 Mahnken, A.H., Buecker, A., Wildberger, J.E., *et al.* (2004) Coronary artery stents in multislice computed tomography: in vitro artifact evaluation. *Inv Rad* **39**(1): 27–33.

38 Van Mieghem, C.A., Cademartiri, F., Mollet, N.R., *et al.* (2006) Multislice spiral computed tomography for the evaluation of stent patency after left main coronary artery stenting: a comparison with conventional coronary angiography and intravascular ultrasound. *Circulation* **114**(7): 645–653.

39 Ehara, M., Kawai, M., Surmely, J.-F., *et al.* (2007) Diagnostic accuracy of coronary in-stent restenosis using 64-slice computed tomography: comparison with invasive coronary angiography. *J Am Coll Cardiol* **49**(9): 951–959.

40 Cademartiri, F., Schuijf, J.D., Pugliese, F., *et al.* (2007) Usefulness of 64-slice multislice computed tomography coronary angiography to assess in-stent restenosis. *J Am Coll Cardiol* **49**(22): 2204–2210.

41 Patel, M.R., Albert, T.S., Kandzari, D.E., *et al.* (2006) Acute myocardial infarction: safety of cardiac MR imaging after percutaneous revascularization with stents. *Radiology* **240**(3): 674–680.

42 Syed, M.A., Carlson, K., Murphy, M., *et al.* (2006) Long-term safety of cardiac magnetic resonance imaging performed in the first few days after bare-metal stent implantation. *J Magn Reson Imaging* **24**(5): 1056–1061.

43 Porto, I., Selvanayagam, J., Ashar, V., *et al.* (2005) Safety of magnetic resonance imaging one to three days after bare metal and drug-eluting stent implantation. *Am J Cardiol* **96**(3): 366–368.

44 Gerber, T.C., Fasseas, P., Lennon, R.J., *et al.* (2003) Clinical safety of magnetic resonance imaging early after coronary artery stent placement. *J Am Coll Cardiol* **42**(7): 1295–1298.

45 Hug, J., Nagel, E., Bornstedt, A., *et al.* (2000) Coronary arterial stents: safety and artifacts during MR imaging. *Radiology* **216**(3): 781–787.

46 Maintz, D., Kugel, H., Schellhammer, F., Landwehr, P. (2001) In vitro evaluation of intravascular stent artifacts in three-dimensional MR angiography. *Inv Rad* **36**(4): 218–224.

47 Maintz, D., Botnar, R.M., Fischbach, R., *et al.* (2002) Coronary magnetic resonance angiography for assessment of the stent lumen: a phantom study. *J Cardiovasc Magn Reson* **4**(3): 359–367.

48 Buecker, A., Spuentrup, E., Ruebben, A., Gunther, R.W. (2002) Artifact-free in-stent lumen visualization by standard magnetic resonance angiography using a new metallic magnetic resonance imaging stent. *Circulation* **105**(15): 1772–1775.

49 Sharir, T., Germano, G., Kavanagh, P.B., *et al.* (1999) Incremental prognostic value of post-stress left ventricular ejection fraction and volume by gated myocardial perfusion single photon emission computed tomography. *Circulation* **100**(10): 1035–1042.

50 Sugeng, L., Mor-Avi, V., Weinert, L., *et al.* (2006) Quantitative assessment of left ventricular size and function: side-by-side comparison of real-time three-dimensional echocardiography and computed tomography with magnetic resonance reference. *Circulation* **114**(7): 654–661.

51 Kwong, R.Y., Chan, A.K., Brown, K.A., *et al.* (2006) Impact of unrecognized myocardial scar detected by cardiac magnetic resonance imaging on event-free survival in patients presenting with signs or symptoms of coronary artery disease. *Circulation* **113**(23): 2733–2743.

52 Yan, A.T., Shayne, A.J., Brown, K.A., *et al.* (2006) Characterization of the peri-infarct zone by contrast-enhanced cardiac magnetic resonance imaging is a powerful predictor of post-myocardial infarction mortality. *Circulation* **114**(1): 32–39.

53 Schmidt, A., Azevedo, C.F., Cheng, A., *et al.* (2007) Infarct tissue heterogeneity by magnetic resonance imaging identifies enhanced cardiac arrhythmia susceptibility in patients with left ventricular dysfunction. *Circulation* **115**(15): 2006–2014.

Chapter 8

Evaluating the Patient with LV Dysfunction for Potential Revascularization

Michael Salerno, Han W. Kim, and Raymond J. Kim

In the United States, heart failure affects approximately 5.2 million people and is responsible for more than 57,000 deaths annually [1]. Despite major advances in therapy, patients with heart failure have a poor prognosis, particularly those with a low left ventricular ejection fraction (LVEF) [2]. Coronary artery disease (CAD) is believed to be the underlying cause in over two-thirds of patients with heart failure and low LVEF [3]. Therefore, a common clinical scenario is the patient with left ventricular dysfunction who needs evaluation for possible coronary revascularization.

Multiple studies have shown that coronary artery bypass grafting (CABG) can improve the prognosis in patients with CAD and low LVEF as compared to medical therapy. Data from the Coronary Artery Surgery Study (CASS) registry demonstrated a five-year survival rate of 63% versus 43% in those treated with CABG versus medical therapy [4]. An analysis of 1454 patients from the Duke Cardiovascular Database with an LVEF less than 40% and one or more coronary arteries with at least 75% stenosis demonstrated a survival advantage favoring CABG over medical therapy independent of the number of diseased coronary arteries [5].

Despite the long-term survival advantage of CABG in patients with left ventricular systolic dysfunction, there is significant perioperative mortality in this population. In 6630 patients who underwent CABG in the CASS registry, the average operative mortality was 1.9% in patients with an LVEF greater than 50% and 6.7% in patients with LVEF of less than 19% [6]. Moreover, perioperative mortality may be substantially higher (up to 30%) in patients with severe left ventricular dysfunction who are also older and have several comorbid

Novel Techniques for Imaging the Heart, 1st edition. Edited by M. Di Carli and R. Kwong.
© 2008 American Heart Association, ISBN: 9-781-4051-7533-3.

conditions [7]. Thus, a crucial step prior to proceeding with surgery is identifying those patients who are most likely to benefit from revascularization.

Importance of Viability Testing

Guidelines for revascularization are provided by the American College of Cardiology and American Heart Association (ACC/AHA) [3,8]. In patients with poor left ventricular (LV) function, surgical revascularization is given a Class I recommendation (evidence/agreement that treatment is useful/efficacious) for patients with the following coronary anatomy: significant left main stenosis; left main equivalent disease, i.e., greater than 70% stenosis of proximal left anterior descending (LAD) and proximal left circumflex (LCx) arteries; and proximal LAD stenosis with two- or three-vessel disease. These recommendations are based largely upon data from older randomized trials that focused primarily on the angiographic appearance of CAD, and did not take other factors such as myocardial viability into consideration. Although these studies showed a benefit in the overall population with severe angiographic disease, from a mechanistic point of view one would expect that additional information such as the presence or absence of extensive viable myocardium could improve patient risk stratification for revascularization.

The potential importance of myocardial viability testing was evaluated by Allman *et al.* in a meta-analysis of 24 studies that included 3088 patients with a mean LVEF of 32% [9]. In patients with significant viability (as determined by thallium perfusion imaging, F-18 fluorodeoxyglucose metabolic imaging, or dobutamine echocardiography), revascularization was associated with a 79.6% reduction in annual mortality compared with medical treatment (3.2% versus 16%, $p < 0.0001$). Conversely, in patients without viability mortality rates were similar for revascularization and medical therapy (7.7% versus 6.2%, $p = $ NS).

Based on data such as these, the ACC/AHA guidelines state that CABG may be performed in patients with poor LV function without any of the previously stated coronary anatomic patterns if there is significant viable myocardium, a Class IIa recommendation (weight of evidence/opinion is in favor of usefulness/efficacy) [8]. In contrast, CABG is not recommended in patients without evidence of intermittent ischemia and significant viable myocardium, a Class III recommendation (evidence/agreement that treatment is not useful/efficacious or may be harmful) [8]. Thus, there is general agreement that viability assessment can play an important role in the preoperative evaluation of patients with LV dysfunction. Additionally, with the improvements provided by newer imaging techniques, viability assessment is expected to become more accurate and reproducible.

However, as a caveat we note at the outset that there are no prospective trials, randomized or otherwise, that have evaluated the role of viability testing in patients who are potential candidates for revascularization. All published studies to date represent small retrospective, observational series of patients.

Hence, an important goal of future investigation should be to further validate the clinical role of viability testing, in addition to refining the technology.

In this chapter, we will discuss the pathophysiological basis of viability imaging and explore what might constitute an "ideal" technique. We will not provide an extensive review of the literature but rather focus on newer imaging techniques such as cardiovascular magnetic resonance (CMR) and multidetector computed tomography (MDCT). In tandem with discussing the potential advantages of these newer techniques, we will re-examine some fundamental concepts and assumptions in the assessment of myocardial viability.

Physiological Basis of Viability Imaging Techniques

Myocardial Morphology

Simple morphological characteristics of the left ventricle can provide useful information about viability. For instance, ventricular wall thinning, as assessed by either echocardiography or cine magnetic resonance imaging (MRI), has been used as a marker for the absence of viability based on the hypothesis that a thinned region represents scar tissue and chronic myocardial infarction (MI). Cwajg *et al.* studied 45 patients with stable CAD and LV dysfunction using echocardiography and concluded that "a simple measurement of end-diastolic wall thickness less than or equal to 6 mm virtually excludes the potential for recovery of function" [10]. Similarly, Baer *et al.* studied 43 patients with chronic MI and LV dysfunction with CMR and concluded that "the depiction of significantly reduced end-diastolic wall thickness [<5.5 mm] excludes a clinically relevant amount of persistent viable myocardium" [11].

However, there are some limitations with this approach. First, it is not intended to examine viability in the setting of acute MI where wall thickness may be normal or even increased by as much as 50% despite the lack of viable myocytes [12]. Second, the time required for acute myocardial necrosis to heal and turn into collagenous scar with resultant wall thinning can be substantial and in the order of six to eight weeks. Third, even in the chronic setting, although it is clear that transmural infarction is frequently associated with myocardial thinning, there is less data in the setting of nontransmural infarction, and the transmurality of infarction that is necessary for wall thinning is unknown.

Myocardial Function

By definition, the presence of contraction or systolic wall thickening in a region demonstrates substantial viable myocardium. However, the converse may not be true. Absent resting contraction does not necessarily mean that the myocardium is dead. Obvious examples of this include the phenomena of myocardial "stunning" and "hibernation," in which contraction is absent despite preserved viability.

Clinically, dysfunctional but viable myocardium can be differentiated from infarction by assessing contractile reserve, as only viable myocardium will respond to inotropic stimulation by demonstrating enhanced contraction and systolic thickening. Based on this principle, both CMR and echocardiography have been used to assess contractile reserve and thus viability. For example, Baer *et al.* performed low-dose dobutamine CMR in 43 patients with mild LV dysfunction (LVEF 42 ± 10%) and demonstrated a sensitivity of 82% and specificity of 81% for predicting regional improvement [11]. Gunning *et al.* used dobutamine CMR to study 30 patients with more severe LV dysfunction (LVEF 24 ± 8%) and found a similar specificity (81%) but worse sensitivity (50%) for functional improvement [13]. Likewise, Sandstede *et al.* found a low sensitivity (61%) but high specificity (90%) for improved segmental wall motion [14]. The latter two studies are consistent with the dobutamine echocardiography literature, which also demonstrate lower sensitivity than specificity for predicting functional improvement [15].

The observation that contractile reserve might have relatively modest sensitivity for predicting functional improvement highlights the indirect relationship between contractile reserve and viability. Experimental studies of chronic low-flow ischemia have shown that some viable regions are so delicately balanced between reductions in flow and function, with exhausted coronary flow reserve, that any inotropic stimulation merely results in ischemia and precludes the ability to enhance contractility [16].

Myocardial Perfusion

Myocardial perfusion is related to myocardial viability in that the chronic absence of blood flow is incompatible with viability. However, it is important to recognize that perfusion does not have a direct one-to-one relationship with viability. For example, myocardial ischemia is caused by reduced perfusion but this pathophysiological state, by definition, requires viable myocardium. Reperfused acute infarction is another pathophysiological state where perfusion and viability are dissociated. The entire infarcted region is by definition non-viable; however, tissue perfusion can range from nearly zero in central regions of the infarct with profound microvascular damage to nearly normal in other regions in which the microvasculature is intact [17]. The heterogeneity of perfusion in reperfused infarction has been demonstrated in humans using contrast echocardiography and measured in animal models using radioactive microspheres [18,19]. Additionally, the pathophysiology of hibernating myocardium itself suggests a discordance. Although there is some conflicting data, hibernating myocardium — which represents viable tissue — is believed to be due to chronically reduced perfusion. These discrepancies in the relationship between perfusion and viability underscore the potential limitations in using a technique that measures perfusion for assessing viability.

Myocardial Metabolism and Cell Membrane Integrity

Techniques that examine the metabolic activity or cell membrane integrity of myocytes should at least theoretically provide the most direct means for determining whether myocytes are alive or dead. Scintigraphic techniques using positron emission tomography (PET) or single photon emission computed tomography (SPECT) are examples of such methods [20]. Specifically, preserved glucose metabolism can be examined by F18-fluorodeoxyglucose (FDG) PET, cell membrane integrity by thallium-201 SPECT, and intact mitochondria by technetium-99m sestamibi SPECT. However, for the latter two techniques myocardial perfusion probably also affects tracer activity to some degree.

Overall, radionuclide techniques demonstrate moderate to good sensitivity (81 to 93%) but poor specificity (50 to 66%) for predicting functional improvement [15]. In general, SPECT has lower diagnostic accuracy than PET and is more prone to underestimate viability, most likely because of technical limitations such as lower spatial resolution, the use of lower energy tracers, and the lack of built-in attenuation correction [21]. The poor specificity of both techniques may also relate to technical limitations, but the use of functional improvement after revascularization as the truth standard for viability may result in an artificially low specificity, as will be discussed later in the chapter.

Delayed-enhancement CMR (DE-CMR) is another technique that can index cell membrane integrity. Although the gadolinium-based contrast media used for DE-CMR is inert and active transport processes across cell membranes for thallium are not present, there appears to be a direct but inverse relationship between gadolinium concentration and the percentage of viable myocytes within any given region of myocardial tissue. The mechanism is likely based on the following: First, tissue volume in normal myocardium is predominantly intracellular (75 to 80% of the water space); and second, currently available gadolinium contrast media are "extracellular" agents because they do not cross cell membranes [22,23]. Thus, the volume of distribution of gadolinium contrast in normal myocardium is quite small (about 20% of the water space), and one can consider viable myocytes as actively excluding contrast media [24]. Pathophysiological states that result in a reduced density of viable myocytes will then have an increased volume of distribution of gadolinium and a higher concentration [25]. Note that this mechanism is independent of the cause or etiology for nonviable myocardium. Whether the tissue consists of contraction-band necrosis in the setting of acute MI, collagenous scar in chronic MI, or fibrosis in various nonischemic cardiomyopathies, the region will have an increased gadolinium concentration if there is a reduced density of viable myocytes [24].

There is a wealth of data in animal models of myocardial injury that have directly compared DE-CMR to histopathology [25–27]. These data demonstrate that DE-CMR can delineate between reversible and irreversible myocardial injury independent of wall motion, infarct age, or reperfusion status. Figure 8.1a

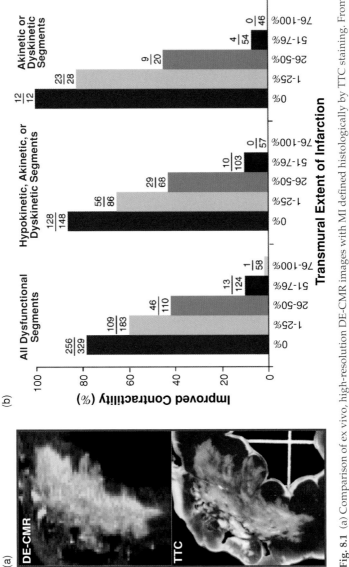

Fig. 8.1 (a) Comparison of ex vivo, high-resolution DE-CMR images with MI defined histologically by TTC staining. From Kim *et al.*, with permission [26]. (b) The relation between the transmural extent of infarction determined by DE-CMR before revascularization and the likelihood of improved contractility after revascularization. From Kim *et al.*, with permission [30].

shows an example of a comparison between DE-CMR and histopathology, demonstrating the nearly exact match between the hyperenhanced (bright) region on DE-CMR and the infarcted region delineated by histopathology. In patients, DE-CMR has been shown to be highly effective in identifying the presence, location, and extent of MI in both the acute and chronic settings [28,29]. Additionally, it has been used to predict reversible myocardial dysfunction in those undergoing revascularization procedures [30–32]. Figure 8.1b demonstrates that for any given myocardial region, there is an inverse relationship between the transmural extent of infarction determined by DE-CMR and the likelihood of improved contractility after revascularization.

Recently, the delayed-enhancement concept has been extended to MDCT. The interpretation of contrast-enhancement patterns on MDCT appears quite similar to that for DE-CMR, and is likely based on the same underlying mechanism because the iodinated contrast media used for MDCT has nearly identical pharmacokinetics as that of "extra-cellular" gadolinium contrast [33]. Likewise, in animal models delayed-enhancement MDCT assessment of acute and chronic MI has been shown to accurately reflect true infarct size and morphology, as determined by histopathology [34]. Although currently there are few studies in humans, these have demonstrated an excellent agreement between delayed-enhancement MDCT and CMR, albeit with reduced contrast-to-noise ratio and image quality for MDCT [33,35]. Figure 8.2 shows a comparison between DE-MDCT and DE-CMR in three patients.

The "Ideal" Technique

Knowing How Much Is Alive Is Not Enough

A useful exercise is to consider what might constitute an "ideal" technique for assessing viability. Certainly, it would be important for the technique to be fast, safe, and provide reproducible results. However, what might not be so apparent is that even if a technique were available that could offer precise quantification of viability without technical limitations (infinite spatial resolution, no artifacts, and so on), this would still be insufficient to provide a complete characterization of viability, and thus insufficient to provide the highest accuracy in predicting wall motion improvement or clinical benefit after coronary revascularization [36]. Certainly, there are additional factors that are not related to limitations in noninvasive testing that could reduce accuracy in predicting functional improvement. These have been well described and include peri- or postoperative occult MI, incomplete revascularization as a result of diffuse disease, or tethering of regions with extensive scarring adjacent to viable regions [37–39]. For the purposes of this section, we will not consider these clinical factors but instead focus on issues related to the noninvasive assessment of viability and examine the concept that "knowing how much is alive is not enough."

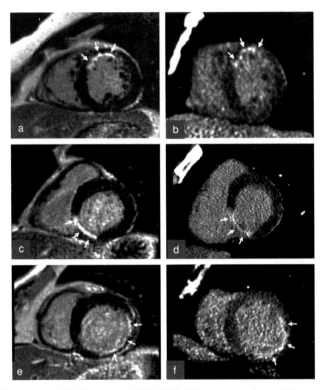

Fig. 8.2 Short-axis DE-CMR (a,c,e) and MDCT (b,d,f) images in three different patients with acute MI attributable to (a,b) left anterior descending, (c,d) right coronary artery, and (e,f) left circumflex artery occlusion after successful revascularization. There is excellent agreement between hyperenhanced regions (arrows) on the two techniques. Adapted from Mahnken *et al.*, with permission [35].

A central tenet of this concept is that a technique that offers even a perfect assessment of what is alive (viable) has substantial and practical limitations compared with a technique that offers both an assessment of what is alive and what is dead (nonviable). This tenet may be counterintuitive because it would seem that by knowing exactly how much is alive, by deductive logic, one should know how much is dead. However, this is an incorrect assumption, and the patient examples in Figure 8.3a might be illustrative.

The left panel in the top row (Patient A) shows a mid-ventricular, short-axis DE-CMR image of a normal heart in diastole. With DE-CMR, nonviable regions such as infarction appear bright (hyperenhanced), whereas viable regions appear black. First, consider only a "nonviability" or bright region assessment. A quick visual inspection shows no evidence of myocardial bright

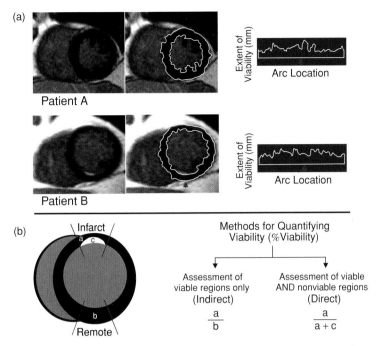

Fig. 8.3 (a) Left panels show delayed-enhancement images of a normal subject (Patient A) and a patient with a subendocardial, inferior wall MI (Patient B). The center panels show the tracing of the borders of viable myocardium. The right panels plot the extent of viability (thickness) as a function of LV location. Note that there is significant regional variation in the extent of viable myocardium. See text for details. Adapted from Kim and Shah, with permission [36]. (b) A cartoon highlighting differences between an indirect and direct method of quantifying regional viability. The indirect method is based on assessment of viable regions only. The direct method is based on assessment of viable and nonviable regions. Viable myocardium is black, and infarct is white. "Remote" zone represents segment with maximum amount of viability. From Fuster *et al.*, with permission [63].

regions, thus one rapidly concludes that no infarction is present. In comparison, now consider only a "viability" or black region assessment. One can trace the endocardial and epicardial borders of viable myocardium (center panel), and then plot the transmural extent of viability as a function of position starting from the anterior wall at the top and moving counterclockwise around the LV (right panel). From the plot, it is obvious that there is marked heterogeneity in the transmural extent of viability, with as much as 12 mm of viable myocardium in the portion of the inferior wall adjacent to the posterior papillary muscle, and as little as 7 mm in the anteroseptal wall at the right ventricle insertion site. Concerning this finding, it is important to note that it has been long known that there can be significant variation in diastolic wall thickness at different points around the LV, even if papillary muscles are excluded and healthy volunteers are studied [40]. This observation then naturally proceeds to the conclusion that there can be significant variability in the transmural extent of viable myocardium at different locations of the normal LV, as was found in Patient A.

The principle that normal hearts can have significant heterogeneity in the extent of viable myocardium has direct clinical implications. For example, a region with 70% of the maximum amount of viability might represent either a normal region with 70% the wall thickness of the thickest region or a region with a subendocardial MI. The images from Patient B (Figure 8.3a) underscore this concept. This particular patient had a clinically documented MI due to occlusion of the right coronary artery (RCA), which was reopened during primary angioplasty. Again, consider first only a "nonviability" assessment. From a quick visual perusal (left panel), one can determine that there is a subendocardial bright region in the inferoseptal wall consistent with the patient's prior MI in the RCA perfusion territory. Next, consider only a "viability" assessment, similar to that performed in Patient A. Again, endocardial and epicardial contours are traced (center panel), but one difference should be noted. The endocardial contour is along the border of viable (black) myocardium, and the infarcted region is not included. The plot showing the extent of viable myocardium (right panel) once more shows marked regional variability, and from this assessment the presence and location of infarction is not evident. Thus, in this patient the intrinsic variation in the extent of viable myocardium for noninfarcted regions is greater than the reduction in viable myocardium for the region with subendocardial infarction. This renders the subendocardial infarction "invisible" for any technique that can assess only viable myocardium, even if the technique has perfect accuracy and has infinite spatial resolution.

These two patient examples highlight the differences between techniques that can visualize only viable myocardium as opposed to techniques that can visualize viable and nonviable myocardium. Additionally, it is important to recognize that the use of different techniques often leads to differences in the way in which viability is quantified, although the nomenclature used may be the same. For instance, when only viable myocardium can be visualized, the percentage of viability in any given segment is assessed indirectly and generally refers to the amount of viability in the segment normalized to the segment with the maximum amount of viability or to data from a gender-specific database of controls. Conversely, when both viable and nonviable myocardium can be visualized, the percentage of viability can be assessed directly and expressed as the amount of viability in the segment normalized to the amount of viability plus infarction in the same segment (Figure 8.3b). These differences in the way in which viability is measured can alter clinical interpretation. For the normal heart in Patient A, the indirect method would show that there is significant regional variability in the extent of viable myocardium (60 to 100% of maximum viability), whereas

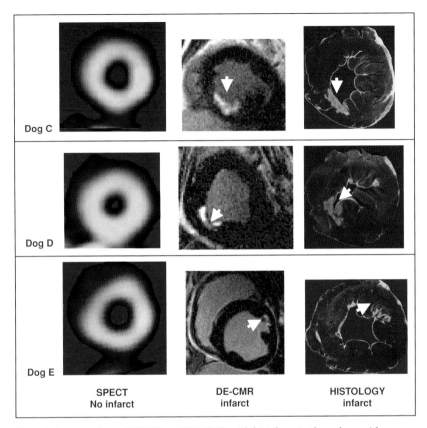

Fig. 8.4 A comparison of SPECT and DE-CMR with histology in three dogs with subendocardial infarcts (arrows). Note that the infarcts are not evident on SPECT. Adapted from Wagner *et al.*, with permission [41].

the direct method would show essentially no variability because all segments would be classified as 100% viable. Likewise for Patient B, the indirect method would not be able to identify the region of subendocardial infarction because the extent of viable myocardium in this sector is within the normal variation. The direct method would clearly identify the region with subendocardial infarction because this region would be the only region with less than 100% viable myocardium.

These patient examples also clarify the mechanism by which subendocardial infarcts are routinely missed by techniques such as SPECT and PET (Figure 8.4) [41–43]. Although it is often reported that limited spatial resolution is the reason, it should be evident that even infinite spatial resolution would not improve the detection of subendocardial infarction by these or other methodologies based

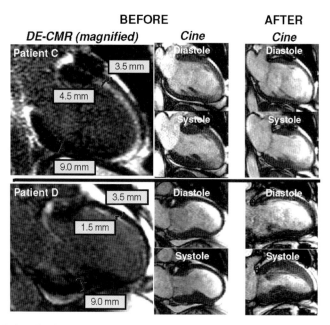

Fig. 8.5 Delayed-enhancement and cine CMR images of two patients (C and D) before coronary revascularization, and cine images two months after revascularization. See text for details. Adapted from Kim and Shah, with permission [36].

on assessing only viable myocardium. Conversely, a methodology with poor spatial resolution (e.g., a single voxel across the LV wall) would still be able to detect subendocardial infarction if it had the ability to assess both living and dead tissue.

Is "Thinned" Myocardium Always Dead?

As discussed previously, prior studies report that in patients with coronary disease and LV dysfunction, regions with thinned myocardium represent scar tissue and cannot improve in contractile function after revascularization [10]. However, the ability of delayed-enhancement imaging to directly visualize both living and dead myocardium has led to some recent observations that appear to refute this concept [10,44,45].

Figure 8.5 shows CMR images of two patients (C and D) who have severe CAD and chronic LV dysfunction. The left panels represent long-axis views acquired before coronary revascularization, and two points should be noted on the cine images. First, both patients have severe contractile dysfunction of the anterior wall. Second, Patient D has an associated thinning of the anterior wall (diastolic wall thickness, 5.0 mm) whereas Patient C does not (diastolic wall thickness, 8.0 mm). Based on these cine images and the existing literature, one might expect that there is more viable myocardium in the anterior wall of Patient C than in Patient D, and in fact question the need for viability testing at all in Patient D as the thinned, akinetic anterior wall must undoubtedly be scar tissue and thus nonviable. However, the DE-CMR images acquired before revascularization indicate a different clinical interpretation. In Patient C, there is a bright endocardial rim of hyperenhancement (infarction) that measures on average 4.5 mm in thickness. The remaining epicardial rim of tissue that is black (viable) measures 3.5 mm in thickness (total thickness, 8 mm). In Patient D, there is also an endocardial rim of hyperenhancement but it measures on average only 1.5 mm in thickness. The epicardial rim that is viable measures 3.5 mm in thickness (total thickness, 5 mm). Note that in both patients the absolute amount of viable myocardium is the same (3.5 mm), but when the extent of viability is expressed as a percentage of the total amount of myocardium in the segment, Patient C has less than 50% viable myocardium ($3.5/8 = 44\%$) whereas Patient D has greater than 50% viable myocardium ($3.5/5 = 70\%$). The right-most panels represent cine images acquired two months after coronary revascularization. Patient C exhibits no improvement in contractile function in the anterior wall, and in fact develops diastolic wall thinning in this region. Conversely, Patient D exhibits not only significant improvement in anterior wall contractile function but also recovery of diastolic wall thickness in this region (from 5 to 9 mm).

Three fundamental points are raised by these patient examples. First, it is apparent that a method that can quantify only viable myocardium, even if technically flawless (infinite spatial resolution, no artifacts, and so on), provides insufficient information to allow a comprehensive assessment of myocardial viability. Because both patients had the same reduced amount of viable myocardium (3.5 mm thick), we would have predicted — incorrectly, as it turns out — that both patients would not improve in contractile function following revascularization. Second, it is evident that the absolute amount of viable myocardium in a given region is dynamic and can increase or decrease as a result of ventricular remodeling. Although it is common knowledge that myocardial viability can decrease — for example, due to MI with associated wall thinning — the reverse process in which regions of thin myocardium become thick with an absolute increase in the transmural extent of viability (as in patient D) has not been previously described. Third, it appears that quantification of nonviable in addition to viable myocardium is important in predicting contractile improvement following revascularization. For instance, incorporating information regarding nonviable myocardium into a ratio of viable to total myocardium (viable plus nonviable) within the same region would lead to the conclusion that the anterior wall of Patient D has a higher percentage of viable myocardium (70%) than Patient C (44%) and thus is more likely to improve in contractile function. The follow-up cine images in Figure 8.5 demonstrate that this prediction is correct.

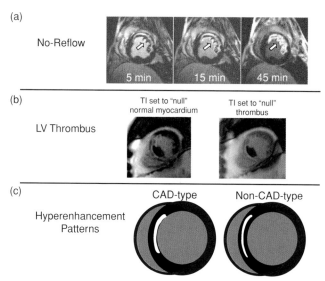

Fig. 8.6 (a) The "no-reflow" phenomenon revealed by DE-CMR. Labels refer to time after administration of gadolinium contrast. The subendocardial black zone surrounded by hyperenhancement corresponds to the region of no-reflow (arrow) within the acute infarction. This region can be distinguished from normal myocardium because it is encompassed in 3D space by hyperenhanced myocardium or the LV cavity, and by the fact that it slowly becomes hyperenhanced over time. From Kim *et al.*, In: Higgins, deRoos, eds. Cardiovascular MRI & MRA. Philadelphia: Lippincott Williams & Wilkins, 2003; 209–237, with permission. (b) DE-CMR images in a patient with an LV thrombus adjacent to the interventricular septum. Note that increasing the inversion time (TI) from that needed to "null" normal myocardium (about 300 ms) to "null" thrombus (about 600 ms) results in increased image intensity for all myocardial regions, whereas the thrombus is now homogeneously black. (c) Cartoon images of hyperenhancement patterns consistent with an ischemic and a nonischemic etiology. See text for details.

Additional Characterization of Scar Tissue

It may be important clinically to provide a characterization of dead tissue in addition to measuring its extent. For example, rather than simply identifying a region of acute infarction as nonviable, DE-CMR and MDCT have the ability to differentiate between acute infarcts with necrotic myocytes and acute infarcts with necrotic myocytes and damaged microvasculature (Figure 8.6a) [19,34,46]. The latter, termed the "no-reflow phenomenon," indicates compromised tissue perfusion despite restoration of epicardial artery patency. The incidence and extent of early no-reflow appears to be associated with worse LV remodeling and outcome [47,48].

There is increased propensity for thrombus formation near infarcted regions with impaired contractility and stagnant LV cavity blood flow (Figure 8.6b). If the thrombus protrudes into the LV cavity, it is easily identified by cine CMR or echocardiography, but layered mural thrombus can often be mistaken as akinetic, nonviable myocardium. Recent data indicate that DE-CMR has an improved sensitivity for detecting LV thrombus compared to transthoracic or transesophageal echocardiography [49,50]. Importantly, the diagnosis of LV thrombus will likely affect patient management and prognosis.

The specific location and shape of dead myocardium within the ventricular wall may shed light on its etiology. Myocardial cell death from ischemic injury progresses as a "wavefront" from the subendocardium to the epicardium [51]. Correspondingly, hyperenhancement patterns that spare the subendocardium and are limited to the middle or epicardial portion of the LV wall are clearly in a non-CAD pattern [52]. Figure 8.6c shows stylized images of two hearts that have the same absolute amount of both viable and nonviable myocardium in the interventricular septum. However, sparing of the subendocardium in the second heart indicates a nonischemic etiology. The importance of this — specifically, regarding potential revascularization decisions — is that even if both hearts have coronary disease and LV dysfunction, the latter may not benefit from revascularization because the injury is not from an ischemic process and the CAD may be incidental. Determination of the pattern of dead myocardium within the ventricular wall requires not only the ability to directly visualize both viable and nonviable myocardium but also high spatial resolution.

Common Assumptions and Clinical Implications

Intermediate Levels of Viability

The reports of predicting functional recovery with DE-CMR have shown that for any given myocardial region, there is a smooth progressive relationship between the transmural extent of viability and the likelihood of functional recovery [30–32,37]. In other words, with each increase in the amount of viability (or decrease in the amount of nonviability) there is a corresponding increment in the likelihood for functional recovery (Figure 8.1b). Two questions are often raised regarding this relationship. The first is with regard to intermediate levels of viability (transmural extent, 50 to 75%), a situation where DE-CMR appears to have limited predictive value in that only about 50% of these regions will have functional recovery. In this case, would viability assessment be improved by considering additional information such as provided by dobutamine contractile reserve testing? The second question is related: Because other techniques such as radionuclide imaging can also demonstrate a smooth progressive relationship between the amount of viability (tracer activity) and the likelihood for functional recovery, in what way exactly does DE-CMR with all of its technical advantages provide an improved diagnosis for the clinician [53]?

In part, the questions are a consequence of some common assumptions regarding functional recovery. First, it is important to distinguish between what would

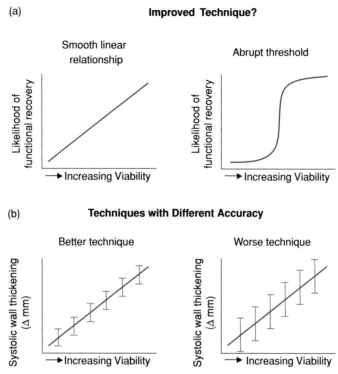

Fig. 8.7 Assumptions in evaluating viability techniques. (a) A technique that demonstrates a smooth, linear relationship between viability and functional recovery may be considered limited in that intermediate levels of viability predict intermediate likelihood for functional recovery. With an abrupt threshold relationship between viability and functional recovery, the problem of predicting intermediate likelihood for functional recovery is greatly minimized. See text for details. (b) Two techniques with different diagnostic capability can show a similar overall relationship between viability and functional improvement. However, if functional improvement is expressed as a continuous rather than binary variable, the better technique may reduce the variability (smaller error bars) in predicting the absolute amount of functional improvement. See text for details.

be desirable clinically from what can actually occur physiologically. Although we may ask for an improved technique with better predictive value, perhaps in reality we are asking for a different physiological relationship — an abrupt threshold of viability, below which there is virtually no chance for functional recovery, and above which nearly all have functional recovery. Figure 8.7a demonstrates that with an abrupt threshold, the problem of predicting an intermediate likelihood for functional recovery is greatly minimized. Unfortunately, this physiological relationship may not exist. Second, it is essential to remember that functional recovery is a continuum (as is viability itself) and not simply a binary (yes or no) function. Thus, part of the problem with intermediate levels of viability is expecting that these regions will or will not have functional recovery in this binary fashion. Because it more closely reflects reality, it might be better to consider most regions with intermediate levels of viability as having a high chance for an intermediate amount of improvement, rather than 50% likely to have complete recovery and the other 50% no improvement whatsoever.

Complicating this issue is the belief that a threshold phenomenon exists between the transmural extent of infarction and systolic thickening. This assumption is based primarily on results by Lieberman *et al.*, who demonstrated in a canine model of acute infarction that akinesia is expected if infarction involves greater than or equal to 20% of the wall thickness [54]. However, evaluation by DE-CMR in humans suggests that a threshold phenomenon does not exist [55,56]. These data suggest that it is unwise to extrapolate the results of Lieberman *et al.*, who did not consider the effects of stunning or ongoing ischemia, to humans following revascularization in whom substantial stunning, ischemia, or hibernation may no longer be present.

The finding that two techniques can demonstrate a similar relationship between the amount of viability and the likelihood of functional recovery does not mean that the techniques have the same diagnostic capability. For example, both an accurate and a less accurate technique can show that for a given intermediate level of viability, on average 50% of segments recover function. However, part of the problem again is defining functional recovery as a binomial variable. Figure 8.7b demonstrates the utility of expressing functional recovery as a continuous variable (e.g., millimeters of improvement in systolic wall thickening). Although the overall relationship is the same, for any given level of viability the better technique will provide a smaller variability (smaller error bars) in the absolute amount of functional improvement than the worse technique.

Functional Recovery as the Standard of Truth

The ideal reference standard for evaluating viability imaging techniques would be histopathological examination. However, for the vast majority of clinical studies this is not feasible, and functional recovery following revascularization has become the de facto standard. This clinical endpoint makes sense for a variety of reasons. Because LV dysfunction portends poor prognosis, one would expect that functional recovery would be an important and beneficial clinical outcome of revascularization. Additionally, if a myocardial region recovers function, then one might confidently assume that the region has a substantial amount of viable myocytes. Indeed, this has been confirmed by histopathological examination. In 33 patients with LAD disease, Maes *et al.* took transmural needle biopsies from the LV anterior wall during CABG [57]. The biopsies from regions that were dysfunctional prior to revascularization but recovered afterward showed $89 \pm 6\%$ of the volume consisted of viable cells. Similarly, Dakik *et al.* reported that among 21 biopsied dyssynergic myocardial segments, the 11 that recovered function after CABG had $93 \pm 4\%$ viability by volume [58].

However, a common misconception is that if a region does not have functional improvement, then this region is nonviable. In fact, Maes and Dakik observed that biopsy specimens from regions that did not improve after revascularization still had $65 \pm 25\%$ and $69 \pm 21\%$ viability by volume, respectively [57,58]. There are several reasons why regions that are predominantly viable might not recover function following revascularization. First, revascularization can often be incomplete in patients with extensive atherosclerosis [38]. Therefore, there may be persistent areas of hibernating myocardium. Second, viable myocardium can be juxtaposed to regions with extensive scarring and unable to respond to revascularization because of tethering [39]. Third, the use of a single evaluation of ventricular function soon after revascularization can lead to an underestimation of the true rate of functional recovery. Bax *et al.* evaluated functional recovery in 26 patients at 3 and 14 months following CABG [59]. At 3 months, only 31% of hibernating segments recovered, whereas at 14 months an additional 61% recovered.

Even with these limitations, one could argue that functional recovery is an appropriate truth standard for viability because without recovery, there can be no benefit to the patient for undergoing revascularization. On this point, the results by Samady *et al.* are instructive [60]. Of 104 consecutive patients that underwent pre- and post-CABG LVEF assessment, 68 had improvement in LVEF (greater than 5% increase) and 36 had no significant change. Surprisingly, the two groups had similar postoperative improvement in angina and heart failure scores, and there was no difference in cardiovascular mortality with a mean follow-up of 32 months. The authors concluded that a lack of improvement in LVEF after CABG is not associated with poorer outcome, and speculated that many patients without improvement in LVEF can nonetheless have substantial viable myocardium that can respond to effective revascularization with beneficial effects on prognosis.

Thus, functional recovery is a flawed truth standard for evaluating viability imaging techniques. The primary problem is that regions (or patients) without functional recovery can have substantial viability that may be important to detect clinically. This has implications for the published studies that have used functional recovery as the standard for evaluating tests of viability. Poor specificity (for functional recovery) should be considered less important than poor sensitivity because for the former, a number of "false positives" (test showed viability but there was no functional recovery) can represent a problem with the truth standard rather than the technique. Further work must be completed to determine how various assessments of viability predict other clinically relevant endpoints such as improvement in symptoms of angina and heart failure, improvement in exercise tolerance, and reduction in future MI, arrhythmias, and death.

Overview of Clinical Interpretation

For clinical purposes, we interpret DE-CMR scans for viability assessment using a standard 17-segment model recommended by the AHA [61]. The extent of hyperenhanced or nonviable tissue within each segment is graded using a five-point scale: $0 = 0\%$; $1 = 1$ to 25% volume; $2 = 26$ to 50% volume; $3 = 51$ to 75% volume; and $4 = 76$ to 100% volume. Although the interpretation is visual and thus rapid, note that the LV myocardium can have a total of 85 (17×5) different levels of nonviable tissue, and one can approach viability as a continuum rather than in a binary manner.

We do not use low-dose dobutamine cine CMR to improve the assessment of viability. For dysfunctional regions with greater than or equal to 50% scar by DE-CMR, the negative predictive value for functional improvement is quite high (92% in the initial report by Kim *et al.*) and likely will be higher than that found by dobutamine CMR [30,62]. For regions with less than 25% scar, it is possible that dobutamine CMR can provide a higher positive predictive value than DE-CMR. However, in this group there is such a large amount of viability and the potential for benefit is so great, it is sensible to be concerned about the possibility of a false negative dobutamine CMR result. Thus in this group, with all other clinical issues being equal, it is usually preferable to err on the side of overestimating rather than underestimating the clinical benefit of revascularization. For regions with 25% to 50% scar, one should recognize that this group represents only a small portion of dysfunctional segments — 14% in the initial report by Kim *et al.* Nonetheless, it is likely that if one dichotomizes this group into those that are contractile reserve positive and those that are negative, these two groups will have differences in the rate of functional improvement after revascularization [32]. But in this case, recall from the previous section that functional improvement is a flawed truth standard for viability. The question whether one can predict a subgroup with a high likelihood of functional improvement is only part of the issue. Perhaps a more important question is whether a substantial amount of viability (e.g., 50 to 75%) might be sufficient to provide clinical benefit even without functional improvement after revascularization. The results of Samady *et al.* strongly suggest that there may be an intermediate level of viability that increases the likelihood of a good clinical outcome but is, meanwhile, insufficient to provide improved resting function [60]. It is likely that improved clinical outcome is related to a number of factors including prevention or even reversal of adverse remodeling, improved contractile response under stress, prevention of recurrent myocardial ischemia/infarction, or prevention of arrhythmias.

The decision for revascularization is dependent on several factors besides the amount of viability, including specifics regarding the coronary anatomy, the presence of angina or ischemia, and patient comorbidities. Additionally, viable myocardium can be in different states (i.e., normal, ischemic, hibernating, cardiomyopathic from a nonischemic process, and so on) and it is likely that differentiating between these states may be important for revascularization decisions in some patients. Thus, although we do not perform low-dose dobutamine CMR, we often incorporate stress-testing with viability assessment to determine whether the dysfunction in viable regions is clearly due to ischemic heart disease. As discussed earlier, it is important to remember that the pattern of nonviable myocardium on DE-CMR can also shed light on the state of viable myocardium. For stress-testing, we prefer adenosine perfusion-CMR over high-dose dobutamine cine CMR because of logistic issues, including scan time, ease of patient monitoring, and staffing [63].

Conclusions

The pathophysiological basis of imaging techniques for assessing viability is varied and can include processes that are only indirectly related to whether myocytes are living or dead. Delayed-enhancement imaging via CMR or MDCT appears to index cell membrane integrity and may be a direct means for evaluating viability. Importantly, delayed-enhancement imaging provides visualization of both living and dead myocardium. Although perhaps counterintuitive, a technique that offers a perfect assessment of what is living (infinite spatial resolution, no artifacts, and so on) has substantial and practical limitations compared with a technique that offers both an assessment of what is living and dead. In particular, the setting of subendocardial infarction and myocardial "thinning" highlights this concept. Additionally, the assessment of the "pattern" of dead myocardium may shed light regarding the etiology of the cardiomyopathic process.

There are many assumptions regarding viability testing. Several arise, in part, from considering viability and functional recovery as a simple binary (yes or no) function rather than as a continuum, the latter of which better reflects reality. Although an important clinical endpoint, functional recovery after revascularization is a flawed truth standard for evaluating viability techniques because myocardium that does not recover may be predominantly viable rather than nonviable. The decision for revascularization involves many factors besides the amount of viability (and nonviability), and incorporating adenosine stress perfusion-CMR may be helpful in selected patients.

References

1 Rosamond, W., Flegal, K., Friday, G., *et al.* (2007) Heart disease and stroke statistics—2007 update: a report from the American Heart Association Statistics Committee and Stroke Statistics Subcommittee. *Circulation* **115**(5): e69–171.
2 White, H.D., Norris, R.M., Brown, M.A., *et al.* (1987) Left ventricular end-systolic volume as the major determinant of survival after recovery from myocardial infarction. *Circulation* **76**(1): 44–51.

3 Hunt, S.A., Abraham, W.T., Chin, M.H., *et al.* (2005) ACC/AHA 2005 guideline update for the diagnosis and management of chronic heart failure in the adult: a report of the American College of Cardiology/American Heart Association Task Force on Practice Guidelines (writing committee to update the 2001 guidelines for the evaluation and management of heart failure): developed in collaboration with the American College of Chest Physicians and the International Society for Heart and Lung Transplantation: endorsed by the Heart Rhythm Society. *Circulation* **112**(12): e154–235.

4 Alderman, E.L., Fisher, L.D., Litwin, P., *et al.* (1983) Results of coronary artery surgery in patients with poor left ventricular function (CASS). *Circulation* **68**(4): 785–795.

5 O'Connor, C.M., Velazquez, E.J., Gardner, L.H., *et al.* (2002) Comparison of coronary artery bypass grafting versus medical therapy on long-term outcome in patients with ischemic cardiomyopathy (a 25-year experience from the Duke Cardiovascular Disease Databank). *Am J Cardiol* **90**(2): 101–107.

6 Kennedy, J.W., Kaiser, G.C., Fisher, L.D., *et al.* (1981) Clinical and angiographic predictors of operative mortality from the collaborative study in coronary artery surgery (CASS). *Circulation* **63**(4): 793–802.

7 Baker, D.W., Jones, R., Hodges, J., *et al.* (1994) Management of heart failure, III: the role of revascularization in the treatment of patients with moderate or severe left ventricular systolic dysfunction. *JAMA* **272**(19): 1528–1534.

8 Eagle, K.A., Guyton, R.A., Davidoff, R., *et al.* (2004) ACC/AHA 2004 guideline update for coronary artery bypass graft surgery: a report of the American College of Cardiology/American Heart Association Task Force on Practice Guidelines (committee to update the 1999 guidelines for coronary artery bypass graft surgery). *Circulation* **110**(14): e340–437.

9 Allman, K.C., Shaw, L.J., Hachamovitch, R., Udelson, J.E. (2002) Myocardial viability testing and impact of revascularization on prognosis in patients with coronary artery disease and left ventricular dysfunction: a meta-analysis. *J Am Coll Cardiol* **39**(7): 1151–1158.

10 Cwajg, J.M., Cwajg, E., Nagueh, S.F., *et al.* (2000) End-diastolic wall thickness as a predictor of recovery of function in myocardial hibernation: relation to rest-redistribution T1-201 tomography and dobutamine stress echocardiography. *J Am Coll Cardiol* **35**(5): 1152–1161.

11 Baer, F.M., Theissen, P., Schneider, C.A., *et al.* (1998) Dobutamine magnetic resonance imaging predicts contractile recovery of chronically dysfunctional myocardium after successful revascularization. *J Am Coll Cardiol* **31**(5): 1040–1048.

12 Haendchen, R.V., Corday, E., Torres, M., *et al.* (1984) Increased regional end-diastolic wall thickness early after reperfusion: a sign of irreversibly damaged myocardium. *J Am Coll Cardiol* **3**(6): 1444–1453.

13 Gunning, M.G., Anagnostopoulos, C., Knight, C.J., *et al.* (1998) Comparison of 201Tl, 99mTc-tetrofosmin, and dobutamine magnetic resonance imaging for identifying hibernating myocardium. *Circulation* **98**(18): 1869–1874.

14 Sandstede, J.J., Bertsch, G., Beer, M., *et al.* (1999) Detection of myocardial viability by low-dose dobutamine cine MR imaging. *Magn Res Imag* **17**(10): 1437–1443.

15 Bax, J.J., Poldermans, D., Elhendy, A., *et al.* (2001) Sensitivity, specificity, and predictive accuracies of various noninvasive techniques for detecting hibernating myocardium. *Curr Prob Cardiol* **26**(2): 147–186.

16 Sansoy, V., Glover, D.K., Watson, D.D., *et al.* (1995) Comparison of thallium-201 resting redistribution with technetium-99m-sestamibi uptake and functional response to dobutamine for assessment of myocardial viability. *Circulation* **92**(4): 994–1004.

17 Ambrosio, G., Weisman, H.F., Mannisi, J.A., Becker, L.C. (1989) Progressive impairment of regional myocardial perfusion after initial restoration of postischemic blood flow. *Circulation* **80**(6): 1846–1861.

18 Ito, H., Tomooka, T., Sakai, N., *et al.* (1992) Lack of myocardial perfusion immediately after successful thrombolysis: a predictor of poor recovery of left ventricular function in anterior myocardial infarction. *Circulation* **85**(5): 1699–1705.

19 Judd, R.M., Lugo-Olivieri, C.H., Arai, M., *et al.* (1995) Physiological basis of myocardial contrast enhancement in fast magnetic resonance images of 2-day-old reperfused canine infarcts. *Circulation* **92**(7): 1902–1910.

20 Dilsizian, V., Bonow, R.O. (1993) Current diagnostic techniques of assessing myocardial viability in patients with hibernating and stunned myocardium. *Circulation* **87**(1): 1–20.

21 Brunken, R.C., Mody, F.V., Hawkins, R.A., *et al.* (1992) Positron emission tomography detects metabolic viability in myocardium with persistent 24-hour single-photon emission computed tomography 201Tl defects. *Circulation* **86**(5): 1357–1369.

22 Polimeni, P.I. (1974) Extracellular space and ionic distribution in rat ventricle. *Am J Physio* **227**(3): 676–683.

23 Weinmann, H.J., Brasch, R.C., Press, W.R., Wesbey, G.E. (1984) Characteristics of gadolinium-DTPA complex: a potential NMR contrast agent. *AJR* **142**(3): 619–624.

24 Shah, D.J., Kim, R.J. (2005) Magnetic resonance of myocardial viability. In: Edelman, R.R. (ed.). *Clinical Magnetic Resonance Imaging*, 3rd ed. Elsevier, New York.

25 Rehwald, W.G., Fieno, D.S., Chen, E.L., *et al.* (2002) Myocardial magnetic resonance imaging contrast agent concentrations after reversible and irreversible ischemic injury. *Circulation* **105**(2): 224–229.

26 Kim, R.J., Fieno, D.S., Parrish, T.B., *et al.* (1999) Relationship of MRI delayed contrast enhancement to irreversible injury, infarct age, and contractile function. *Circulation* **100**(19): 1992–2002.

27 Fieno, D.S., Kim, R.J., Chen, E.L., *et al.* (2000) Contrast-enhanced magnetic resonance imaging of myocardium at risk: distinction between reversible and irreversible injury throughout infarct healing. *J Am Coll Cardiol* **36**(6): 1985–1991.

28 Choi, K.M., Kim, R.J., Gubernikoff, G., *et al.* (2001) Transmural extent of acute myocardial infarction predicts long-term improvement in contractile function. *Circulation* **104**(10): 1101–1107.

29 Wu, E., Judd, R.M., Vargas, J.D., *et al.* (2001) Visualisation of presence, location, and transmural extent of healed Q-wave and non-Q-wave myocardial infarction. *Lancet* **357**(9249): 21–28.

30 Kim, R.J., Wu, E., Rafael, A., *et al.* (2000) The use of contrast-enhanced magnetic resonance imaging to identify reversible myocardial dysfunction. *N Engl J Med* **343**(20): 1445–1453.

31 Schvartzman, P.R., Srichai, M.B., Grimm, R.A., *et al.* (2003) Nonstress delayed-enhancement magnetic resonance imaging of the myocardium predicts improvement of function after revascularization for chronic ischemic heart disease with left ventricular dysfunction. *Am Heart J* **146**(3): 535–541.

32 Wellnhofer, E., Olariu, A., Klein, C., *et al.* (2004) Magnetic resonance low-dose dobutamine test is superior to SCAR quantification for the prediction of functional recovery. *Circulation* **109**(18): 2172–2174.

33 Gerber, B.L., Belge, B., Legros, G.J., *et al.* (2006) Characterization of acute and chronic myocardial infarcts by multidetector computed tomography: comparison with contrast-enhanced magnetic resonance. *Circulation* **113**(6): 823–833.

34 Lardo, A.C., Cordeiro, M.A., Silva, C., *et al.* (2006) Contrast-enhanced multidetector computed tomography viability imaging after myocardial infarction: characterization of myocyte death, microvascular obstruction, and chronic scar. *Circulation* **113**(3): 394–404.

35 Mahnken, A.H., Koos, R., Katoh, M., *et al.* (2005) Assessment of myocardial viability in reperfused acute myocardial infarction using 16-slice computed tomography in comparison to magnetic resonance imaging. *J Am Coll Cardiol* **45**(12): 2042–2047.

36 Kim, R.J., Shah, D.J. (2004) Fundamental concepts in myocardial viability assessment revisited: when knowing how much is "alive" is not enough. *Heart (Br Card Soc)* **90**(2): 137–140.

37 Selvanayagam, J.B., Kardos, A., Francis, J.M., *et al.* (2004) Value of delayed-enhancement cardiovascular magnetic resonance imaging in predicting myocardial viability after surgical revascularization. *Circulation* **110**(12): 1535–1541.

38 Ragosta, M., Beller, G.A., Watson, D.D., *et al.* (1993) Quantitative planar rest-redistribution 201Tl imaging in detection of myocardial viability and prediction of improvement in left ventricular function after coronary bypass surgery in patients with severely depressed left ventricular function. *Circulation* **87**(5): 1630–1641.

39 Force, T., Kemper, A., Perkins, L., *et al.* (1986) Overestimation of infarct size by quantitative two-dimensional echocardiography: the role of tethering and of analytic procedures. *Circulation* **73**(6): 1360–1368.

40 Helak, J.W., Reichek, N. (1981) Quantitation of human left ventricular mass and volume by two-dimensional echocardiography: in vitro anatomic validation. *Circulation* **63**(6): 1398–1407.

41 Wagner, A., Mahrholdt, H., Holly, T.A., *et al.* (2003) Contrast-enhanced MRI and routine single photon emission computed tomography (SPECT) perfusion imaging for detection of subendocardial myocardial infarcts: an imaging study. *Lancet* **361**(9355): 374–379.

42 Klein, C., Nekolla, S.G., Bengel, F.M., *et al.* (2002) Assessment of myocardial viability with contrast-enhanced magnetic resonance imaging: comparison with positron emission tomography. *Circulation* **105**(2): 162–167.

43 Ibrahim, T., Bulow, H.P., Hackl, T., *et al.* (2007) Diagnostic value of contrast-enhanced magnetic resonance imaging and single-photon emission computed tomography for detection of myocardial necrosis early after acute myocardial infarction. *J Am Coll Cardiol* **49**(2): 208–216.

44 John, A.S., Dreyfus, G.D., Pennell, D.J. (2005) Images in cardiovascular medicine. Reversible wall thinning in hibernation predicted by cardiovascular magnetic resonance. *Circulation* **111**(3): e24–25.

45 Shah, D.J., Kim, H.W., Elliott, M., *et al.* (2003) Contrast MRI predicts reverse remodeling and contractile improvement in akinetic thinned myocardium. *Circulation* **108**(17 Suppl): IV–697.

46 Albert, T.S., Kim, R.J., Judd, R.M. (2006) Assessment of no-reflow regions using cardiac MRI. *Basic Res Cardiol* **101**(5): 383–390.

47 Wu, K.C., Zerhouni, E.A., Judd, R.M., *et al.* (1998) Prognostic significance of microvascular obstruction by magnetic resonance imaging in patients with acute myocardial infarction. *Circulation* **97**(8): 765–772.

48 Hombach, V., Grebe, O., Merkle, N., *et al.* (2005) Sequelae of acute myocardial infarction regarding cardiac structure and function and their prognostic significance as assessed by magnetic resonance imaging. *Eur Heart J* **26**(6): 549–557.

49 Mollet, N.R., Dymarkowski, S., Volders, W., *et al.* (2002) Visualization of ventricular thrombi with contrast-enhanced magnetic resonance imaging in patients with ischemic heart disease. *Circulation* **106**(23): 2873–2876.

50 Srichai, M.B., Junor, C., Rodriguez, L.L., *et al.* (2006) Clinical, imaging, and pathological characteristics of left ventricular thrombus: a comparison of contrast-enhanced magnetic resonance imaging, transthoracic echocardiography, and transesophageal echocardiography with surgical or pathological validation. *Am Heart J* **152**(1): 75–84.

51 Reimer, K.A., Jennings, R.B. (1979) The "wavefront phenomenon" of myocardial ischemic cell death, II: transmural progression of necrosis within the framework of ischemic bed size (myocardium at risk) and collateral flow. *Lab Invest* **40**(6): 633–644.

52 Mahrholdt, H., Wagner, A., Judd, R.M., *et al.* (2005) Delayed enhancement cardiovascular magnetic resonance assessment of non-ischaemic cardiomyopathies. *Eur Heart J* **26**(15): 1461–1474.

53 Perrone-Filardi, P., Pace, L., Prastaro, M., *et al.* (1996) Assessment of myocardial viability in patients with chronic coronary artery disease: rest-4-hour-24-hour 201Tl tomography versus dobutamine echocardiography. *Circulation* **94**(11): 2712–2719.

54 Lieberman, A.N., Weiss, J.L., Jugdutt, B.I., *et al.* (1981) Two-dimensional echocardiography and infarct size: relationship of regional wall motion and thickening to the extent of myocardial infarction in the dog. *Circulation* **63**(4): 739–746.

55 Mahrholdt, H., Wagner, A., Parker, M., *et al.* (2003) Relationship of contractile function to transmural extent of infarction in patients with chronic coronary artery disease. *J Am Coll Cardiol* **42**(3): 505–512.

56 Nelson, C., McCrohon, J., Khafagi, F., *et al.* (2004) Impact of scar thickness on the assessment of viability using dobutamine echocardiography and thallium single-photon emission computed tomography: a comparison with contrast-enhanced magnetic resonance imaging. *J Am Coll Cardiol* **43**(7): 1248–1256.

57 Maes, A., Flameng, W., Nuyts, J., *et al.* (1994) Histological alterations in chronically hypoperfused myocardium: correlation with PET findings. *Circulation* **90**(2): 735–745.

58 Dakik, H.A., Howell, J.F., Lawrie, G.M., *et al.* (1997) Assessment of myocardial viability with 99mTc-sestamibi tomography before coronary bypass graft surgery: correlation with histopathology and postoperative improvement in cardiac function. *Circulation* **96**(9): 2892–2898.

59 Bax, J.J., Visser, F.C., Poldermans, D., *et al.* (2001) Time course of functional recovery of stunned and hibernating segments after surgical revascularization. *Circulation* **104**(12 Suppl 1): I314–318.

60 Samady, H., Elefteriades, J.A., Abbott, B.G., *et al.* (1999) Failure to improve left ventricular function after coronary revascularization for ischemic cardiomyopathy is not associated with worse outcome. *Circulation* **100**(12): 1298–1304.

61 Cerqueira, M.D., Weissman, N.J., Dilsizian, V., *et al.* (2002) Standardized myocardial segmentation and nomenclature for tomographic imaging of the heart: a statement for healthcare professionals from the Cardiac Imaging Committee of the Council on Clinical Cardiology of the American Heart Association. *Circulation* **105**(4): 539–542.

62 Kim, R.J., Manning, W.J. (2004) Viability assessment by delayed enhancement cardiovascular magnetic resonance: will low-dose dobutamine dull the shine? *Circulation* **109**(21): 2476–2479.

63 Fuster, V., Kim, R.J. (2005) Frontiers in cardiovascular magnetic resonance. *Circulation* **112**(1): 135–144.

Chapter 9

Role of Hybrid Imaging: PET/CT and SPECT/CT

Marcelo F. Di Carli

The integration of nuclear medicine cameras with multidetector computed tomography (CT) scanners — e.g., positron emission tomography (PET/CT) and single photon emission computed tomography (SPECT/CT) — provides a unique opportunity to delineate cardiac and vascular anatomic abnormalities and their physiologic consequences in a single setting. For the evaluation of the patient with known or suspected coronary artery disease (CAD), it allows the detection and quantification of the burden of the extent of calcified and noncalcified plaques — coronary artery calcium (CAC) and coronary angiography — quantification of vascular reactivity and endothelial health, identification of flow-limiting coronary stenoses, and assessment of myocardial viability. Consequently, by revealing the burden of anatomic CAD and its physiologic significance, hybrid imaging can provide unique information that may improve noninvasive diagnosis, risk assessment, and management of CAD. In addition, by integrating the detailed anatomic information from CT with the high sensitivity of radionuclide imaging to evaluate targeted molecular and cellular abnormalities, hybrid imaging may play a key role in shaping the future of molecular diagnostics and therapeutics. The discussion that follows will review current and future applications of hybrid imaging in cardiovascular disease.

Strengths and Weaknesses of Individual Components of the Hybrid Imaging Approach

CT Imaging

As discussed in Chapters 5 and 15, using state-of-the-art technology in carefully selected patients, it is possible to obtain high-quality images of the coronary

Novel Techniques for Imaging the Heart, 1st edition. Edited by M. Di Carli and R. Kwong.
© 2008 American Heart Association, ISBN: 9-781-4051-7533-3.

arteries. The available evidence suggests that on a per-patient basis, the average weighted sensitivity for detecting at least one coronary artery with greater than 50% stenosis is 94% (range: 75 to 100%), whereas the average specificity is 77% (range: 49 to 100%) [1]. The corresponding average positive predictive value (PPV) and negative predictive value (NPV) are 84% (range: 50 to 100%) and 87% (range: 35 to 100%), respectively, and the overall diagnostic accuracy is 89% (range: 68 to 100%). On a per-segment basis, the average weighted sensitivity for detecting at least one coronary artery with greater than 50% stenosis is 83% (range: 30 to 99%), whereas the average specificity is 92% (range: 64 to 98%). The corresponding average PPV and NPV are 67% (range: 14 to 91%) and 97% (range: 83 to 99%), respectively, and the overall diagnostic accuracy is 92% (range: 66 to 98%) [1]. Data from the Coronary Artery Evaluation Using 64-Row Multidetector Computed Tomography Angiography (Core64) trial, the first multicenter evaluation of the diagnostic performance of 64-slice computed tomography angiography (CTA) for the detection of CAD, provides yet new evidence that seems to temper the initial optimistic results from single-center studies [2]. The results confirmed the robustness of CTA-64 for the complete visualization of the coronary tree: 95% of segments and 98% of vessels were evaluable, and 97% of patients had all coronary segments evaluable. On a per-patient basis, the sensitivity for detecting at least one coronary artery with greater than 50% stenosis was 85%, lower than in single-center studies using similar technology, whereas the specificity was 90%. The corresponding average PPV and NPV were 91% and 83%, respectively. On a per-vessel basis, the reported sensitivity for detecting coronary arteries with greater than 50% stenosis was 76%, whereas the specificity was 93%. The corresponding PPV and NPV were 82% and 89%, respectively.

These reported accuracies of CTA to date should be interpreted in light of the relatively narrow range of CAD likelihood in patients examined (i.e., high or intermediate–high), as evidenced by the high prevalence of obstructive CAD in these series (62%) [1,2]. Further, results are generally limited to relatively large vessel sizes (greater than or equal to 1.5 mm), excluding the results of smaller or uninterpretable vessels (generally, distal vessels and side branches), the inclusion of which lowers sensitivity. An ongoing problem with CT is that high-density objects such as calcified coronary plaques and stent struts limit its ability to accurately delineate the degree of coronary luminal narrowing. As the bright (blooming) signal from such high-density objects extends beyond their true size into neighboring volume voxels, it generally leads to the overestimation of stenosis severity and an overall reduction in test specificity and PPV [3,4]. Of note, the Core64 trial excluded patients with high calcium scores (greater than 600) [2]. From a clinical perspective, a normal CTA is helpful as it effectively excludes the presence of obstructive CAD and the need for further testing, defines a low clinical risk, and makes management decisions straightforward. However, because of its limited accuracy to define stenosis severity and predict flow-limiting disease, abnormal CTA results are more problematic to interpret and to use as the basis for defining the potential need of invasive coronary angiography and myocardial revascularization [5,6].

Myocardial Perfusion Scintigraphy

As discussed in Chapter 10, myocardial perfusion scintigraphy represents a robust approach to diagnose obstructive CAD, quantify the magnitude of jeopardized myocardium, and assess the extent of myocardial viability. The extensive published literature with SPECT suggests that its average sensitivity for detecting greater than 50% angiographic stenosis is 87% (range: 71 to 97%), whereas the average specificity is 73% (range: 36 to 100%) [7]. With the use of attenuation correction methods, the specificity improves, especially among patients undergoing exercise stress testing [7]. With PET perfusion imaging, the reported average sensitivity for detecting greater than 50% angiographic stenosis is 91% (range: 83 to 100%), whereas the average specificity is 89% (range: 73 to 100%) [8].

Although the relative assessment of myocardial perfusion with radionuclide imaging remains a sensitive means for diagnosing obstructive CAD, this approach often uncovers only that territory supplied by the most severe stenosis. This result is based on the fact that in patients with CAD, coronary vasodilator reserve is often abnormal even in territories supplied by noncritical angiographic stenoses, thereby reducing the heterogeneity of flow between "normal" and "abnormal" zones, and limiting the ability to delineate the presence of multivessel CAD [9,10]. This fact is true for both SPECT and PET myocardial perfusion imaging.

One advantage of PET over SPECT is its unique ability to assess left ventricular function at rest and during peak stress (as opposed to post-stress with SPECT) [11]. Data suggest that in normal subjects, left ventricular ejection fraction (LVEF) increases during peak vasodilator stress [11]. However, in patients with obstructive CAD the rise in LVEF (from baseline to peak stress) is inversely related to the extent of significant angiographic CAD. Indeed, patients with multivessel disease or left main disease show a frank drop in LVEF during peak stress even in the absence of apparent perfusion defects. In contrast, those without significant CAD or with one-vessel disease show a normal increase in LVEF. Consequently, the diagnostic sensitivity of gated PET for correctly ascertaining the presence of multivessel disease increases from 50 to 79% [11].

Alternatively, absolute measurements of myocardial blood flow (in ml/min/g) and coronary vasodilator reserve could also help improve the detection of multivessel CAD. In patients with so-called "balanced" ischemia or diffuse CAD, measurements of coronary vasodilator reserve would uncover areas of myocardium at risk that would generally be missed by performing only relative assessments of myocardial perfusion [12].

Despite the strengths of stress myocardial perfusion scintigraphy to identify flow-limiting CAD, define its extent and severity, and identify its associated risks of adverse events, it fails to describe the presence and extent of subclinical atherosclerosis (Figure 9.1) [13,14]. This limitation is not unexpected because the myocardial perfusion imaging method is designed and targeted on the identification of flow-limiting stenoses. Although myocardial perfusion imaging will likely continue to define the need for revascularization, the objective assessment of atherosclerotic burden (both calcified and noncalcified plaques) by CT might be able to play a role in individualizing the intensity and goals of medical therapy.

Clinical Value Added of the Hybrid Imaging Approach

Diagnosing Obstructive CAD

As discussed previously, CTA provides excellent diagnostic sensitivity for stenoses in the proximal and mid-segments (greater than 2 mm in diameter) of the main coronary arteries. Due to its relatively limited spatial resolution (compared to invasive angiography), the sensitivity of this approach is reduced substantially in more distal coronary segments and side branches [1]. This limitation can be offset by the scintigraphic information that is generally not affected by the location of coronary stenoses. More importantly, the stress perfusion information provides valuable clinical information regarding the physiologic significance of anatomic stenoses for the identification of patients in need of potential revascularization (Figure 9.2). The quantification of coronary blood flow can extend this approach by demonstrating the extent of reduction of vasodilator reserve to identify patients with abnormal endothelial function and microvascular disease [15,16]. This modification takes on added relevance given the greater recognition of premature risk in patients with diabetes mellitus, obesity, and metabolic syndrome in whom evaluation of atherosclerotic burden alone can under-recognize the extent of jeopardized myocardium. Alternatively, CTA improves the detection of multivessel CAD, which as discussed previously is one of the main pitfalls of stress perfusion scintigraphy.

Assessing Prognosis

The potential to acquire and quantify rest and stress myocardial perfusion (in ml/min/g, and derive estimates of coronary vasodilator reserve) and CT information from a single study using hybrid imaging opens the door to expand the prognostic potential of stress imaging. Recent data from our laboratory suggest that the quantification of CAC scores at the time of stress myocardial perfusion PET imaging using a hybrid approach can enhance risk predictions in patients with suspected CAD [17]. In a consecutive series of 621 patients undergoing stress PET imaging and CAC scoring in the same clinical setting, risk-adjusted analysis demonstrated a stepwise increase in cardiac event rates with increasing levels of CAC score for any level of perfusion abnormality. This finding was observed in patients with and without evidence of ischemia on PET/MPI

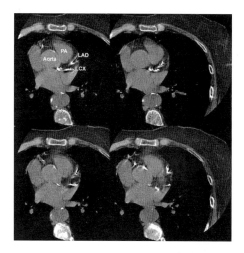

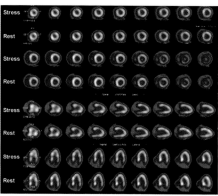

Fig. 9.1 Integrated myocardial perfusion PET and CT calcium scoring in a 67-year-old woman with a history of hypertension being evaluated for dystnea. Dipyridamole-stress and rest rubidium-82 images in corresponding short axis, vertical long, and horizontal long axis slices. The short axis slices represent progression from the apical (above) to the basal (below) part of the heart, and are oriented with the anterior wall on the top, the lateral wall to the right, the inferior wall at the bottom, and the interventricular septum to the left. The vertical long axis slices represent progression from the septum (left) to the lateral (right) walls, and are oriented with the anterior wall on top, inferior wall at the bottom, and the left ventricular apex to the right. The horizontal long axis slices represent progression from the inferior (left) to the anterior (right) walls, and are oriented with the septal wall on the left, lateral wall to the right, and the left ventricular apex on the top. The images demonstrate normal myocardial perfusion throughout the left ventricle. The axial CT images demonstrate extensive calcification of the distal left main, proximal left anterior descending, first diagonal branch, and the distal right coronary arteries. The Agatston coronary calcium score was 2540. This score is greater than the 904th percentile rank for [men] aged 66–70 years. Reprinted with permission from Raff, G.L., Gallagher, M.J., O'Neill, W.W., Goldstein, J.A. (2005) *J Am Coll Cardiol* **46**: 552–557.

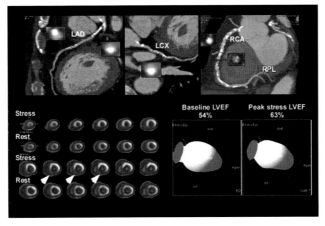

Fig. 9.2 Integrated PET/CTA study. There is extensive calcified plaque burden throughout the coronary arteries. The left anterior descending and left circumflex arteries show multiple calcified plaques in their proximal and midsegments. The dominant right coronary artery shows multiple calcified plaques, with a severe noncalcified plaque in its midsegment. However, the rest and peak dobutamine stress myocardial perfusion PET study (lower left panel) demonstrates only moderate ischemia in the inferior wall (arrows). In addition, LVEF was normal at rest and demonstrated a normal rise during peak stress. Reproduced from Di Carli and Hachamovitch, with permission [1].

(Figure 9.3). Indeed, the annualized event rate in patients with normal PET/MPI and a CAC score <1000 was substantially lower than among those with normal PET/MPI and a CAC score greater than or equal to 1000. Likewise, the annualized event rate in patients with ischemia on PET/MPI and no CAC score was lower than among those with ischemia and a CAC score greater than or equal to 1000. These findings suggest an incremental risk stratification by incorporating information regarding the anatomic extent of atherosclerosis to conventional models using myocardial perfusion alone, a finding that may serve as a more rational basis for personalizing the intensity and goals of medical therapy in a more cost-effective manner. Importantly, CTA as an adjunct to PET perfusion imaging could expand the opportunities to identify patients at a greater risk of adverse cardiovascular events. Indeed, recent limited data suggest that the quantification of CAD extent and severity by CTA can provide estimates of risk similar to those obtained with invasive coronary angiography [18].

Guiding Patient Management

One of the most compelling arguments supporting a clinical role of hybrid imaging is its potential ability for optimizing and personalizing management decisions. The importance of stress perfusion imaging in the integrated strategy

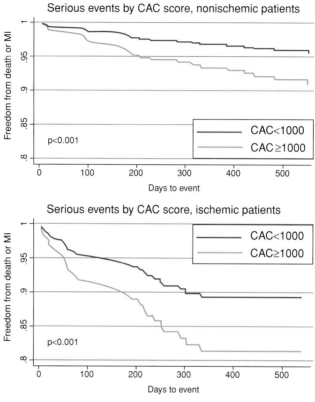

Fig. 9.3 Adjusted survival curves for freedom from death or myocardial infarction adjusted for age, gender, symptoms, and conventional CAD risk factors in patients without ischemia (top panel) and with ischemia (lower panel). Reproduced from Schenker *et al.*, with permission [17].

is the ability of noninvasive estimates of jeopardized myocardium to identify which patients may benefit from revascularization — that is, differentiating high-risk patients with extensive scars from those with extensive ischemia. The advantages of this approach are clear — the avoidance of unnecessary catheterizations that expose patients to risk and the potential for associated cost savings [19]. Multiple studies have shown the value of ischemia information for optimizing clinical decision-making. The nonrandomized Coronary Artery Surgery Study (CASS) registry reported that surgical revascularization in patients with CAD improved survival only among those with three-vessel disease with severe ischemia on exercise stress testing, whereas medical therapy was a superior initial therapy in patients without this finding [20]. Nonrandomized observational data using risk-adjustment techniques and propensity scores has also demonstrated the ability of stress perfusion imaging to identify which patients may accrue a survival benefit from revascularization [21]. The benefit of an ischemia-guided approach to management is further supported by invasive estimates of flow-limiting CAD (e.g., fractional flow reserve, FFR) [22]. In the setting of an FFR greater than 0.75, revascularization can be safely deferred without increased patient risk despite the presence of what visually appears to be a significant stenosis [22]. Indeed, cardiac event rates are extremely low in these patients, even lower than predicted if treated with PCI, and this differential risk appears to be sustained at the time of a five-year follow-up [23,24]. Importantly, in patients with visually defined left main coronary disease, an FFR greater than 0.75 was associated with an excellent three-year survival rate and freedom from major adverse cardiovascular events [23]. Conversely, event rates are increased when lesions with FFR less than 0.75 are not revascularized [25]. Thus, by identifying which patients have sufficient ischemia to merit revascularization, it appears that stress perfusion imaging may play a significant role in the selection of patients for catheterization within a strategy based on the identification of patient benefit. This physiologic data may have a greater clinical impact than visually defined coronary anatomy for revascularization decision making.

As discussed previously, the hybrid imaging approach can also facilitate the identification of patients without flow-limiting disease (i.e., normal perfusion) who have extensive, albeit subclinical, CAD. Recent data from multiple laboratories suggest that as many as 50% of patients with normal stress perfusion imaging may show extensive (non-flow limiting) coronary atherosclerosis (both calcified and noncalcified plaques) [13,14]. Although these patients do not require revascularization due to the absence of ischemia, patients with extensive atherosclerosis are at higher risk of adverse events, and thus probably warrant more aggressive medical therapy [17,26,27]. Consequently, it may be possible to tailor antithrombotic, cholesterol-reduction, and anti-inflammatory pharmacotherapy on the basis of CT findings. The major challenge for future developments will be to identify which patients will benefit from a combined hybrid approach as opposed to a single modality approach with stepped testing. It is undefined whether all patients will require all pieces of information that can be acquired to optimize their care.

Molecular Imaging: Potential Future Role of Hybrid Imaging

By integrating the detailed anatomic information from CT with the high sensitivity of radionuclide imaging to evaluate targeted molecular and cellular abnormalities in the myocardium and vasculature, hybrid imaging may play a key role in shaping the future of molecular diagnostics and therapeutics [28–30].

One of the areas of greatest research interest has been centered on the evaluation of inflammation within an atheroma. As discussed in greater detail in

Chapter 16, there is marked heterogeneity in the composition of human atherosclerotic plaques. It would be clinically desirable to have reliable noninvasive imaging tools that can characterize the composition of such plaques, thereby allowing one to determine their risk for complications (e.g., erosion and rupture). Such imaging tools would provide mechanistic insights into atherothrombotic processes, better risk stratification, an optimal selection of therapeutic targets, and the means for monitoring therapeutic responses. Several imaging modalities have been employed to study atherosclerotic plaques and their composition. PET/CT appears attractive because it allows the image fusion of structure and function (biology), thereby allowing the characterization of plaques. Several studies in experimental and human models of atherosclerosis have demonstrated a relationship between the intensity of FDG uptake and the number of macrophage infiltrations within plaques, suggesting that the FDG signal measured noninvasively by PET may reflect the inflammatory burden in an atheroma [29–32]. The intensity of the FDG signal is reproducible, appears to correlate with risk factors of atherosclerosis, and seems to change in response to statin therapy [33–36]. If confirmed and further validated by future studies, hybrid imaging approaches such as PET/CT might expand our ability for the early detection of patients at risk and provide a more personalized guide to therapeutic intervention.

Conclusions

Innovation in noninvasive cardiovascular imaging is rapidly advancing our ability to image in great detail the structure and function in the heart and vasculature, and hybrid PET/CT and SPECT/CT techniques represent clear examples of this innovation. By providing concurrent quantitative information about myocardial perfusion and metabolism with coronary and cardiac anatomy, hybrid imaging offers the opportunity for a comprehensive noninvasive evaluation of the burden of atherosclerosis and its physiologic consequences in the coronary arteries and the myocardium. This integrated platform for assessing anatomy and biology offers a great potential for translating advances in molecularly targeted imaging into humans. The goals of future investigation should be to refine these technologies, establish standard protocols for image acquisition and interpretation, address the issue of cost-effectiveness, and validate a range of clinical applications in large-scale clinical trials.

References

1 Di Carli, M.F., Hachamovitch, R. (2007) New technology for noninvasive evaluation of coronary artery disease. *Circulation* **115**: 1464–1480.
2 Miller, J.M., Rochitte, C.E., Dewey, M., *et al.* (2007) Coronary artery evaluation using 64-row multidetector computed tomography angiography (CORE-64): results of a

multicenter, international trial to assess diagnostic accuracy compared with conventional coronary angiography. *Circulation* **116**: 2630.

3 Hoffmann, U., Moselewski, F., Cury, R.C., *et al.* (2004) Predictive value of 16-slice multidetector spiral computed tomography to detect significant obstructive coronary artery disease in patients at high risk for coronary artery disease: patient versus segment-based analysis. *Circulation* **110**: 2638–2643.

4 Mollet, N.R., Cademartiri, F., van Mieghem, C.A., *et al.* (2005) High-resolution spiral computed tomography coronary angiography in patients referred for diagnostic conventional coronary angiography. *Circulation* **112**: 2318–2323.

5 Leber, A.W., Becker, A., Knez, A., *et al.* (2006) Accuracy of 64-slice computed tomography to classify and quantify plaque volumes in the proximal coronary system: a comparative study using intravascular ultrasound. *J Am Coll Cardiol* **47**: 672–677.

6 Raff, G.L., Gallagher, M.J., O'Neill, W.W., Goldstein, J.A. (2005) Diagnostic accuracy of noninvasive coronary angiography using 64-slice spiral computed tomography. *J Am Coll Cardiol* **46**: 552–557.

7 Klocke, F.J., Baird, M.G., Lorell, B.H., *et al.* (2003) ACC/AHA/ASNC guidelines for the clinical use of cardiac radionuclide imaging—executive summary: a report of the American College of Cardiology/American Heart Association Task Force on Practice Guidelines (ACC/AHA/ASNC committee to revise the 1995 guidelines for the clinical use of cardiac radionuclide imaging). *J Am Coll Cardiol* **42**: 1318–1333.

8 Di Carli, M.F., Dorbala, S., Meserve, J., *et al.* (2007) Clinical myocardial perfusion PET/CT. *J Nucl Med* **48**: 783–793.

9 Uren, N.G., Crake, T., Lefroy, D.C., *et al.* (1994) Reduced coronary vasodilator function in infarcted and normal myocardium after myocardial infarction. *N Engl J Med* **331**: 222–227 (see comments).

10 Yoshinaga, K., Katoh, C., Noriyasu, K., *et al.* (2003) Reduction of coronary flow reserve in areas with and without ischemia on stress perfusion imaging in patients with coronary artery disease: a study using oxygen 15-labeled water PET. *J Nucl Cardiol* **10**: 275–283.

11 Dorbala, S., Vangala, D., Sampson, U., *et al.* (2007) Value of vasodilator left ventricular ejection fraction reserve in evaluating the magnitude of myocardium at risk and the extent of angiographic coronary artery disease: a 82Rb PET/CT study. *J Nucl Med* **48**: 349–358.

12 Parkash, R., deKemp, R.A., Ruddy, T.D., *et al.* (2004) Potential utility of rubidium 82 PET quantification in patients with 3-vessel coronary artery disease. *J Nucl Cardiol* **11**: 440–449.

13 Schuijf, J.D., Wijns, W., Jukema, J.W., *et al.* (2006) Relationship between noninvasive coronary angiography with multi-slice computed tomography and myocardial perfusion imaging. *J Am Coll Cardiol* **48**: 2508–2514.

14 Di Carli, M.F., Dorbala, S., Curillova, Z., *et al.* (2007) Relationship between CT coronary angiography and stress perfusion imaging in patients with suspected ischemic heart disease assessed by integrated PET-CT imaging. *J Nucl Cardiol* **14**: 799–809.

15 Campisi, R., Di Carli, M.F. (2004) Assessment of coronary flow reserve and microcirculation: a clinical perspective. *J Nucl Cardiol* **11**: 3–11.

16 Camici, P.G., Crea, F. (2007) Coronary microvascular dysfunction. *N Engl J Med* **356**: 830–840.

17 Schenker, M.P., Dorbala, S., Hong, E.C.T., *et al.* Relationship between coronary calcification, myocardial ischemia, and outcomes in patients with intermediate likelihood of coronary artery disease: a combined positron emission tomography/computed tomography study. *Circulation* (in press).

18 Min, J.K., Shaw, L.J., Devereux, R.B., *et al.* (2007) Prognostic value of multidetector coronary computed tomographic angiography for prediction of all-cause mortality. *J Am Coll Cardiol* **50**: 1161–1170.

19 Shaw, L.J., Hachamovitch, R., Berman, D.S., *et al.* (1999) The economic consequences of available diagnostic and prognostic strategies for the evaluation of stable angina patients: an observational assessment of the value of precatheterization ischemia. Economics of Noninvasive Diagnosis (END) Multicenter Study Group. *J Am Coll Cardiol* **33**: 661–669.

20 Weiner, D.A., Ryan, T.J., McCabe, C.H., *et al.* (1986) The role of exercise testing in identifying patients with improved survival after coronary artery bypass surgery. *J Am Coll Cardiol* **8**: 741–748.

21 Hachamovitch, R., Hayes, S.W., Friedman, J.D., *et al.* (2003) Comparison of the short-term survival benefit associated with revascularization compared with medical therapy in patients with no prior coronary artery disease undergoing stress myocardial perfusion single photon emission computed tomography. *Circulation* **107**: 2900–2907.

22 Kern, M.J., Lerman, A., Bech, J.W., *et al.* (2006) Physiological assessment of coronary artery disease in the Cardiac Catheterization Laboratory: a scientific statement from the American Heart Association Committee on Diagnostic and Interventional Cardiac Catheterization, Council on Clinical Cardiology. *Circulation* **114**: 1321–1341.

23 Bech, G.J., De Bruyne, B., Pijls, N.H., *et al.* (2001) Fractional flow reserve to determine the appropriateness of angioplasty in moderate coronary stenosis: a randomized trial. *Circulation* **103**: 2928–2934.

24 Pijls, N.H., van Schaardenburgh, P., Manahoran, G., *et al.* (2007) Percutaneous coronary intervention of functionally nonsignificant stenosis: 5-year follow-up of the DEFER study. *J Am Coll Cardiol* **49**: 2105–2111.

25 Chamuleau, S.A.J., Meuwissen, M., Koch, K.T., *et al.* (2002) Usefulness of fractional flow reserve for risk stratification of patients with multivessel coronary artery disease and an intermediate stenosis. *Am J Cardiol* **89**: 377–380.

26 Budoff, M.J., Shaw, L.J., Liu, S.T., *et al.* (2007) Long-term prognosis associated with coronary calcification: observations from a registry of 25,253 patients. *J Am Coll Cardiol* **49**: 1860–1870.

27 Greenland, P., Bonow, R.O., Brundage, B.H., *et al.* (2007) ACCF/AHA 2007 clinical expert consensus document on coronary artery calcium scoring by computed tomography in global cardiovascular risk assessment and in evaluation of patients with chest pain: a report of the American College of Cardiology Foundation Clinical Expert Consensus Task Force (ACCF/AHA writing committee to update the 2000 expert consensus document on electron beam computed tomography) developed in collaboration with the Society of Atherosclerosis Imaging and Prevention and the Society of Cardiovascular Computed Tomography. *J Am Coll Cardiol* **49**: 378–402.

28 Wagner, B., Anton, M., Nekolla, S.G., *et al.* (2006) Noninvasive characterization of myocardial molecular interventions by integrated positron emission tomography and computed tomography. *J Am Coll Cardiol* **48**: 2107–2115.

29 Rudd, J.H., Warburton, E.A., Fryer, T.D., *et al.* (2002) Imaging atherosclerotic plaque inflammation with [18F]-fluorodeoxyglucose positron emission tomography. *Circulation* **105**: 2708–2711.

30 Tawakol, A., Migrino, R.Q., Bashian, G.G., *et al.* (2006) In vivo 18F-fluorodeoxyglucose positron emission tomography imaging provides a noninvasive measure of carotid plaque inflammation in patients. *J Am Coll Cardiol* **48**: 1818–1824.

31 Tawakol, A., Migrino, R.Q., Hoffmann, U., *et al.* (2005) Noninvasive in vivo measurement of vascular inflammation with F-18 fluorodeoxyglucose positron emission tomography. *J Nucl Cardiol* **12**: 294–301.

32 Zhang, Z., Machac, J., Helft, G., *et al.* (2006) Non-invasive imaging of atherosclerotic plaque macrophage in a rabbit model with F-18 FDG PET: a histopathological correlation. *BMC Nucl Med* **6**: 3.

33 Rudd, J.H., Myers, K.S., Bansilal, S., *et al.* (2007) (18)Fluorodeoxyglucose positron emission tomography imaging of atherosclerotic plaque inflammation is highly reproducible: implications for atherosclerosis therapy trials. *J Am Coll Cardiol* **50**: 892–896.

34 Tahara, N., Kai, H., Yamagishi, S., *et al.* (2007) Vascular inflammation evaluated by [18F]-fluorodeoxyglucose positron emission tomography is associated with the metabolic syndrome. *J Am Coll Cardiol* **49**: 1533–1539.

35 Ogawa, M., Magata, Y., Kato, T., *et al.* (2006) Application of 18F-FDG PET for monitoring the therapeutic effect of antiinflammatory drugs on stabilization of vulnerable atherosclerotic plaques. *J Nucl Med* **47**: 1845–1850.

36 Tahara, N., Kai, H., Ishibashi, M., *et al.* (2006) Simvastatin attenuates plaque inflammation: evaluation by fluorodeoxyglucose positron emission tomography. *J Am Coll Cardiol* **48**: 1825–1831.

Chapter 10

Critical Review of Imaging Approaches for the Diagnosis and Prognosis of CAD

Rory Hachamovitch and George A. Beller

The reader may wonder why a chapter on older stress imaging techniques is included in a text focused on newer, cutting-edge imaging modalities. It is important to preface the discussion of newer modalities, such as cardiac magnetic resonance (CMR) imaging and cardiac computed tomography (CT), with a review of stress imaging for several reasons. As imaging modalities that preceded these newer technologies, stress single photon emission computed tomography (SPECT) and echocardiography are de facto benchmarks and serve as methodological "case studies" for test validation. Newer modalities will need to accrue data regarding their performance characteristics in a manner similar to that of older imaging techniques, hence it is useful to understand the methodological approaches to validating stress imaging and recognize the potential pitfalls along the way. The validation of newer technologies will also require the identification of a newer modality's optimal role within a testing strategy — which tests should precede and follow the newer modality, and which patients undergo which form of testing. The goals of this chapter are to review the diagnostic and prognostic performance characteristics of the established stress imaging modalities, outline the methodological issues and limitations of these approaches, and to review (with CTA as an example) the potential limitations and hurdles of accepting newer technologies into testing strategies.

Anatomic Validation of Diagnostic Testing

Traditionally, coronary artery disease (CAD) has been categorized on the basis of anatomic criteria (e.g., absent, present, single vessel, multivessel). Hence, the

Novel Techniques for Imaging the Heart, 1st edition. Edited by M. Di Carli and R. Kwong.
© 2008 American Heart Association, ISBN: 9-781-4051-7533-3.

accuracy of stress testing has been based on the accuracy of identifying the presence of flow-limiting epicardial stenosis (usually 50 and 70% epicardial stenoses by angiography). Consequently, initial reports of new modalities assess diagnostic accuracy — the amount of agreement between the results of a test and those of a reference standard, as expressed in terms of sensitivity and specificity, likelihood ratios, diagnostic odds ratios, and areas under a receiver-operator characteristic curve.

Numerous studies have assessed the relative accuracies of stress imaging using either nuclear cardiology techniques or echocardiographic methods, and a number of studies have reported pooled data. For stress SPECT, pooled sensitivity was reported to be 87 and 89%, and average specificity estimates to be 73 and 75%, respectively, for exercise and pharmacologic stress [1]. For stress positron emission tomography (PET), pool analysis reported 94% sensitivity and 89% specificity for CAD detection [2]. The addition of post-stress wall motion abnormalities or an abnormal post-stress ejection fraction and end-systolic volume enhances the sensitivity and overall accuracy for predicting underlying multi-vessel disease [3,4]. For stress echocardiography, pooled sensitivity and specificity estimates in patients undergoing exercise echocardiography were found to be 86 and 81%, respectively, with an overall accuracy of 85%. With dobutamine stress, the corresponding values were 82, 84, and 83%, respectively [5]. Although ranges of values have been reported for both modalities, both stress echocardiography and SPECT are mature modalities with excellent reported sensitivities and specificities.

Various studies have also reported the accuracies of these two modalities in a variety of relevant clinical subgroups (patients undergoing exercise or pharmacologic stress, men versus women, young versus old, normal versus abnormal resting electrocardiogram, and so on), again finding reasonable success in identifying obstructive CAD [6,7]. Both modalities depend on adequate image quality, reader expertise, and adequate stress performed, as well as other factors, for optimal test performance. Further, the "quality of local expertise and facilities should be important considerations when the referring physician recommends a cardiac stress imaging test for a patient" [5]. Currently, this criterion holds true for both modalities and although differences between these modalities may exist, interlaboratory and inter-reader variability probably outweigh any intermodality differences.

A quality evaluation process for nuclear cardiology has been proposed at a consensus conference [8]. This process includes appropriate patient selection and the acquisition of images using reproducible imaging protocols and well-functioning equipment with trained and accredited laboratory staff. Ideally, this will yield diagnostic-quality images optimized for individual patients that will be interpreted with a high degree of accuracy and reproducibility, and communicated to referral physicians in a lucid, comprehensive, clinically relevant, and timely manner to optimize patient therapy with the ultimate objective of improving health outcomes. The Appropriateness Criteria Working Group of the American College of Cardiology (ACC) has recommended standards to guide the ordering physician in understanding when stress myocardial perfusion imaging (MPI) is deemed appropriate in specific clinical scenarios [9,10].

In recent years, advances have been made in SPECT imaging that have improved quality and provided quantitative computer-assisted techniques aimed at objective quantitative image analysis for interpreting stress and rest SPECT studies [11–14]. Presently, indices of left ventricular size as well as regional and global function can be assessed on gated SPECT imaging. Quantitative defect extent and magnitude can be measured with good reproducibility and accuracy. Quantitative measures of transient ischemic dilation (TID) can enhance the identification of multivessel CAD. A correction for attenuation has been purported to reduce artifacts and improve specificity of SPECT images [15].

Limitations to the Use of Diagnostic Metrics

Although diagnostic-based assessment of testing is ubiquitous, it is increasingly appreciated that the limitations of this approach compromise its validity. The diagnostic accuracies reported previously are overwhelmingly limited by the numerous limitations and pitfalls associated with the use of diagnostic metrics. In particular, the pre- and post-test biases introduced by patient selection and referral to a gold-standard method after testing merit review and are crucial for clinicians to understand and recognize [16–18].

In practice, referral to catheterization is proportional to the degree of abnormality reported on stress imaging [19,20]. Albeit appropriate, this pattern is problematic when these patients constitute the cohorts of studies investigating stress imaging's accuracy due to the *partial verification bias* that results. This bias is associated with a lowered specificity and increased sensitivity compared to a nonbiased sample. The magnitude of this bias' impact is generally underappreciated [18]. For example, when radionuclide ventriculography shifted from a new to an accepted modality (with a concomitant increase in the likelihood and prevalence of CAD in patients undergoing testing), its specificity fell from a range of 78–94% to 31–49% [16]. A discussion of possible approaches to address this limitation has been published elsewhere [18]. Given the frequency of design-related bias in studies of diagnostic testing, it follows that one must be interpreting cautious of reports expressing test accuracies in the absence of either elimination of (by study design) or correction for (by formulae) the biases present [21].

Normalcy Rate

In light of this bias, the *normalcy rate*, the frequency of normal results among a very low (generally defined as less than 5%) pre-test likelihood of CAD patients was developed as a surrogate for specificity [22]. The normalcy rate for stress SPECT imaging in 8964 patients from a pooled analysis of studies in the literature was 89% compared to 74% for the specificity value [1]. Although used in the imaging literature, normalcy has not been formally validated, does not appear in the mainstream epidemiologic literature, and has a number of limitations. The selection of patients for this metric is challenging [23]. Further, these patients are problematic. Why would low-likelihood patients be referred to MPI? Are they generalizable to low-likelihood patients or non-low-likelihood patients? Finally, whether an association exists between normalcy and specificity rates, and whether it persists as the likelihood of disease increases, is as yet undefined.

Understanding the Limitations of Meta-Analysis

Stress imaging data are often subject to meta-analyses and yield pooled estimates of test accuracy with greater power. Meta-regression permits a meta-analysis to risk-adjust the results for possible confounders between studies or to examine a study's potential confounders. However, the validity and generalizability of a meta-analysis' results are intrinsically limited by the data that is included. Consequently, a meta-analysis of stress imaging for CAD detection does not adjust for intersite variability in patient characteristics, test usage, or referral biases. Hence, meta-analyses do not estimate the impact or the relative magnitude and direction of the biases associated with each site, and their results ignore and potentially magnify the individual biases.

Outcome-Based Validation of Diagnostic Testing

The use of a risk- or outcome-based approach for the assessment of testing has gained widespread support over the past decade due to its advantages over traditional anatomy-based approaches [24]. This approach is directly applicable to patient care, from the perspective of the physician formulating treatment decisions, the patient attempting to understand their disease, and the health care system seeking optimal resource utilization. Further, with improved understanding of the relationship between test results and outcomes, the test's application can be enhanced with respect to an optimal selection of patients for testing as well as interfacing post-test therapeutics and test results.

The basis of risk stratification after stress imaging is defined by several concepts and, generally, these principles hold true for both stress SPECT and echocardiography. First, optimal risk stratification is based on the concept that the risk associated with a normal stress imaging study is sufficiently low that revascularization is unlikely to improve patient outcome. Hence, catheterization is an unlikely option after testing. Patients with abnormal stress imaging results are at greater risk of adverse events, and thus are potential candidates for intervention [19,20,25]. Their risk is proportional to the magnitude of the imaging abnormalities. Based on this premise, outcome data from an imaging modality should initially be examined for two patterns: the risk of adverse events after a normal study, and the relationship between risk and increasing test abnormality.

Risk of Adverse Events after a Normal Imaging Study

To date, an extensive body of literature supports the concept of a normal stress SPECT study being associated with a low risk of hard events (cardiac death or nonfatal myocardial infarction). Pooled data from 16 studies involving 27,855 patients reported a hard event rate of 0.6% per year over a mean follow-up of 26.8 months [1]. Although it has been proposed that normal SPECT results are associated with a very low likelihood (less than 1%) of hard events for at least 12 months independent of gender, age, symptom status, past history of CAD, presence of anatomic CAD, and imaging technique or isotope, a recent follow-up study of patients with normal SPECT revealed that risk varies widely as a function of patients' underlying clinical risk [26,27]. Although normal stress SPECT studies are generally associated with low risk, a number of stress SPECT and echocardiography studies have reported hard event rates exceeding 1% per year in higher-risk cohorts (e.g., prior CAD, diabetics, elderly, pharmacologic stress), as previously discussed [6,28,29].

With stress echocardiography, a similar pattern emerges with rates of cardiac death and hard events generally less than 1% per year among those with normal test results, with greater risk following pharmacologic compared to exercise stress [29]. The guidelines conclude that a "negative stress echocardiographic study generally denotes a low rate of adverse cardiovascular events" [5]. When considering larger cohorts, especially of routine intermediate-risk patients presenting for testing, the results here will hold true. However, despite the previous statements from several prominent societies, these claims, as discussed later, probably have somewhat limited generalizability.

Relationship between Risk and the Extent and Severity of Imaging Results

Increasing risk has been found to be associated with worsening test abnormalities, whether using SPECT or echocardiography (Figures 10.1 and 10.2) [19,20,30,31]. This relationship was first defined for the relationship between defect extent and severity for both exercise and pharmacologic SPECT, but has since been shown to be the case for exercise and pharmacologic stress echocardiography defect extent as well [6,29]. In addition, both forms of stress imaging have shown that even after patients are stratified by pre-imaging data, the imaging results further risk-stratify patients into low-risk versus higher-risk subgroups (Figures 10.3 and 10.4), a demonstration of clinical incremental prognostic value [19,31]. Nonperfusion SPECT imaging variables such as

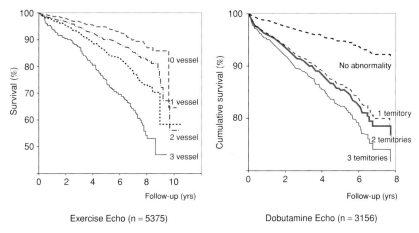

Fig. 10.1 Event-free survival with exercise (left) and dobutamine (right) stress echocardiography as a function of the number of vascular territories with wall motion abnormalities. There is a significant difference in survival across a number of territories in both panels ($p < 0.001$). Reprinted with permission from Marwick, T.H., (2003) *Stress Echocardiography: Clinical Application in the Diagnosis and Management of Coronary Artery Disease*. 2nd ed. Kluwer Academic Publishers, Norwell, MA, 167–206.

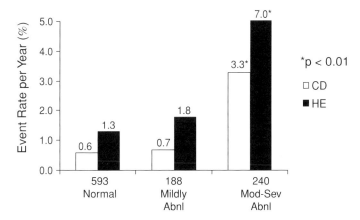

Fig. 10.2 Event rates per year in patients with high (greater than 0.80) pre-test likelihood of CAD but without prior CAD undergoing stress SPECT with normal, mild, and moderately to severe abnormal scans. Numbers under columns represent the number of patients in each subgroup. There is a significant difference in event rates across scan categories ($p < 0.01$) for both cardiac death (white bars) and hard events (black bars). Reprinted with permission from Hachamovitch, R., Hayes, S., Friedman, J.D., *et al.* (2004) *J Am Coll Cardiol* **43**: 200–208.

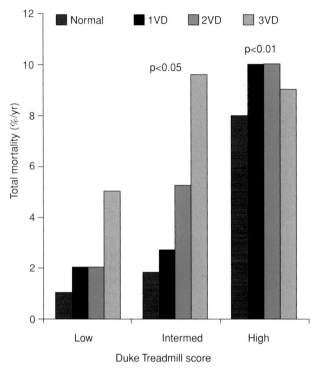

Fig. 10.3 Rates of total mortality after exercise stress echocardiography in patients with low, intermediate, and high Duke treadmill scores. Patients are further stratified by the stress echocardiography results (normal, one, two, or three vessels with abnormality). There is a significant difference in survival across echocardiographic results in patients with intermediate ($p < 0.05$) and high ($p < 0.01$) Duke treadmill score categories. Reprinted with permission from Marwick, T.H., (2003) *Stress Echocardiography: Clinical Application in the Diagnosis and Management of Coronary Artery Disease*. 2nd ed. Kluwer Academic Publishers, Norwell, MA, 167–206.

transient ischemic cavity dilation and variables reflecting regional and global left ventricular (LV) function add useful prognostic information to a sole assessment of extent and severity of perfusion defects [28].

Certain subsets of patients appear to benefit significantly from stress perfusion imaging or stress echocardiography. Diabetics with an abnormal perfusion scan or an abnormal stress echo have a greater subsequent event rate than nondiabetic patients with the same extent or severity of abnormality [6,28,32]. Similarly, patients with chronic renal disease can be well risk-stratified by either stress perfusion imaging or stress echocardiography in the absence of symptoms of CAD [33]. Accelerated CAD is a frequent complication of renal disease, and the use of noninvasive imaging for prognostication avoids the risk of administering contrast, which is necessary with CT angiography or coronary angiography.

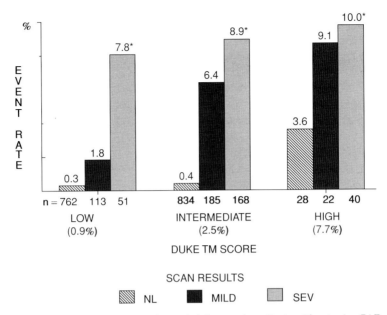

Fig. 10.4 Hard event rates over a 19-month follow-up in patients without prior CAD undergoing stress SPECT. Patients are separated into low, intermediate, and high Duke treadmill scores. Patients are further stratified by the stress SPECT results (normal, mild, and moderately to severe abnormal scans). Numbers under columns represent the number of patients in each subgroup, and event rates in Duke treadmill score categories are shown under the category labels. A significant difference in event rates across scan categories ($p < 0.01$) is present in the intermediate and high Duke treadmill score subgroups as a function of scan result. Reprinted with permission from Hachamovitch, R., Berman, D.S., Kiat, H., *et al.* (1996) *Circulation* **93**(5): 905–914.

Identifying Treatment Benefit

Virtually all prognostic studies of stress imaging to date have focused on medically treated patients. This approach identifies which patients are likely to experience adverse events but not necessarily which patients may benefit from medical therapy versus revascularization. For example, two patients with equally sized perfusion defects are at similarly high risk. However, if one patient has no evidence of viability while the second manifests demonstrable ischemia without evidence of scar, the latter patient is far more likely to benefit from a revascularization strategy than the former.

The paradigm of stress imaging's prognostic role was expanded by a study evaluating the relationship between perfusion defects, post-MPI treatment, and patient survival [20]. Using multivariable modeling, including a propensity score to adjust for nonrandomized treatment assignment, an interaction between patient treatment and ischemia was found such that in the setting of no or mild ischemia, patients undergoing medical therapy as their initial treatment

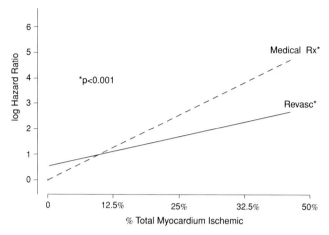

Fig. 10.5 Natural log of the hazard function (based on Cox proportional hazards model) versus percent of the myocardium ischemic on stress SPECT. Separate lines depicting the relationship between risk and ischemia are shown for patients treated with medical therapy (Medical Rx) and revascularization (Revasc). There is a significant difference across ischemia for risk and between treatment groups (interaction from multivariable model, $p < 0.01$). Reprinted with permission from Hachamovitch, R., Hayes, S.W., Friedman, J.D., et al. (2003) Circulation **107**(23): 2900–2907.

had superior survival rates compared to patients referred to revascularization. In the setting of moderate to severe ischemia (greater than 10% of the total myocardium), patients undergoing revascularization had an increased survival benefit compared to patients undergoing medical therapy (Figure 10.5). At these levels of ischemia, patients at greater clinical risk (elderly, women, diabetics, and pharmacologic stress patients) had greater absolute benefit with revascularization over medical therapy. A subsequent study incorporating gated SPECT data extended these results to show that although gated LV ejection fraction (LVEF) best predicted cardiac mortality, only ischemia could identify enhanced survival with a specific treatment strategy [34]. These results have not yet been reproduced in the echocardiography literature.

Understanding and Estimating Post-test Risk

The Need for Imaging Scores in Risk Estimation and Reporting
Many clinicians use a risk-based approach to patient management, particularly with respect to the application of imaging results [19,20,24]. However, incorporating pre-imaging data into their post-imaging estimates of patient risk is a significant challenge facing physicians. This problem is exemplified by the wide range of post-test risk at any level of test abnormality (Figure 10.6). For

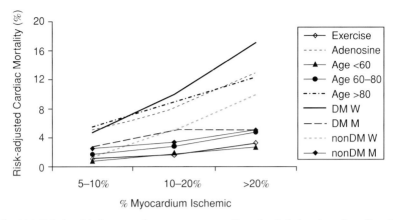

Fig. 10.6 Relationship between the percent myocardium that is ischemic and predicted risk. These risk-adjusted results demonstrate the wide variability in cardiac death risk associated with any amount of ischemia due to the confounding effects of clinical and demographic data. The risk for any amount of ischemia increases in the setting of diabetes mellitus, increased age, or pharmacologic stress, whereas in patients who are younger, nondiabetic, or able to exercise, the risk for any amount of ischemia decreases (based on data from Hachamovitch *et al.* [20]).

example, a SPECT study demonstrating 10 to 20% of the myocardium ischemic may be associated with an anticipated cardiac mortality of 2 to 10%, varying with patient characteristics. A similar pattern emerges when closely examining outcomes after normal studies.

Prognostic Post-test Referral Bias

The partial verification bias that obfuscates our ability to measure diagnostic test accuracy has a prognostic counterpart. As stated previously, post-test resource utilization is driven by the imaging results. From a prognostic perspective, greater reductions in post-test risk occur in patients with abnormal studies due to the greater intervention rate. Hence, a prognostic study that includes all patients would misestimate the risk associated with the imaging result because risk is reduced by revascularization that occurs in proportion to the test result. Accepted methods for prognostic analyses include the exclusion (censoring) of patients referred to revascularization early after testing in an attempt to avoid this underestimation. Unfortunately, with the increased dependence on imaging results in formulating resource utilization decisions, it is now recognized that this censoring of patients undergoing early revascularization (and more abnormal test results) from outcome studies has resulted in a relative underestimation of risk and a flattening of the test abnormality-risk relationship [35]. Other more complicated biases can also develop when data elements associated with risk and those associated with referral to revascularization become disparate [36].

Consequently, prognostic studies limited to medically treated patients result in the misestimation of risk, with the error increasing as a function of increasing test-related resource utilization rates. This error can be ameliorated by all patients analyzed using multivariable techniques to account for treatment decisions [20,34].

The impact of referral biases and pre-imaging data on post-imaging outcomes indicate that they must be considered along with the imaging results in the estimation of patient risk. This result can be achieved by the use of validated scores for estimating the patient likelihood of CAD or the risk of adverse events. Such multiple scores exist and have been validated for the exercise treadmill test (ETT) [37]. Recently, Elhendy and colleagues validated a score combining clinical, stress test, and echocardiographic parameters that permitted estimates of cardiac mortality risk in medically treated patients [38]. This score also risk-stratified patients with respect to hard events. Similarly, a prognostic score for stress SPECT has been derived that also accounts for post-test therapy, thus "correcting" for the possible referral bias [39]. In light of the significant variability in referral patterns to stress imaging, a putative score must be validated in a variety of populations with varying composition, risk, geography, and other factors before it can be applied clinically with confidence.

Limitations of Stress MPI and Stress Echocardiography

When compared with stress echocardiography, the limitations of stress SPECT perfusion imaging, among those already cited previously, are:
- Longer imaging protocols that may take many hours;
- Greater equipment expense and the necessity of injecting radiopharmaceuticals with radiation exposure;
- Less than desirable specificity in many laboratories because of a failure to distinguish attenuation artifacts (e.g., breast, diaphragmatic) from myocardial scarring;
- High visceral activity, particularly with the use of technetium-99m labeled pharmaceuticals during vasodilator stress, which may interfere with the evaluation of the inferior/posterior wall;
- An inability to visualize the heart in a real-time approach;
- Lower spatial resolution than seen with echocardiography;
- Higher costs to patients; and
- An inability to quantitate flow reserve or regional flow in ml/min/g.

The last limitation can potentially be overcome by PET perfusion imaging, although quantitation of flow reserve or absolute flow measurements are not routinely performed in most PET laboratories.

Limitations of stress echocardiography include the following:
- Images are difficult to acquire at peak exercise because of exertional hyperpnoea and cardiac excursion.

- An ischemic response is required for the elucidation of regional abnormal wall motion, whereas mere detection of flow heterogeneity is a positive test for stress perfusion imaging.
- Dobutamine echocardiography requires an adequate heart-rate response or else sensitivity is reduced.
- The rapid recovery of motion abnormalities can be seen with mild ischemia, particularly with one-vessel disease, which could lead to a false negative test result if a substantial delay occurs between image acquisition and cessation of exercise.
- The detection of residual ischemia within an infarct zone is difficult because of resting akinesis.
- The technique is highly operator-dependent for the acquisition of echocardiographic data and the analysis of images, with interindividual variability reported for interpreting stress echocardiograms.
- Complete high-quality images viewing all myocardial segments occurs in only 85% of patients.
- Quantitative assessment of wall motion thickening and LVEF is not well validated, and the visual assessment of the ejection fraction is rather operator-dependent.

Validating New Modalities for Daily Practice: Do Prettier Pictures Result in Better Outcomes?

Although the introduction of a new imaging modality is accompanied by claims that older imaging modalities will be replaced, the usual case is that these tests undergo further testing and their optimal application is determined over time. The integration of newer imaging modalities into clinical practice and testing algorithms can occur in two distinct patterns. First, a newer modality can be shown to be sufficiently superior in addressing a specific clinical question that it directly replaces an older modality.

Alternatively, a new modality may be sufficiently unique that it permits imaging of a particular structure or phenomenon that previously could not be assessed. Although new tests are usually compared to an accepted gold standard, often also in comparison to an "older" test, occasionally a test can be said to be first in its class. For example, magnetic resonance spectroscopy has no previously validated test to which it can be compared, hence its validation in patients would be problematic. Alternatively, computed tomography angiography (CTA), although "first in its class" with respect to noninvasive imaging of atherosclerotic burden, morphology, structure, and so on, can be compared to invasive angiography for detecting epicardial coronary stenoses or invasive intravascular ultrasound (IVUS) for the assessment of atherosclerosis. Although CTA has significant potential as a test of atherosclerosis (see discussion in Chapter 15), most of its validation has been as a noninvasive alternative to invasive catheterization, and will be discussed later.

As discussed in several chapters throughout this textbook, two examples of newer modalities with potential application to the diagnostic or prognostic assessment of CAD are CMR and CTA. Both these modalities have the potential to yield new insights into the disease process and aid in identifying patients with disease and greater risk. Further, these modalities produce images of a quality that far surpasses that of older imaging modalities. However, to date there is insufficient data to support their use as routine testing. It is vital to review the type of data necessary to determine what role a new test will need to establish a clinical niche, and we will use CTA as an example.

The Use of CTA: Evaluating a New Addition to a Testing Strategy

Advocates of an imaging-based (or physiologic approach) to the evaluation of patients with intermediate to high likelihood (or risk) have claimed the superior clinical- and cost-effectiveness and efficiency of a conservative, sequential testing strategy that includes the use of stress imaging prior to referral to catheterization, the latter being an invasive test with potential risks, hazards, and costs. With the development of CTA, an anatomy-based approach to patient evaluation can be performed noninvasively. Hence, whether to pursue anatomy- or physiology-based testing strategies will have to be re-evaluated.

With respect to CTA, the question facing investigators and clinicians is where it can best fit in future testing algorithms for known or suspected CAD. This evaluation includes the determination of whether CTA is a replacement for stress imaging or a test that would precede (or follow) stress imaging, and in what application CTA may enhance cost-effectiveness. The dissemination of CTA in the United States has been accompanied by claims that its superior accuracy for anatomic CAD justifies its role in testing strategies as a replacement for stress imaging. We address this claim using a series of questions addressing CTA's accuracy, the relationship between imaging and patient benefit, and comparing the roles of stress imaging and CTA. The other major consideration with respect to considering CTA as the first noninvasive test for patients with suspected CAD is radiation exposure, particularly in higher pretest likelihood patients where the finding of intermediate severity stenoses (30 to 70%) may require additional testing, as with stress perfusion imaging. In the first randomized study of 64-slice CTA versus stress perfusion imaging in clinically low- to intermediate-risk patients presenting with acute chest pain, 25% of patients in the CTA group also had to undergo stress MPI, owing to either lesions of unclear significance (26 to 70% stenoses) or nondiagnostic-quality scans [40].

Can CTA Define the Extent of Anatomic CAD, and Thus Estimate the Extent of Jeopardized Myocardium?

The estimation of jeopardized myocardium plays a central role in achieving optimal anatomy-based risk stratification, which is enhanced by incorporating stenosis severity, location, and LAD involvement in addition to the number of vessels with CAD [41]. Given the importance of jeopardized myocardium in defining optimal revascularization candidates, it is vital to define whether CTA replicates invasive angiography results or is a cruder estimate of anatomic CAD, thus limiting CTA's application [42].

Many studies have reported outstanding CTA accuracies for CAD detection; pooled data from 1653 patients estimated sensitivity and specificity as 93 and 81%, respectively [2]. These studies are based on patients referred for elective catheterization and recruited to CTA, resulting in a high prevalence of disease (63%); recalculation of the reported positive and negative predicative values (86 and 88%, respectively) for lower-prevalence populations reveals more modest values for positive and negative predicative values (30% prevalence: 68 and 96%, respectively; 15% prevalence: 46 and 98%, respectively) [2].

Importantly, direct comparisons of CTA to quantitative coronary angiography reveal suboptimal agreement, thus potentially limiting CTA's ability to accurately estimate jeopardized myocardium [43]. Multiple limitations of this technology and associated interpretative issues may explain this discrepancy, including limitations in visualizing smaller vessels (less than 2.0 mm), exclusion of nonvisualized vessels and various CTA artifacts, and especially beam hardening caused by perivascular calcification [2]. To summarize, CTA appears to be an accurate means to exclude the presence of CAD due to an outstanding negative predictive value; however, its ability to accurately predict the presence of anatomic stenosis and its severity may be limited with current technology. Consequently, whether CTA will permit the accurate estimation of jeopardized myocardium is currently unproven and is likely to be the focus of numerous future investigations.

Is Anatomic Data Enough for Identifying Optimal Candidates for Revascularization?

If one of the newer modalities can accurately estimate jeopardized myocardium as well as invasive catheterization, will this information allow us to identify revascularization candidates, thus obviating the need for stress imaging? A number of concepts regarding the identification of optimal revascularization candidates have been identified by RCT to date. As summarized by Yusuf and colleagues, "the general concept [is] that the greater the amount of myocardium jeopardized (i.e., more extensive or proximal coronary disease), the greater the improvement in prognosis" with coronary artery bypass grafting (CABG) [42]. Consequently, revascularization enhances survival in patients with anatomic disease subtending extensive amounts of myocardium (left main, three vesse, or proximal LAD artery CAD) independently of LV function [42]. Although LV function did not influence relative benefit with surgery, a greater absolute benefit was noted with increased patient risk (e.g., reduced LV function) — "the absolute benefit of surgery depends on inherent patient risk as well as the relative benefits conferred by the procedure." Hence, although the relative benefit was only identified by the extent of anatomic CAD and not by clinical risk score, LV dysfunction, prior CAD, abnormal ETT, or patient age, these latter factors all influenced the absolute benefit of this procedure by altering the underlying patient risk.

In this context, the results of the recent COURAGE trial, comparing strategies of percutaneous coronary intervention (PCI) and medical therapy versus medical therapy alone in stable patients with known CAD (and evidence of ischemia by noninvasive testing) must be mentioned as well [44]. Although the results of this study indicate no survival advantage to a PCI strategy, it is unclear whether imaging should be performed to identify the high-risk patient because revascularization would not be advantageous with respect to any conventional endpoint. However, it is unclear how much ischemia was present in the COURAGE patients, and whether the absence of demonstrable therapeutic benefit is related to insufficient amounts of ischemia in recruited patients. Patients with severe ischemia were excluded from this trial, as were patients whose anatomy was not suitable for PCI. However, of the patients reported the frequencies of single reversible defects and multiple defects were similar in the PCI and medical groups. To date, no RCT of stable CAD has examined a strategy that originates with testing as a first step with treatment based on test results, although this type of trial is clearly needed. Finally, it must be noted that the results of COURAGE are generalizable to patients with known CAD but not to patients being evaluated with suspected CAD, a patient group with a very different hazard function in whom very different results may have occurred.

Is Identification of Ischemia Important?

The justification of stress imaging in testing strategies has hinged on the identification of which patients may benefit from a revascularization strategy by means of noninvasive estimates of jeopardized myocardium rather than catheterization-derived anatomy. Although with its advantages — avoidance of excess catheterizations, their associated cost and risk, the potential "occulostenotic reflex," differentiation of high-risk patients into those with extensive scar versus extensive ischemia, and so on — only indirect evidence supports its use, as no RCT to date has compared medical therapy to revascularization on the basis of noninvasive ischemia estimates in stable patients [7,45].

Nonetheless, revascularization in patients with three-vessel CAD was associated with enhanced survival only in those patients with ischemic ETT results, whereas medical therapy was a superior initial therapy in patients without this finding [46]. In the setting of reduced LVEF, CABG improved survival in most subsets of patients with the exception of patients with a preserved exercise capacity [47]. Further, patients without prior CAD accrued a survival benefit from revascularization over medical therapy only when significant ischemia was present, with the absolute benefit varying with underlying patient risk and LVEF [20,34].

Can CTA Identify the Presence of Ischemia in Addition to Atherosclerosis?

Although a normal CTA convincingly excludes the presence of inducible ischemia (negative predictive value greater than 90%), well under half of patients with abnormal CTA have demonstrable ischemia [2]. In one study, the positive predictive value of CTA alone was 31% for detecting hemodynamically significant lesions, and rose to 77% when SPECT information was added, with maintenance of a 99% negative predictive value [48]. Hence, although CTA can identify with great accuracy which patients are not in need of further evaluation (high negative predictive value) and will likely guide antithrombotic, cholesterol-reduction, and anti-inflammatory pharmacotherapy, it has insufficient accuracy to identify candidates for catheterization or revascularization (poor positive predictive value for identifying ischemia). For the present, the pattern of test performance described here suggests that CTA may perform well as a test placed earlier in a strategy, e.g., atherosclerosis testing, the identification of patients at intermediate likelihood who might be stress imaging candidates, rather than a test to identify patients with significant ischemia who may benefit from catheterization. Initial data suggest that CTA might also be a good alternative to coronary angiography for the identification of CAD in patients with dilated cardiomyopathy of unknown etiology [49].

Are Current Stress Imaging Modalities Adequate?

The most profound limitation of current stress imaging modalities is their inability to assess coronary flow reserve. For SPECT in particular, it is not unusual for the extent and severity of perfusion abnormalities to underestimate the anatomic disease present, especially in comparison to approaches directly measuring flow reserve [50]. Unfortunately, the flow-perfusion relationship for SPECT varies with the extent and severity of the underlying anatomic CAD such that in patients with multivessel CAD, the agreement decreases to less than 80% [50,51]. SPECT imaging underestimates the extent of CAD because only relative tracer uptake is assessed, rather than attaining quantitative measurements of myocardial blood flow in ml/min/g under rest and stress conditions. In one study, 25% of patients with anatomic three-vessel disease (greater than or equal to 50% stenosis in the three major coronary vessels) had vascular perfusion or function abnormalities in the supply zones of the three stenotic arteries [3]. Twelve percent had totally normal SPECT studies. Similarly, only 56% of patients with left main CAD had greater than 10% myocardial ischemia on stress SPECT [4]. Thus, if stress SPECT or PET imaging is performed as the first test and an unexpected "normal" perfusion scan is encountered, CTA may be useful as the next test to identify patients with multivessel disease and balanced ischemia or diffusely exhausted flow reserve. In this context, stress PET might be the stress imaging modality of choice over SPECT or stress echocardiography due to its ability to routinely acquire flow reserve data in all patients [2]. This approach can also permit the routine assessment of endothelial function in appropriate patients as well.

Thus, although stress imaging might be superior to CTA as a gatekeeper to the catheterization laboratory, this superiority may necessitate the use of PET as the stress imaging approach. However, whether stress perfusion CMR or CT will also be able to capture this information is unclear and may develop as well. First-pass CMR, particularly using a 3-T magnet, appears promising for perfusion imaging of CAD detection [52]. It is very likely that future patient assessments may permit the combined assessment of stress and rest perfusion and function, as well as anatomy/atherosclerosis and flow characteristics. The challenge for the future will be to identify which patients will benefit from a combined hybrid approach as opposed to a single modality approach with stepped testing. It is unclear which patients will require all pieces of information that can be acquired to optimize their care. How cost-effective strategies can be pieced together from these more advanced imaging approaches and the consideration of radiation exposure will require close scrutiny.

Conclusions

Considerable evidence exists supporting the use of stress SPECT and stress echocardiography for both diagnostic and prognostic applications. As reviewed, the evaluation of testing in a diagnostic context is compromised, and the prognostic data are more robust and applicable to daily practice. Although prior emphasis was on risk stratification with these modalities, increasing evidence suggests that estimates of patient risk are feasible, and that the identification of which patients can benefit from revascularization will be the new basis to judge testing modalities in the future. Application of a new modality such as CTA is promising, but its optimal role in a testing strategy is as yet undefined. Molecular imaging of vulnerable atherosclerotic plaques may also prove useful in identifying patients at high risk for acute coronary events, and such "hotspot" imaging data can be used to enhance coronary anatomic images as obtained by CT or CMR [53].

References

1 Klocke, F.J., Baird, M.G., Bateman, T.M., *et al.* (2003) ACC/AHA/ASNC guidelines for the clinical use of cardiac radionuclide imaging: a report of the American 1995 guidelines for the clinical use of radionuclide imaging. *Circulation* **108**(11): 1404–1418.

2 Di Carli, M.F., Hachamovitch, R. (2007) New technology for non-invasive evaluation of coronary artery disease. *Circulation* **115**: 1464–1480.

3 Lima, R.S., Watson, D.D., Goode, A.R., *et al.* (2003) Incremental value of combined perfusion and function over perfusion alone by gated SPECT myocardial perfusion imaging for detection of severe three-vessel coronary artery disease. *J Am Coll Cardiol* **42**: 64–70.

4 Berman, D.S., Kang, X., Slomka, P.J., *et al.* (2007) Underestimation of extent of ischemia by gated SPECT myocardial perfusion imaging in patients with left main coronary artery disease. *J Nucl Cardiol* **14**: 521–528.

5 Cheitlin, M.D., Armstrong, W.F., Aurigemma, G.P., *et al*. (2003) A report of the American College of Cardiology/American Heart Association Task Force on Practice Guidelines. ACC/AHA/ASE committee to update the 1997 guidelines for the clinical application of echocardiography.

6 Marwick, T.H. (2003) Application of stress echocardiography to the prediction of outcomes. In: Marwick, T.H. (ed.), *Stress Echocardiography: Clinical Application in the Diagnosis and Management of Coronary Artery Disease*, 2nd ed. Kluwer Academic Publishers, Norwell, MA, 167–206.

7 Berman, D.S., Wong, N.D., Gransar, H., *et al*. (2004) Relationship between stress-induced myocardial ischemia and atherosclerosis measured by coronary calcium tomography. *J Am Coll Cardiol* **44**: 923–930.

8 Douglas, P.S., Iskandrian, A.E., Krumholz, H.M., *et al*. (2006) American College of Cardiology; American College of Radiology; American Heart Association; American Society of Echocardiography; American Society of Nuclear Cardiology; Heart Failure Society of America; Heart Rhythm Society; Society of Atherosclerosis Imaging and Prevention; Society for Cardiovascular Angiography and Interventions; Society of Cardiovascular Computed Tomography; Society for Cardiovascular Magnetic Resonance; Society for Vascular Medicine and Biology. Achieving quality in cardiovascular imaging: proceedings from the American College of Cardiology-Duke University Medical Center Think Tank on Quality in Cardiovascular Imaging. *J Am Coll Cardiol* **48**: 2141–2151.

9 Patel, M.R., Spertus, J.A., Brindis, R.G., *et al*. (2005) American College of Cardiology Foundation. ACCF proposed method for evaluating the appropriateness of cardiovascular imaging. *J Am Coll Cardiol* **46**: 1606–1613.

10 Brindis, R.G., Douglas, P.S., Hendel, R.C., *et al*. (2005) American College of Cardiology Foundation Quality Strategic Directions Committee Appropriateness Criteria Working Group; American Society of Nuclear Cardiology; American Heart Association. ACCF/ASNC appropriateness criteria for single-photon emission computed tomography myocardial perfusion imaging (SPECT MPI): a report of the American College of Cardiology Foundation Quality Strategic Directions Committee Appropriateness Criteria Working Group and the American Society of Nuclear Cardiology endorsed by the American Heart Association. *J Am Coll Cardiol* **46**: 1587–1605.

11 Garcia, E.V., Faber, T.L., Cooke, C.D., *et al*. (2007) The increasing role of quantification in clinical nuclear cardiology: the Emory approach. *J Nucl Cardiol* **14**: 420–432.

12 Germano, G., Kavanagh, P.B., Slomka, P.J., *et al*. (2007) Quantitation in gated perfusion SPECT imaging: the Cedars-Sinai approach. *J Nucl Cardiol* **14**: 433–454.

13 Ficaro, E.P., Lee, B.C., Kritzman, J.N., Corbett, J.R. (2007) Corridor4DM: the Michigan method for quantitative nuclear cardiology. *J Nucl Cardiol* **14**: 455–465.

14 Watson, D.D., Smith, W.H., II. (2007) The role of quantitation in clinical nuclear cardiology: the University of Virginia approach. *J Nucl Cardiol* **14**: 466–482.

15 Thompson, R.C., Heller, G.V., Johnson, L.L., *et al*. (2005) Value of attenuation correction on ECG-gated SPECT myocardial perfusion imaging related to body mass index. *J Nucl Cardiol* **12**: 195–202.

16 Rozanski, A., Diamond, G.A., Berman, D.S., *et al*. (1983) The declining specificity of exercise radionuclide ventriculography. *N Engl J Med* **309**: 518–522.

17 Hennekens, C.H., Buring, J.E. (1987) Analysis of epidemiological studies: evaluating the role of bias. In: *Epidemiology in Medicine*. Little, Brown and Co., Boston, 272–286.

18 Zhou, X.H., Obuchowski, N.A., McClish, D.K. (2002) Methods for correcting verification bias. In: *Statistical Methods in Diagnostic Medicine.* John Wiley and Sons, New York, 307–358.

19 Hachamovitch, R., Berman, D.S., Kiat, H., *et al.* (1996) Exercise myocardial perfusion SPECT in patients without known coronary artery disease: incremental prognostic value and use in risk stratification. *Circulation* **93**(5): 905–914.

20 Hachamovitch, R., Hayes, S.W., Friedman, J.D., *et al.* (2003) Comparison of the short-term survival benefit associated with revascularization compared with medical therapy in patients with no prior coronary artery disease undergoing stress myocardial perfusion single photon emission computed tomography. *Circulation* **107**(23): 2900–2907.

21 Whiting, P., Rutjes, A.W., Reitsma, J.B., *et al.* (2004) Sources of variation and bias in studies of diagnostic accuracy. *Ann Intern Med* **140**: 189–202.

22 Maddahi, J., Garcia, E.V., Berman, D.S., *et al.* (1980) Improved noninvasive assessment of coronary artery disease by quantitative analysis of regional stress myocardial distribution and washout of thallium-201. *Circulation* **64**: 924–935.

23 Rozanski, A., Diamond, G.A., Forrester, J.S., *et al.* (1984) Alternate referent standards for cardiac normality: implications for diagnostic imaging. *Ann Intern Med* **101**(2): 164.

24 Califf, R.M., Armstrong, P.W., Carver, J.R., *et al.* (1996) 27th Bethesda Conference: matching the intensity of risk factor management with the hazard for coronary disease events. Task Force 5: stratification of patients into high, medium and low risk subgroups for purposes of risk factor management. *J Am Coll Cardiol* **27**(5): 1007–1019.

25 Hachamovitch, R., Shaw, L., Berman, D.S. (2000) Methodological considerations in the assessment of noninvasive testing using outcomes research: pitfalls and limitations. *Prog Cardiovasc Dis* **43**(3): 215–230.

26 Bateman, T.M. (1997) Clinical relevance of a normal myocardial perfusion scintigraphic study. *J Nucl Cardiol* **4**: 172–173.

27 Hachamovitch, R., Hayes, S., Friedman, J.D., *et al.* (2003) Determinants of risk and its temporal variation in patients with normal stress myocardial perfusion scans: what is the warranty period of a normal scan? *J Am Coll Cardiol* **41**(8): 1329–1340.

28 Berman, D.S., Hachamovitch, R., Shaw, L.J., *et al.* (2004) Nuclear cardiology. In: Fuster, V.A.R., King, S., O'Rourke, R.A., Wellens, H.J.J. (eds.), *Hurst's The Heart.* McGraw-Hill Companies, New York, 525–565.

29 Armstrong, W.F., Zoghbi, W.A. (2005) Stress echocardiography: current methodology and clinical applications. *J Am Coll Cardiol* **45**: 1739–1747.

30 Marwick, T.H., Case, C., Sawada, S., *et al.* (2001) Prediction of mortality using dobutamine echocardiography. *J Am Coll Cardiol* **37**: 754–760.

31 Marwick, T.H., Case, C., Vasey, C., *et al.* (2001) Prediction of mortality by exercise echocardiography: a strategy for combination with the Duke treadmill score. *Circulation* **103**: 2566–2571.

32 Giri, S., Shaw, L.J., Murthy, D.R., *et al.* (2002) Impact of diabetes on the risk stratification using stress single-photon emission computed tomography myocardial perfusion imaging in patients with symptoms suggestive of coronary artery disease. *Circulation* **105**: 32–40.

33 Rakhit, D.J., Armstrong, K.A., Beller, E., *et al.* (2006) Risk stratification of patients with chronic kidney disease: results of screening strategies incorporating clinical risk scoring and dobutamine stress echocardiography. *Am Heart J* **152**: 363–370.

34 Hachamovitch, R., Hayes, S., Friedman, J.D., *et al.* Relative role of inducible ischemia versus ejection fraction in the prediction of survival benefit with revascularization compared to medical therapy in patients with no prior revascularization undergoing stress myocardial perfusion SPECT. *J Nucl Cardiol* (in press).

35 Hachamovitch, R., Hayes, S., Friedman, J., *et al.* (2004) Stress myocardial perfusion SPECT is clinically effective and cost-effective in risk-stratification of patients with a high likelihood of CAD but no known CAD. *J Am Coll Cardiol* **43**: 200–208.

36 Hachamovitch, R., Hayes, S.W., Friedman, J.D., *et al.* (2003) Is there a referral bias against revascularization of patients with reduced LV ejection fraction? influence of ejection fraction and inducible ischemia on post-SPECT management of patients without history of CAD. *J Am Coll Cardiol* **42**(7): 1286–1294.

37 Mark, D.B., Hlatky, M.A., Harrell, F.E., Jr., *et al.* (1987) Exercise treadmill score for predicting prognosis in coronary artery disease. *Ann Intern Med* **106**(6).

38 Elhendy, A., Mahoney, D.W., McCully, R.B., *et al.* (2004) Use of a scoring model combining clinical, exercise test, and echocardiographic data to predict mortality in patients with known or suspected coronary artery disease. *Am J Cardiol* **93**(10): 1223–1228.

39 Hachamovitch, R., Hayes, S., Friedman, J., *et al.* (2005) A prognostic score for prediction of cardiac mortality risk after adenosine stress myocardial perfusion scintigraphy. *J Am Coll Cardiol* **45**: 722–729.

40 Goldstein, J.A., Gallagher, M.J., O'Neill, W.W., *et al.* (2007) A randomized controlled trial of multi-slice coronary computed tomography for evaluation of acute chest pain. *J Am Coll Cardiol* **49**: 863–871.

41 Califf, R.M., Phillips, H.R., III, Hindman, M.C., *et al.* (1985) Prognostic value of a coronary artery jeopardy score. *J Am Coll Cardiol* **5**: 1055–1063.

42 Yusuf, S., Zucker, D., Peduzzi, P., *et al.* (1994) Effect of coronary artery bypass graft surgery on survival: overview of 10-year results from randomised trials by the Coronary Artery Bypass Graft Surgery Trialists Collaboration. *Lancet* **344**(8922): 563–570 (see comments). Published erratum appears in *Lancet* **344**(8934): 1446.

43 Leber, A.W., Knez, A., von Ziegler, F., *et al.* (2005) Quantification of obstructive and nonobstructive coronary lesions by 64-slice computed tomography: a comparative study with quantitative coronary angiography and intravascular ultrasound. *J Am Coll Cardiol* **46**: 147–154.

44 Boden, W.E., O'Rourke, R.A., Teo, K.K., *et al.* (2007) Optimal medical therapy with or without PCI for stable coronary disease. *N Engl J Med* **356**.

45 Shaw, L.J., Hachamovitch, R., Berman, D.S., *et al.* (1999) The economic consequences of available diagnostic and prognostic strategies for the evaluation of stable angina patients: an observational assessment of the value of precatheterization ischemia. Economics of Noninvasive Diagnosis (END) Multicenter Study Group. *J Am Coll Cardiol* **33**(3): 661–669.

46 Weiner, D.A., Ryan, T.J., McCabe, C.H., *et al.* (1986) The role of exercise testing in identifying patients with improved survival after coronary artery bypass surgery. *J Am Coll Cardiol* **8**(4): 741–748.

47 Weiner, D.A., Ryan, T.J., McCabe, C.H., *et al.* (1987) Value of exercise testing in determining the risk classification and the response to coronary artery bypass grafting in three-vessel coronary artery disease: a report from the Coronary Artery Surgery Study (CASS) registry. *Am J Cardiol* **60**(4): 262–266.

48 Rispler, S., Keidar, Z., Ghersin, E., *et al.* (2007) Integrated single-photon emission computed tomography and computed tomography coronary angiography for the assessment of hemodynamically significant coronary artery lesions. *J Am Coll Cardiol* **49**: 1059–1067.

49 Andreini, D., Pontone, G., Pepi, M., *et al.* (2007) Diagnostic accuracy of multidetector computed tomography coronary angiography in patients with dilated cardiomyopathy. *J Am Coll Cardiol* **49**: 2044–2050.

50 Ragosta, M., Bishop, A.H., Lipson, L.C., *et al.* (2007) Comparison between angiography and fractional flow reserve versus single-photon emission computed tomographic myocardial perfusion imaging for determining lesion significance in patients with multivessel coronary disease. *Am J Cardiol* **99**: 896–902.

51 Kern, M.J., Lerman, A., Bech, J.W., *et al.* (2006) Physiological assessment of coronary artery disease in the Cardiac Catheterization Laboratory: a scientific statement from the American Heart Association Committee on Diagnostic and Interventional Cardiac Catheterization, Council on Clinical Cardiology. *Circulation* **114**: 1321–1341.

52 Cheng, A.S., Pegg, T.J., Karamitsos, T.D., *et al.* (2007) Cardiovascular magnetic resonance perfusion imaging at 3-Tesla for the detection of coronary artery disease: a comparison with 1.5-Tesla. *J Am Coll Cardiol* **49**: 2440–2449.

53 Jaffer, F.A., Libby, P., Weissleder, R. (2006) Molecular and cellular imaging of atherosclerosis: emerging applications. *J Am Coll Cardiol* **47**: 1328–1338.

Chapter 11

Evaluating the Patient with New Onset Heart Failure

Joseph B. Selvanayagam and Theodoros D. Karamitsos

Heart failure is described as left ventricular (LV) dysfunction leading to congestion and reduced systemic perfusion, most often manifesting clinically as dyspnea. The pathophysiology of this syndrome is complex due to the wide spectrum of underlying etiologic processes including ischemic heart disease, hypertension, valvular heart disease, myocarditis, primary myocardial disease, and acquired infiltrative and pericardial disorders. The differentiation of these conditions is paramount to the appropriate prescription of care within this population. The final common pathway morphologically involves progressive LV dilatation or hypertrophy, often leading to spherical remodeling. These changes further adversely affect the myocardium by increasing wall tension and cause or exacerbate mitral regurgitation, which in turn results in further adverse remodeling [1].

The American College of Cardiology/American Heart Association (ACC/AHA) guidelines place special emphasis on detecting subclinical LV systolic and diastolic dysfunction [1,2]. Routine physical examination maneuvers have been found to be suboptimal in detecting either systolic or diastolic LV dysfunction [3,4]. Although echocardiography will remain the mainstay of initial assessment of patients presenting in heart failure, cardiovascular magnetic resonance (CMR) by virtue of its multiparametric nature has the potential to be the principal noninvasive imaging modality for both the diagnosis and prognosis of the patient with new onset heart failure.

Novel Techniques for Imaging the Heart, 1st edition. Edited by M. Di Carli and R. Kwong.
© 2008 American Heart Association, ISBN: 9-781-4051-7533-3.

Assessment of Cardiac Morphology, Right and Left Ventricular Function

CMR has rapidly become the imaging method of choice and the gold standard in the assessment of cardiac function of both normal and abnormal ventricles [5–8]. With regard to measurement of global LV function, given its 3D nature and order of magnitude greater signal-to-noise ratio, CMR is highly superior to 2D echocardiography [5]. This imaging is typically performed in — although not limited to — the conventional serial short-axis views and the three cardinal long-axis views. The ability of CMR to image in any plane without the need for optimal imaging windows allows for unprecedented flexibility for the interrogation of abnormal heart structures. CMR is also considered to be the most accurate imaging method for the evaluation of right ventricular (RV) volumes. CMR measurement of RV volumes has been validated with a close correlation between RV and LV stroke volumes, and between RV stroke volumes and tricuspid flow measurements [9]. The inherent 3D nature of CMR makes it particularly well suited to study the RV, given its complex and variable morphology (even in normal volunteers) [10]. CMR measurements of the RV volumes can either be acquired in a transverse (axial) orientation or in an axis aligned along the LV short axis.

Cine images are obtained using steady state free precession (SSFP) sequence, which provides images of higher signal-to-noise ratio (than older sequences such as FLASH), and hence exceptional delineation of the blood-myocardium interface. This method allows for the accurate and reproducible quantitative assessment of chamber dimensions and systolic function using manual or semi-automated planimetry techniques.

Visual inspection of the LV and RV architecture identifies patterns of regional or diffuse wall thinning and concentric or asymmetric hypertrophy, and provides clues to other myopathic processes such as LV noncompaction [11,12]. Pericardial thickness and calcification can be assessed. The atria and cardiac valves are evaluated for primary or secondary structural abnormalities, and the functional consequences of these morphologic changes are simultaneously evaluated through looped playback of the segmented cine image, making note of regional and global systolic function and valvular flow abnormalities. By providing high resolution, 3D images, CMR can provide ancillary information on the geometry of the LV (Figure 11.1) and the presence of mitral regurgitation or LV thrombus (Figure 11.2). The detailed assessment of LV shape and volume by CMR can be particularly crucial in patients with severe heart failure due to coronary artery disease (CAD), in whom LV reconstruction surgery is contemplated in addition to coronary revascularization.

Tissue Characterization: Ischemic Cardiomyopathy

The development of the late gadolinium enhancement (LGE) CMR technique has revolutionized the role of CMR in clinical and research practice, and has

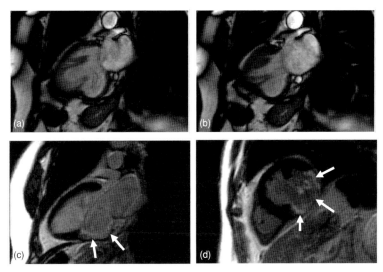

Fig. 11.1 Large LV (basal inferoposterior wall) aneurysm detected pre-CABG in a patient with triple-vessel coronary disease. Panels (a) and (b) demonstrate vertical long-axis cine images (end-diastole and end-systole, respectively) showing basal inferior wall dyskinesia. Panels (c) and (d) demonstrate DE-CMR images showing extensive scar tissue in this region. The size of the aneurysm was underappreciated on the echocardiogram, and the patient underwent CABG and LV aneurysmectomy. Courtesy of the Oxford Centre for Clinical Magnetic Resonance Research (OCMR).

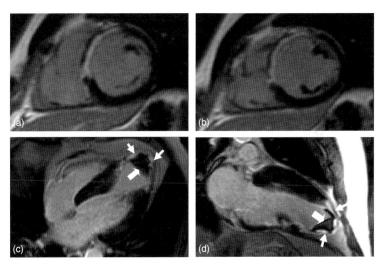

Fig. 11.2 Two patient examples of LGE imaging by CMR in ischemic heart failure. Panels (a) and (b) demonstrate anteroseptal delayed hyperenhancement (DHE) in a patient presenting with two-week-old anterior myocardial infarction and proximal left anterior descending artery (LAD) occlusion. Panels (c) and (d) are from a patient with a history of apical myocardial infarction 12 months prior and mid-LAD occlusion, showing a thinned apical wall with fully transmural LGE (small arrows). Coexistent apical thrombus is also seen in this patient (block arrows). Courtesy of the Oxford Centre for Clinical Magnetic Resonance Research (OCMR).

HYPERENHANCEMENT PATTERNS

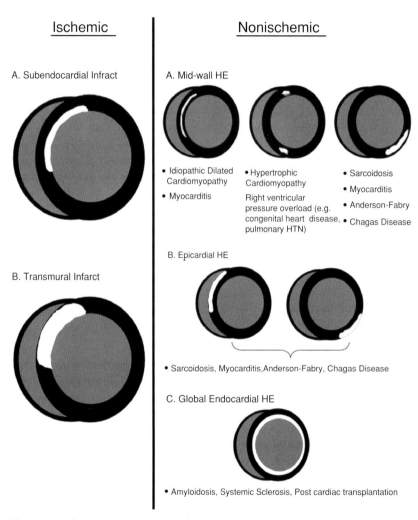

Ischemic

A. Subendocardial Infract

B. Transmural Infarct

Nonischemic

A. Mid-wall HE

- Idiopathic Dilated Cardiomyopathy
- Myocarditis

- Hypertrophic Cardiomyopathy

  Right ventricular pressure overload (e.g. congenital heart disease, pulmonary HTN)

- Sarcoidosis
- Myocarditis
- Anderson-Fabry
- Chagas Disease

B. Epicardial HE

- Sarcoidosis, Myocarditis, Anderson-Fabry, Chagas Disease

C. Global Endocardial HE

- Amyloidosis, Systemic Sclerosis, Post cardiac transplantation

Fig. 11.3 A schematic representation of the various hyperenhancement patterns in ischemic and nonischemic cardiomyopathy. Reprinted with permission from Mahrholdt, H., Wagner, A., Judd, R.M., *et al.* (2005) *Eur Heart J* **26**: 1461–1474.

potential roles in both the diagnosis and prognosis of newly diagnosed heart failure patients [13]. Specific patterns of fibrosis and scarring have been identified in many of the cardiomyopathy states and are summarized in Figure 11.3 [14–17]. Ischemic cardiomyopathy is characterized by subendocardial-based areas of late enhancement that correlate to irreversible myocardial necrosis on

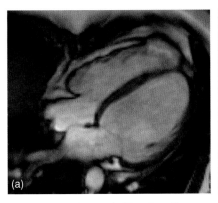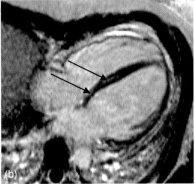

Fig. 11.4 A patient with dilated cardiomyopathy. Panel (a) is an end-diastolic image for the analysis of geometry, myocardial mass, volumes, and function using SSFP sequence. Panel (b) is the corresponding end-diastolic image obtained with the LGE-CMR technique, where signal-intense areas represent fibrotic tissue and the normal myocardium appears dark. Note the mid-wall striae of increased signal in the septum (black arrows). Image courtesy of the Oxford Centre for Clinical Magnetic Resonance Research (OCMR).

histopathology (Figure 11.4), a pattern consistent with the "wave front phenomenon" as described by Reimer and colleagues [18]. Patients who have nonischemic dilated cardiomyopathy may also have delayed-enhancement magnetic resonance imaging (DE-MRI) evidence of scarring in up to 30% of cases; however, this is typically in a noncoronary distribution and frequently appears as a mid-wall striae [16]. (This condition is discussed in more detail in the following section.) Therefore, based on the presence and pattern of myocardial fibrosis, the etiology of the cardiomyopathy can be accurately ascertained. Delineation of the underlying etiology is of clinical value for patients who have heart failure. In patients with ischemic substrate for their heart failure, the delineation of potential areas of myocardial ischemia and viability is crucial to defining clinical management.

CMR Assessment of Myocardial Viability

In the clinical realm, contractile abnormalities in patients with ischemic heart disease can occur as a consequence of stunning, hibernation, and scar, with the relative importance of these factors varying both between and within myocardial segments and dynamically over time. Detecting viable myocardium, whether hibernating or stunned, is of scientific and clinical significance, and there is now a reasonable body of nonrandomized evidence supporting revascularization of hibernating myocardium (reviewed by Rihal *et al.*) [19]. Two CMR techniques have been proposed for the assessment of myocardial viability. LGE-CMR, a technique that defines the transmural extent of scar, and dobutamine CMR, analogous to dobutamine echocardiography, measure the contractile reserve of dysfunctional myocardium and are interpreted by visual analysis. The relative utility of these techniques is discussed in detail in Chapter 8.

Given its ability to visualize myocardial segments accurately, CMR can be used to define ventricular function during pharmacological stress, principally with dobutamine stress magnetic resonance (DSMR). Earlier concerns of patient safety have been alleviated by the introduction of hemodynamic monitoring and wall-motion display software that allows the physician to safely monitor patients during stress testing. Similar to dobutamine stress echocardiography, a lack of increase in either wall motion or systolic wall thickening, a reduction of both, or significant changes in the rotational pattern of the LV myocardium ("tethering") with increasing dobutamine dose are indicative of pathological findings. Nine studies with 250 patients using DSMR to predict recovery of function have been published to date with a mean sensitivity of 74% (range: 50 to 89%) and a specificity of 84% (range: 70 to 95%). Therefore, based on current clinical techniques, the CMR assessment of contractile reserve performs at a moderate sensitivity but a high specificity in the prediction of recovery of segmental function after revascularization.

In the setting of chronic ischemic cardiomyopathy, to date there have been two single-center clinical studies examining the utility of the transmural extent of LGE in predicting the recovery of contractile function. The first was performed by Kim *et al.* in a cohort of 41 patients undergoing revascularization by either percutaneous transluminal coronary angioplasty or coronary artery bypass graft (CABG). They found that the likelihood of improvement in regional function after revascularization decreased progressively as the transmural extent of LGE before revascularization increased [20]. These same authors reported regional functional improvement rates at three months of 78% in segments without LGE, 59% in segments with 1 to 25% LGE, and 2% in segments with more than 75% LGE. When considering only akinetic or dyskinetic segments, regional function improvement occurred in 100% in segments without LGE, 82% in segments with 1 to 25% LGE, 45% in segments with 26 to 50% LGE, and only 4% in segments with more than 50% LGE. These results were subsequently confirmed in a study from our institution, which exclusively examined patients after surgical revascularisation [21]. When only segments with severe preoperative dysfunction (i.e., severe hypokinesia, dyskinesia, or akinesia) were considered in our study, the positive and negative predictive values were higher, at 81 and 72%, respectively. The ability of LGE-CMR to evaluate those segments that have severe dysfunction (and often the most difficult to evaluate with other imaging techniques) with great diagnostic accuracy is one of the strengths of this technique. In addition, with excellent spatial resolution and contrast-to-noise ratio, LGE-CMR has a high sensitivity to detect viable myocardium, and thus may provide a more sensitive prediction of the recovery of segmental function than inotropic contractile reserve.

Tissue Characterization: Nonischemic Cardiomyopathy

CMR has found fertile ground in the field of nonischemic cardiomyopathies mainly because of its intrinsic ability to provide information on myocardial tissue characterization. CMR can characterize the various aspects of myocardial tissue by "weighting" of the T1 or T2 values through manipulation of the repetition time and echo time. Using T1-weighted spin echo techniques, blood appears black, whereas fat appears white. They are mainly useful for high-resolution anatomical imaging. T2-weighted spin echo sequences can identify areas of myocardial inflammation or edema [22]. Contrast-enhanced CMR with gadolinium DTPA can further characterize areas of myocardial necrosis, fibrosis, infiltration, or edema.

Myocarditis

Acute myocarditis has several modes of presentation: it might manifest itself as new onset heart failure, it might masquerade as an acute coronary syndrome, and it might even present with life-threatening arrhythmias, including ventricular tachycardia. Establishing the diagnosis of myocarditis is difficult. The ultimate proof that the patient has myocarditis is provided by endomyocardial biopsy, but the patchy nature of the disease limits its diagnostic role [23]. A combined CMR approach using T2-weighted imaging and contrast-enhanced T1-weighted images yields high diagnostic accuracy and thus, is a useful tool in the diagnosis and assessment of patients with suspected acute myocarditis [24]. Friedrich *et al.* were the first to propose CMR for the noninvasive diagnosis of acute myocarditis [25]. Using T1-weighted images, they found that the myocardium in patients with suspected myocarditis has a greater signal intensity relative to skeletal muscle [25]. T2-weighted images early after symptom onset can show focal increases of subepicardial and mid-wall myocardial signal, defining areas of myocardial edema [24]. LGE-CMR has been shown to have additional value in the detection of active myocarditis as defined by histopathology [26]. LGE in the setting of myocarditis has a "nonischemic" pattern, typically affecting the subepicardium and the midmyocardial wall. This focal enhancement becomes diffuse over a period of days to weeks, then decreases during healing and may become invisible after recovery [26]. Alternatively, large areas of scarring might still be visible after healing, causing distinctive enhancing linear mid-wall striae. CMR-guided endomyocardial biopsy can result in a greater yield of positive findings than routine RV biopsy [26]. The long-term prognostic significance of LGE in myocarditis is not yet explored.

Dilated Cardiomyopathy

Dilated cardiomyopathy (DCM) is characterized by a poorly contracting and dilated left ventricle in the absence of significant CAD. Histologically, it is characterized by the degeneration of myocytes and progressive interstitial fibrosis.

In a prospective CMR study of fibrosis patterns in patients with a clinical diagnosis of DCM and normal coronary angiograms, 59% of patients showed no delayed hyperenhancement and 28% showed patchy or longitudinal striae of mid-wall enhancement [16]. Importantly, this pattern of mid-wall LGE correlated well with autopsy findings on explanted hearts from patients with DCM. In this study, approximately 10% of the patients showed the usual CAD pattern of subendocardial enhancement (despite "noncritical" coronary disease on angiography), suggesting that an ischemic etiology is still likely due to the recanalization of a previously occluded vessel, spasm, or arterial emboli [16]. This finding shows that coronary angiography alone is frequently inadequate in differentiating between heart failure of ischemic or nonischemic etiology.

Notwithstanding its role in diagnosis, potentially the most significant application of the DE-CMR in cardiomyopathy patients is its emerging role in determining prognosis. Recent work from Assomull *et al.* suggest that the presence of LGE in DCM patients might be associated with an adverse outcome over and above traditional risk factors [27]. The authors examined a group of 101 patients with DCM and divided them according to the presence or absence in mid-wall fibrosis. The presence of mid-wall fibrosis was associated with the high rate of all cause mortality and hospitalization. Multivariate analyses also demonstrated that mid-wall fibrosis was the sole significant cause of death and hospitalization when taking into account other factors such as age as well as LV and RV ejection fraction [27]. Further studies with greater numbers of patients are needed to establish the prognostic value of CMR on DCM.

Hypertrophic Cardiomyopathy

Hypertrophic cardiomyopathy (HCM) is characterized by the development of cardiac hypertrophy without an obvious cause, such as pressure or volume overload. Apart from a variable degree of cardiac hypertrophy, the typical pathological features of the disease are the development of myocyte and myofibrillar disarray and increased fibrosis. Pathologically, two types of fibrosis have been identified in HCM-interstitial (so-called "plexiform") fibrosis and replacement fibrosis.

Transthoracic echocardiography is the most commonly used imaging modality to assess HCM. However, recognizing atypical forms of hypertrophy (e.g., on the posterolateral wall or the apex) is particularly difficult using echocardiography [11,28]. CMR is particularly useful in differentiating between hypertrophic cardiomyopathy and other causes of LV hypertrophy, as it allows the precise definition of the site and extent of hypertrophy. Furthermore, using DE-CMR patchy mid-wall or transmural LGE can be demonstrated most commonly in areas of maximal wall thickness (Figure 11.5) [11]. Histopathological-CMR correlation studies strongly relate the presence of LGE in HCM to areas of replacement (rather than interstitial) fibrosis [29]. Clinical studies have reported CMR detected rates of fibrosis in up to 80% of patients studied, with the variation

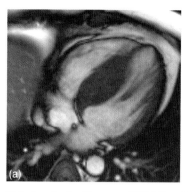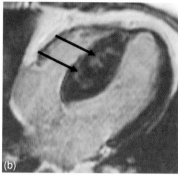

Fig. 11.5 A patient with severe HCM. Panel (a) is an end-diastolic image for the analysis of geometry, myocardial mass, volumes, and function using SSFP sequence. Panel (b) is the corresponding end-diastolic image obtained with the DE-CMR technique, where signal-intense areas represent fibrotic tissue and the normal myocardium appears dark. Note the patchy signal-intense areas in the anteroseptal wall (black arrows).

across studies probably accounted for by the widely variable patient populations studied [15,30]. Further, there is emerging evidence that these areas of replacement fibrosis identified by LGE-CMR might incrementally portend an adverse prognosis over established clinical risk factors [15].

Arrhythmogenic Right-Ventricular Cardiomyopathy

Arrhythmogenic right-ventricular cardiomyopathy (ARVC) is a rare inherited disease characterized by the enlargement, dysfunction, and fibrofatty replacement of the RV. Biventricular dilatation is present in up to 20% of cases, making differentiation from DCM difficult. CMR is well suited to investigate the right ventricle as it obtains 3D images in multiple planes without geometrical assumptions. Structural and functional abnormalities suggestive of ARVC are regional wall motion abnormalities (e.g., early diastolic bulging of RV free wall), the thinning and formation of aneurysms in the RV free wall, RV and LV dilation, and an increased signal on T1-weighted images suggesting fatty infiltration. Recent studies have highlighted the role of CMR in detecting fibrosis in the RV myocardium in patients with ARVC [31,32]. The presence of LGE showed good correlation with histopathology and predicted inducible ventricular tachycardia during electrophysiological studies, which has important implications for risk stratification [31]. The identification of fat within the myocardium by CMR may not be specific and is, in fact, the least reproducible CMR parameter [33]. Importantly, intramyocardial fat detection on CMR is still not a Task Force criterion for ARVC diagnosis. Conversely, regional wall motion abnormalities limited to the RV are highly specific to the disease [33]. Experience is needed and caution should be exercised in interpreting the results — especially in the absence of wall motion abnormalities — because the normal variants of the RV are generally greater than for the LV. Despite the controversies surrounding its role in ARVC, CMR is a valuable diagnostic tool that substantially enhances the sensitivity of clinical diagnosis, particularly in early stages of disease [34].

Restrictive Cardiomyopathy

Restrictive cardiomyopathy (RCM) is the least common of the cardiomyopathies. It is characterized by impaired ventricular filling and can cause symptoms and signs of left- or right-side failure because it may affect both ventricles. CMR can help in differentiating between constrictive pericarditis and restrictive cardiomyopathy on the basis of pericardial thickness [35]. On spin echo T1-sequences, the normal pericardium appears as a hypointense line less than 4 mm thick. Free-breathing real-time cine MRI can easily depict increased ventricular coupling, which can be helpful to better differentiate between constrictive pericarditis and RCM patients [36].

Infiltrative Diseases

Cardiac involvement in systemic amyloidosis is frequent. Characteristic features of cardiac amyloidosis by CMR imaging are concentric hypertrophy with poor contractility, a thickened interatrial septum, and biatrial dilatation [37]. Following gadolinium administration, there may be a circumferential pattern of LGE of the subendocardium or a more patchy transmural pattern [37–39]. An especially unique feature of LGE-MRI appearances in this population is the blood pool appearing atypically dark and reflecting the similar myocardial and blood T1 values due to high myocardial uptake and fast blood-pool washout. Although yet to be proven, imaging with a highly reproducible and quantifiable technique such as CMR might help estimate the prevalence of cardiac involvement in systemic amyloidosis when cardiac morphological changes are not apparent by echocardiography.

Only 5% of patients with sarcoidosis have signs or symptoms of cardiac involvement, even though 20 to 30% of patients have autopsy evidence of cardiac sarcoid [40,41]. Sarcoidosis may cause congestive heart failure, mitral regurgitation or, rarely, pulmonary hypertension [42]. The early diagnosis of cardiac involvement is important, as one manifestation of cardiac sarcoidosis is sudden death due to malignant arrhythmias [43]. Smedema *et al.* have reported CMR sensitivity of 100% and specificity of 78% compared to the Japanese Ministry of Health clinical criteria [44]. However, the actual sensitivity and specificity of CMR in this condition remains unclear, as endomyocardial biopsy is needed to confirm cardiac involvement. CMR can help detect cardiac sarcoid by demonstrating some of its characteristic features: septal thinning, LV/RV dilatation and systolic dysfunction, and pericardial effusion [42,45]. T2-weighted sequences can also help in identifying disease activity [46]. LGE-CMR may show a nonischemic pattern of enhancement isolated to the midmyocardial wall or the epicardium or multiple foci of LGE [14]. However, subendocardial or transmural hyperenhancement has been also observed, mimicking the ischemic pattern. The long-term prognostic implications of LGE in cardiac sarcoidosis are not yet available at this time.

Iron Overload Cardiomyopathy

Myocardial iron overload can be quantitatively assessed by T2* myocardial measurements [47]. This method is useful to guide treatment and monitor response to iron-chelating drug regimens [48].

Other Cardiomyopathies

Other rare cardiomyopathies such as left apical ballooning (Tako-tsubo cardiomyopathy) and LV noncompaction can be investigated and characterized with CMR [12,49].

Role of Cardiac Computed Tomography

Cardiac computed tomography (CT) can have a role in the management of the undifferentiated heart failure patient, principally in excluding the presence of significant obstructive epicardial disease using CT angiography. As discussed in Chapters 5 and 15, current generation 64-slice scanners demonstrate excellent diagnostic accuracy for both proximal coronary vessels and smaller distal vessels [50–52]. These recent studies especially demonstrate a high (greater than 95%) negative predictive value for the exclusion of significant epicardial stenosis. Hence, although it has not been prospectively evaluated in the newly diagnosed heart failure population, the data would indicate that this modality can be used to stratify the patient with heart failure into an ischemic or nonischemic etiology group.

Conclusions

The evaluation and management of patients with heart failure and specific cardiomyopathies remains clinically challenging. Essential to the appropriate care of these patients is not only an understanding of the patient's cardiac morphology and function but also identification of pathologic and modifiable substrate. By virtue of its safety, high degree of accuracy and reproducibility, and multiparametric nature, CMR represents the principal imaging modality that potentially addresses each of these points of care for heart failure patients. However, coronary CT angiography can aid in ruling out epicardial coronary artery stenosis as the cause of LV dysfunction in selected patients presenting with congestive heart failure.

References

1 Hunt, S.A. (2005) ACC/AHA 2005 guideline update for the diagnosis and management of chronic heart failure in the adult: a report of the American College of Cardiology/American Heart Association Task Force on Practice Guidelines. Writing committee to update the 2001 guidelines for the evaluation and management of heart failure. *J Am Coll Cardiol* **46**: e1–82.

2 Ho, K.K., Anderson, K.M., Kannel, W.B., *et al.* (1993) Survival after the onset of congestive heart failure in Framingham Heart Study subjects. *Circulation* **88**: 107–115.

3 Capomolla, S., Ceresa, M., Pinna, G., *et al.* (2005) Echo-Doppler and clinical evaluations to define hemodynamic profile in patients with chronic heart failure: accuracy and influence on therapeutic management. *Eur J Heart Fail* **7**: 624–630.

4 Badgett, R.G., Lucey, C.R., Mulrow, C.D. (1997) Can the clinical examination diagnose left-sided heart failure in adults? *JAMA* **277**: 1712–1719.

5 Bellenger, N.G., Davies, L.C., Francis, J.M., *et al.* (2000) Reduction in sample size for studies of remodeling in heart failure by the use of cardiovascular magnetic resonance. *J Cardiovasc Magn Reson* **2**: 271–278.

6 Grothues, F., Smith, G.C., Moon, J.C., *et al.* (2002) Comparison of interstudy reproducibility of cardiovascular magnetic resonance with two-dimensional echocardiography in normal subjects and in patients with heart failure or left ventricular hypertrophy. *Am J Cardiol* **90**: 29–34.

7 Alfakih, K., Plein, S., Thiele, H., *et al.* (2003) Normal human left and right ventricular dimensions for MRI as assessed by turbo gradient echo and steady-state free precession imaging sequences. *J Magn Reson Imaging* **17**: 323–329.

8 Lorenz, C.H., Walker, E.S., Morgan, V.L., *et al.* (1999) Normal human right and left ventricular mass, systolic function, and gender differences by cine magnetic resonance imaging. *J Cardiovasc Magn Reson* **1**: 7–21.

9 Helbing, W.A., Rebergen, S.A., Maliepaard, C., *et al.* (1995) Quantification of right ventricular function with magnetic resonance imaging in children with normal hearts and with congenital heart disease. *Am Heart J* **130**: 828–837.

10 Helbing, W.A., Bosch, H.G., Maliepaard, C., *et al.* (1995) Comparison of echocardiographic methods with magnetic resonance imaging for assessment of right ventricular function in children. *Am J Cardiol* **76**: 589–594.

11 Rickers, C., Wilke, N.M., Jerosch-Herold, M., *et al.* (2005) Utility of cardiac magnetic resonance imaging in the diagnosis of hypertrophic cardiomyopathy. *Circulation* **112**: 855–861.

12 Petersen, S.E., Selvanayagam, J.B., Wiesmann, F., *et al.* (2005) Left ventricular noncompaction: insights from cardiovascular magnetic resonance imaging. *J Am Coll Cardiol* **46**: 101–105.

13 Simonetti, O.P., Kim, R.J., Fieno, D.S., *et al.* (2001) An improved MR imaging technique for the visualization of myocardial infarction. *Radiology* **218**: 215–223.

14 Mahrholdt, H., Wagner, A., Judd, R.M., *et al.* (2005) Delayed enhancement cardiovascular magnetic resonance assessment of non-ischaemic cardiomyopathies. *Eur Heart J* **26**: 1461–1474.

15 Moon, J.C., McKenna, W.J., McCrohon, J.A., *et al.* (2003) Toward clinical risk assessment in hypertrophic cardiomyopathy with gadolinium cardiovascular magnetic resonance. *J Am Coll Cardiol* **41**: 1561–1567.

16 McCrohon, J.A., Moon, J.C., Prasad, S.K., *et al.* (2003) Differentiation of heart failure related to dilated cardiomyopathy and coronary artery disease using gadolinium-enhanced cardiovascular magnetic resonance. *Circulation* **108**: 54–59.

17 Moon, J.C.C., Sachdev, B., Elkington, A.G., *et al.* (2003) Gadolinium enhanced cardiovascular magnetic resonance in Anderson-Fabry disease: evidence for a disease specific abnormality of the myocardial interstitium. *Eur Heart J* **24**: 2151–2155.

18 Reimer, K.A., Lowe, J.E., Rasmussen, M.M., Jennings, R.B. (1977) The wavefront phenomenon of ischemic cell death, 1: myocardial infarct size vs duration of coronary occlusion in dogs. *Circulation* **56**: 786–794.

19 Rihal, C.S., Raco, D.L., Gersh, B.J., Yusuf, S. (2003) Indications for coronary artery bypass surgery and percutaneous coronary intervention in chronic stable angina: review of the evidence and methodological considerations. *Circulation* **108**: 2439–2445.

20 Kim, R.J., Wu, E., Rafael, A., *et al.* (2000) The use of contrast-enhanced magnetic resonance imaging to identify reversible myocardial dysfunction. *N Engl J Med* **343**: 1445–1453.

21 Selvanayagam, J.B., Kardos, A., Francis, J.M., *et al.* (2004) Value of delayed-enhancement cardiovascular magnetic resonance imaging in predicting myocardial viability after surgical revascularization. *Circulation* **110**: 1535–1541.

22 Abdel-Aty, H., Simonetti, O., Friedrich, M.G. (2007) T2-weighted cardiovascular magnetic resonance imaging. *J Magn Reson Imaging* **26**: 452–459.

23 Chow, L.H., Radio, S.J., Sears, T.D., McManus, B.M. (1989) Insensitivity of right ventricular endomyocardial biopsy in the diagnosis of myocarditis. *J Am Coll Cardiol* **14**: 915–920.

24 Abdel-Aty, H., Boye, P., Zagrosek, A., *et al.* (2005) Diagnostic performance of cardiovascular magnetic resonance in patients with suspected acute myocarditis: comparison of different approaches. *J Am Coll Cardiol* **45**: 1815–1822.

25 Friedrich, M.G., Strohm, O., Schulz-Menger, J., *et al.* (1998) Contrast media-enhanced magnetic resonance imaging visualizes myocardial changes in the course of viral myocarditis. *Circulation* **97**: 1802–1809.

26 Mahrholdt, H., Goedecke, C., Wagner, A., *et al.* (2004) Cardiovascular magnetic resonance assessment of human myocarditis: a comparison to histology and molecular pathology. *Circulation* **109**: 1250–1258.

27 Assomull, R.G., Prasad, S.K., Lyne, J., *et al.* (2006) Cardiovascular magnetic resonance, fibrosis, and prognosis in dilated cardiomyopathy. *J Am Coll Cardiol* **48**: 1977–1985.

28 Moon, J.C., Fisher, N.G., McKenna, W.J., Pennell, D.J. (2004) Detection of apical hypertrophic cardiomyopathy by cardiovascular magnetic resonance in patients with non-diagnostic echocardiography. *Heart* **90**: 645–649.

29 Moon, J.C., Reed, E., Sheppard, M.N., *et al.* (2004) The histologic basis of late gadolinium enhancement cardiovascular magnetic resonance in hypertrophic cardiomyopathy. *J Am Coll Cardiol* **43**: 2260–2264.

30 Choudhury, L., Mahrholdt, H., Wagner, A., *et al.* (2002) Myocardial scarring in asymptomatic or mildly symptomatic patients with hypertrophic cardiomyopathy. *J Am Coll Cardiol* **40**: 2156–2164.

31 Tandri, H., Saranathan, M., Rodriguez, E.R., *et al.* (2005) Noninvasive detection of myocardial fibrosis in arrhythmogenic right ventricular cardiomyopathy using delayed-enhancement magnetic resonance imaging. *J Am Coll Cardiol* **45**: 98–103.

32 Hunold, P., Wieneke, H., Bruder, O., *et al.* (2005) Late enhancement: a new feature in MRI of arrhythmogenic right ventricular cardiomyopathy? *J Cardiovasc Magn Reson* **7**: 649–655.

33 Tandri, H., Castillo, E., Ferrari, V.A., *et al.* (2006) Magnetic resonance imaging of arrhythmogenic right ventricular dysplasia: sensitivity, specificity, and observer variability of fat detection versus functional analysis of the right ventricle. *J Am Coll Cardiol* **48**: 2277–2284.

34 Sen-Chowdhry, S., Prasad, S.K., Syrris, P., *et al.* (2006) Cardiovascular magnetic resonance in arrhythmogenic right ventricular cardiomyopathy revisited: comparison with task force criteria and genotype. *J Am Coll Cardiol* **48**: 2132–2140.

35 Masui, T., Finck, S., Higgins, C.B. (1992) Constrictive pericarditis and restrictive cardiomyopathy: evaluation with MR imaging. *Radiology* **182**: 369–373.

36 Francone, M., Dymarkowski, S., Kalantzi, M., *et al.* (2006) Assessment of ventricular coupling with real-time cine MRI and its value to differentiate constrictive pericarditis from restrictive cardiomyopathy. *Eur Radiol* **16**: 944–951.

37 Selvanayagam, J.B., Hawkins, P.N., Paul, B., *et al.* (2007) Evaluation and management of the cardiac amyloidosis. *J Am Coll Cardiol* **50**: 2101–2110.

38 Maceira, A.M., Joshi, J., Prasad S.K., *et al.* (2005) Cardiovascular magnetic resonance in cardiac amyloidosis. *Circulation* **111**: 186–193.

39 Cheng, A.S., Banning, A.P., Mitchell, A.R., *et al.* (2006) Cardiac changes in systemic amyloidosis: visualisation by magnetic resonance imaging. *Int J Cardiol* **113**: E21–23.

40 Sharma, O.P., Maheshwari, A., Thaker, K. (1993) Myocardial sarcoidosis. *Chest* **103**: 253–258.

41 Silverman, K.J., Hutchins, G.M., Bulkley, B.H. (1978) Cardiac sarcoid: a clinicopathologic study of 84 unselected patients with systemic sarcoidosis. *Circulation* **58**: 1204–1211.

42 Doughan, A.R., Williams, B.R. (2006) Cardiac sarcoidosis. *Heart* **92**: 282–288.

43 Roberts, W.C., McAllister, H.A., Jr., Ferrans, V.J. (1977) Sarcoidosis of the heart. A clinicopathologic study of 35 necropsy patients (group 1) and review of 78 previously described necropsy patients (group 11). *Am J Med* **63**: 86–108.

44 Smedema, J.P., Snoep, G., van Kroonenburgh, M.P., *et al.* (2005) Evaluation of the accuracy of gadolinium-enhanced cardiovascular magnetic resonance in the diagnosis of cardiac sarcoidosis. *J Am Coll Cardiol* **45**: 1683–1690.

45 Serra, J.J., Monte, G.U., Mello, E.S., *et al.* (2003) Images in cardiovascular medicine: cardiac sarcoidosis evaluated by delayed-enhanced magnetic resonance imaging. *Circulation* **107**: e188–189.

46 Vignaux, O., Dhote, R., Duboc, D., *et al.* (2002) Detection of myocardial involvement in patients with sarcoidosis applying T2-weighted, contrast-enhanced, and cine magnetic resonance imaging: initial results of a prospective study. *J Comput Assist Tomogr* **26**: 762–767.

47 Westwood, M., Anderson, L.J., Firmin, D.N., *et al.* (2003) A single breath-hold multiecho T2* cardiovascular magnetic resonance technique for diagnosis of myocardial iron overload. *J Magn Reson Imaging* **18**: 33–39.

48 Tanner, M.A., Galanello, R., Dessi, C., *et al.* (2007) A randomized, placebo-controlled, double-blind trial of the effect of combined therapy with deferoxamine and deferiprone

on myocardial iron in thalassemia major using cardiovascular magnetic resonance. *Circulation* **115**: 1876–1884.

49 Karamitsos, T.D., Bull, S., Spyrou, N., *et al.* (2007) Tako-tsubo cardiomyopathy presenting with features of left ventricular non-compaction. *Int J Cardiol.* Ref Type: E-pub ahead of print.

50 Leber, A.W., Knez, A., von Ziegler, F., *et al.* (2005) Quantification of obstructive and nonobstructive coronary lesions by 64-slice computed tomography: a comparative study with quantitative coronary angiography and intravascular ultrasound. *J Am Coll Cardiol* **46**: 147–154.

51 Raff, G.L., Gallagher, M.J., O'Neill, W.W., Goldstein, J.A. (2005) Diagnostic accuracy of noninvasive coronary angiography using 64-slice spiral computed tomography. *J Am Coll Cardiol* **46**: 552–557.

52 Fine, J.J., Hopkins, C.B., Ruff, N., Newton, F.C. (2006) Comparison of accuracy of 64-slice cardiovascular computed tomography with coronary angiography in patients with suspected coronary artery disease. *Am J Cardiol* **97**: 173–174.

Chapter 12

Evaluating the Patient before Noncardiac Surgery

William O. Ntim, Rahul Aggarwal, and W. Gregory Hundley

Cardiac events complicating noncardiac surgery result in significant perioperative mortality and morbidity [1–4]. Postoperative myocardial infarction (MI) confers an in-hospital mortality rate of 15 to 25% and is an independent risk for cardiovascular death and MI during the six months following surgery [2,5–8]. Preoperative risk assessment therefore presents a unique opportunity to improve perioperative outcomes, as well as determine the need for cardioprotective therapies [9–12]. Consensus guidelines developed by the American College of Cardiology (ACC) and the American Heart Association (AHA) provide a detailed algorithm incorporating clinical markers, functional status, surgery-specific risk, and history of prior coronary evaluation or treatment (Figure 12.1) [13].

Myocardial perfusion scintigraphy and stress echocardiography are often used to risk-stratify patients with intermediate clinical predictors of cardiovascular risk before noncardiac surgery [13,14–20]. However, an estimated 10 to 20% of all routine echocardiograms exhibit suboptimal acoustic windows, leading to difficulty in image interpretation [21–23]. In addition, conventional single photon emission computed tomography (SPECT) is compromised by soft-tissue attenuation artifacts due to prior surgical procedures, chest deformation, breast tissue, or obesity [24–26].

Two relatively new tomographic imaging techniques, cardiovascular magnetic resonance (CMR) and cardiac computed tomography (CCT), do not suffer from these limitations [27–28]. This chapter will focus on the use of CMR and CCT for assessing perioperative cardiac risk for individuals needing noncardiac surgery.

Novel Techniques for Imaging the Heart, 1st edition. Edited by M. Di Carli and R. Kwong.
© 2008 American Heart Association, ISBN: 9-781-4051-7533-3.

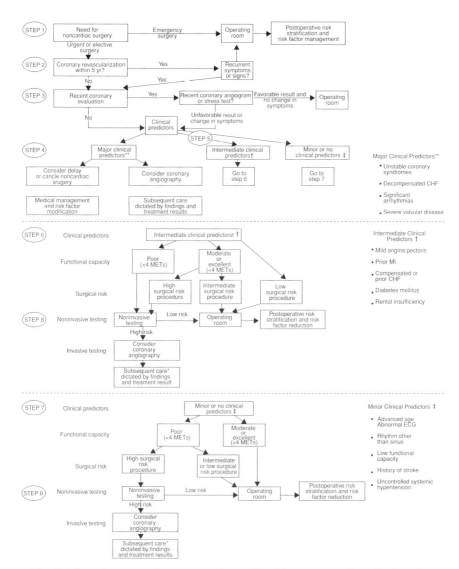

Fig. 12.1 Stepwise approach to preoperative cardiac risk assessment. From Eagle *et al.*, used with permission [13].

Indications for Preoperative Noninvasive Testing

Preoperative Left Ventricular Function

The noninvasive assessment of resting left ventricular (LV) function has been shown to consistently predict perioperative ischemic events, although it may be a useful predictor of long-term survival [18,29–31]. Preoperative noninvasive evaluation of LV function is recommended in patients with current or poorly controlled heart failure [13]. Preoperative congestive heart failure (CHF) is a risk factor for postoperative pulmonary complications after noncardiothoracic surgery [32]. CMR is an acceptable alternate tool for the preoperative assessment of LV function [33,34].

Preoperative Valvular Function

Severe aortic stenosis is considered a significant independent risk factor for perioperative cardiac morbidity and mortality in patients undergoing noncardiac surgery [13,35–38]. Echocardiography plays an important role in the preoperative evaluation of aortic stenosis [38,39]. The accurate determination of aortic valve area can be limited by the inability to measure the LV outflow tract (LVOT) diameter in cases of heavy annular calcification and sequential stenoses from coexistent LVOT obstruction from basal septal hypertrophy or hypertrophic cardiomyopathy [40–42]. A transesophageal echocardiogram, which may be performed in such situations, is a semi-invasive procedure with potential risks [43,44].

CMR is a well-tolerated and appropriate noninvasive test for the evaluation of aortic stenosis. The assessment of transaortic gradients and area by CMR has been extensively validated [45–49]. Thus, for patients in need of valvular assessments that are not well-suited for echocardiography, CMR can serve as a suitable alternative for the determination of transvalvular pressure gradients or valve area. Clinical Case Examples 1 and 2 illustrate the applications of CMR to assess valvular structure and function.

Adult Congenital Heart Disease

Published guidelines on preoperative cardiac risk assessment have predominantly targeted patients with acquired heart disease [13,50–52]. Improvements in cardiac surgery and the care of patients with congenital heart disease (CHD) have led to an enormous growth in adult survivors with CHD [54]. Preoperative risk markers specific to this population must therefore be considered (Tables 12.1 and 12.2) [55,56].

CMR has become an established complementary technique in adults with postsurgical CHD with technically limited echocardiograms from surgical scars and sternal wires [31,57–59]. CMR provides an accurate determination of right and left ventricular function prior to noncardiac surgery [61–63].

Poorly controlled hypertension confers increased perioperative risk [13]. Uncommon but significant secondary causes of hypertension such as hemodynamically significant coarctation and renal artery stenosis may need to be corrected prior to elective noncardiac surgery. CMR is among the preferred noninvasive techniques for the evaluation of coarctation of the aorta and renal vasculature before and after operative or interventional treatment [64].

Table 12.1 Clinical Factors that Predict Greater Risk in Patients with CHD (Patients Undergoing Noncardiac Surgery) [56]

Pulmonary hypertension
Cyanosis
Pulmonary to systemic shunt
Severe ventricular dysfunction
Systemic right ventricle
Fontan circulation
Decompensated congestive heart failure
Poor functional class
Uncontrolled significant arrhythmias
Severe systemic hypertension
Unstable coronary syndrome

Reprinted with permission from Colman, J.M. Noncardiac surgery in Adult Congenital Heart Disease. In: Gatzoulis, M.A., Webb, G.D., Daubeney, P.E.F., eds. Diagnosis and Management of Adult Congenital Heart Disease. Churchill Livingstone; 2003:99–104.

Unrestricted left-to-right shunts result in abnormally high pulmonary blood flow, leading to pulmonary hypertension. Pulmonary hypertension is associated with a greater risk of perioperative events [55,56]. The quantification of the shunt ratio by CMR has a good correlation with echocardiography and cardiac catheterization data [65,66]. Preoperative CMR is also useful for the evaluation of conduits and baffles following palliative surgery of complex CHD [67–69]. Clinical Case Example 3 illustrates the application of CMR to evaluate complex congenital heart disease.

Preoperative Stress Testing

The ACC/AHA guidelines algorithm integrates clinical markers, functional capacity, and surgery-specific risk to determine recommendations for a non-invasive stress testing (Figure 12.1). A simplified method for selecting patients for preoperative stress testing is shown in Table 12.3 [13]. CMR may be considered in patients not well-suited for these established stress modalities.

The diagnostic accuracy and prognostic significance of stress CMR in identifying significant coronary artery disease have been reported in 2005, when a pooled data analysis demonstrated that stress CMR has an accuracy comparable to traditional methods in identifying significant coronary stenosis (stress

Table 12.2 Strategy for Assessment of the CHD Patient through Noncardiac Surgery [56]

- Define the condition
  - Primary lesions
  - Surgical palliation or correction
  - Residual and sequelae

- Assess the surgical risk
  - Global risk: clinical predictors and proposed surgery
  - Specific CHD risk factors
  - Co-morbid conditions

- Complete preoperative information gathering and testing as necessary

Reprinted with permission from Colman, J.M. Noncardiac surgery in Adult Congenital Heart Disease. In: Gatzoulis, M.A., Webb, G.D., Daubeney, P.E.F., eds. Diagnosis and Management of Adult Congenital Heart Disease. Churchill Livingstone; 2003:99–104.

perfusion CMR: mean sensitivity = 84%, specificity = 85%; wall motion CMR: mean sensitivity = 89%, specificity = 84%) [27]. Improvements of image quality in CMR perfusion have been made in the last few years. Recently, Jahnke *et al.* reported the prognosis from 513 patients who underwent stress CMR for the assessment of cardiac symptoms. In this intermediate-risk cohort, a normal stress CMR portends a favorable prognosis (three-year event-free survival for normal CMR stress perfusion and wall motion of 99.2%) [70]. The utility of CMR as a preoperative stress assessment tool is further discussed.

Table 12.3 ACC/AHA Guidelines: Shortcut to Noninvasive Testing in Preoperative Patients if Two or More Factors Are Present [13]

- Intermediate clinical predictors present
  - Canadian class 1 or 2 angina
  - Previous MI based on history or pathologic Q waves
  - Compensated or prior previous congestive heart failure
  - Diabetes mellitus

- Poor functional capacity (less than 4 METs)

- High surgical risk vascular procedure; prolonged surgical procedures with large fluid shifts or blood loss

Reprinted with permission from Eagle, K.A., Berger, P.B., Calkins, H., *et al.* (2002) ACC/AHA guideline update for perioperative cardiovascular evaluation for noncardiac surgery-executive summary. *J Am Coll Cardiol* **39**(3): 542–553.

Dobutamine Stress CMR

Rerkpattanapipat *et al.* studied the utility of dobutamine stress CMR for assessing perioperative cardiovascular risk in patients undergoing noncardiac surgery (Figure 12.2) [71]. One hundred and two patients were followed for the occurrence of cardiac death, MI, or CHF during or after noncardiac surgery. Among 84 patients with intermediate clinical predictors of MI or cardiac death (as defined by the ACC/AHA guidelines), patients with evidence of inducible ischemia had a 20% rate of perioperative cardiac events as compared to a 2% event rate in those without ischemia ($p < 0.008$) [72]. Patients without evidence of ischemia and who achieved a heart rate response of greater than or equal to 80% of the maximum predicted heart rate response for age had no perioperative events. Clinical Case Example 4 illustrates the application of dobutamine stress CMR for preoperative risk evaluation.

Stress Perfusion CMR

Preoperative reversible perfusion defects by nuclear imaging predict an increased risk of perioperative cardiac events in patients with intermediate clinical risk predictors [73–75]. Stress perfusion CMR for the detection of coronary artery disease has a sensitivity and specificity comparable to pharmacologic nuclear stress testing [70,76–78].

Ishida *et al.* conducted a prospective study among 49 patients to evaluate the accuracy of stress perfusion CMR in the detection of significant coronary artery disease prior to the elective repair of an aortic aneurysm [79]. The overall sensitivity, specificity, and accuracy of perfusion CMR for the detection of significant coronary stenosis were 88, 87, and 88%, respectively. This study proved the feasibility of stress perfusion CMR prior to noncardiac surgery. The prognostic value of preoperative stress perfusion CMR has not been fully elucidated. Clinical Case Example 5 illustrates the application of dobutamine stress CMR for preoperative risk evaluation.

Perioperative Myocardial Tissue Characterization

As discussed in detail in Chapter 8, late gadolinium enhancement (LGE) by CMR is a marker of fibrosis, and therefore useful in the diagnosis and risk stratification of patients with cardiomyopathy [80,81]. Scintigraphic fixed perfusion defects, indicative of myocardial infarction, are predictive of late cardiac events [82,83]. LGE is superior to SPECT in the detection of myocardial necrosis [84]. Thus, CMR has the potential for identifying patients who retain preoperative cardiac risk in the postoperative period.

Coronary Computed Tomographic Angiography

As discussed in Chapter 5, multidetector computed tomography (MDCT) scanners have allowed improved noninvasive coronary artery imaging with conventional (invasive) coronary angiography (CCA) accuracy comparable to

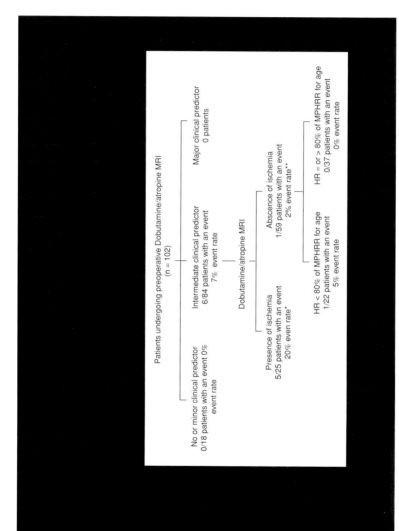

Fig. 12.2 Preoperative evaluation with dobutamine/atropine stress CMR. From Rerkpattanapipat *et al.*, used with permission [70].

(sensitivity 82 to 95%, specificity 86 to 98% for the detection of coronary stenosis) and negative predictive value consistently above 97% [85–90]. Although the incremental prognostic value of coronary calcification independent of traditional coronary artery risk factors is well established, the prognostic information about noncalcified plaque detected by cardiac computed tomographic angiography (CTA) is currently unknown [91,92].

Preoperative coronary angiography is recommended in patients with intermediate to high clinical risk profiles with a nondiagnostic noninvasive stress test undergoing high-risk surgery [13]. CCA has attendant risks [93]. In addition, preoperative coronary revascularization in selected patients with stable cardiac symptoms has not been shown to alter long-term outcomes [94,95]. In patients undergoing valvular heart surgery, published studies for CTA comparing it to CCA have reported sensitivities of 81 to 100%, specificity of 80 to 92%, and negative predicted values of 98 to 100% for the detection of significant coronary stenosis [89,96–99].

The accuracy of CTA prior to noncardiac surgery has not been reported. In a retrospective study of 75 patients undergoing noncardiac thoracic surgery, preoperative coronary artery calcification had sensitivity, specificity, and positive predictive and negative predictive values of 100, 71, 23, and 100%, respectively, for perioperative cardiac complications [100]. Thus, CTA has a potential use in delineating coronary anatomy in selected stable patients prior to high-risk noncardiac surgery. However, further prospective studies are needed to establish the accuracy and prognostic value of CTA performed in patients undergoing noncardiac surgery.

Limitations

Cardiovascular Magnetic Resonance

CMR is presently contraindicated in patients with devices such as pacemakers, implantable defibrillators, and aneurysmal clips. MRI contrast agents for stress perfusion tests or for late gadolinium enhancement imaging may need to be avoided in severe kidney disease or patients on dialysis due to the risk of nephrogenic systemic fibrosis. Dobutamine stress wall motion study can be safely performed in patients with renal disease. The safety considerations of CMR are discussed in greater detail in Chapter 4.

Computed Tomography Angiography

Extreme obesity, uncontrolled arrhythmia, or respiratory motion can limit image quality. Extensive coronary calcification or high calcium scores greater than 1000 Agatston units may limit the assessment of coronary stenosis [89]. The limitations of CTA are discussed in greater detail in Chapter 4.

Conclusions

The usefulness of CMR as a preoperative assessment tool for congenital and acquired heart disease has been demonstrated. Preoperative dobutamine stress

CMR provides additional prognostic information. Further studies are needed to determine the diagnostic and prognostic significance of stress perfusion CMR in the noncardiac surgery setting. CTA offers a potential alternative to invasive angiography in identifying coronary stenosis in selected patients with stable cardiac symptoms. Its role as preoperative risk stratification tool is yet to be determined.

Clinical Case Examples

Example 1. Aortic stenosis

A 73-year-old woman presented with shortness of breath secondary to pulmonary edema. She underwent an adenosine stress CMR, which showed no inducible ischemia. An incidental finding of a stenotic aortic valve was noted. Planimetry calculated the aortic valve area to be 1.1 cm^2. (a) Parasternal mid-systolic cine view: aortic stenosis (video clip 3 ⊙). (b) Short-axis cine view of aortic stenosis (red arrow) during mid-systole. (c) Short-axis mid-diastolic view of the aortic valve. (d) Phase contrast view of stenotic flow (video clip 4 ⊙).

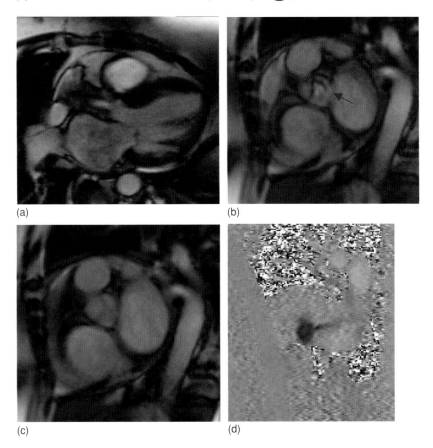

(a)   (b)

(c)   (d)

Example 2. Bicuspid aortic valve

A 59-year-old man presented for the evaluation of chronic shortness of breath. Previous cardiac workups included a cardiac catheterization demonstrating nonobstructive coronary artery disease and a mildly dilated aortic root. A subsequent cardiac MRI was performed to evaluate the aortic root. A bicuspid aortic valve was seen on short-axis cine views. The figures show (a) mid-diastolic and (video clip 5 👁) (b) mid-systolic views.

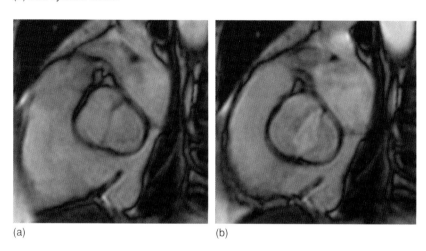

(a)   (b)

Example 3. Complex congenital heart disease

A 35-year-old woman with a dextro-transposition of the great arteries (D-TGA) status-post Mustard procedure at 18 months of age presented with mild fatigue and

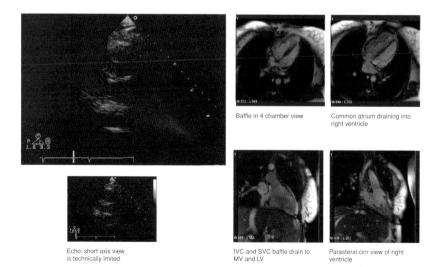

Echo: short axis view   Baffle in 4 chamber view   Common atrium draining into
is technically lmited   right ventricle

                               IVC and SVC baffle drain to Parasteral cinr view of right
                               MV and LV   ventricle

shortness of breath. A prior echo done one year prior was technically limited by poor windows (short axis). Thus, a CMR was performed to evaluate for left ventricular and baffle functions. The superior and inferior vena cava were noted to be baffled to the mitral valve with subsequent flow into the left ventricle and then out the pulmonary artery. A surgically created common atrium drained through the tricuspid valve into the right ventricle and on into the aorta. See video clips 6, 7, 8, 9, 10 👁.

Example 4. Preoperative risk assessment with dobutamine stress CMR

A 63-year-old woman with end-stage renal disease on hemodialysis presented for a preoperative evaluation for renal transplantation. She underwent a dobutamine stress CMR. Following the administration of 20 μg/kg/min of dobutamine along with

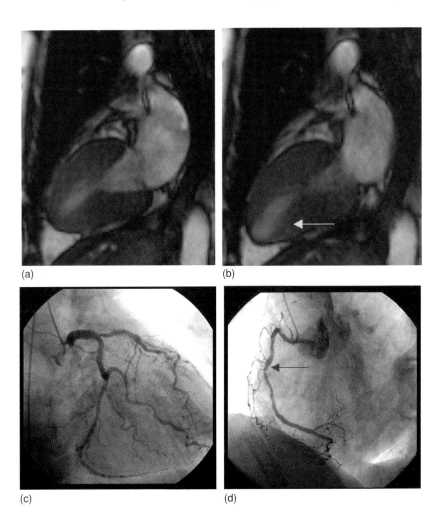

(a)　　　　　　　　　　　　(b)

(c)　　　　　　　　　　　　(d)

0.2 mg of atropine, her heart rate increased to 122/bpm and her blood pressure to 149/96 mmHg. At this juncture, the patient complained of chest and neck pain with associated apical inferior (yellow arrow) and inferolateral wall motion abnormalities. A cardiac catheterization demonstrated significant three-vessel disease, necessitating a successful three-vessel coronary artery bypass graft (CABG). (a) Resting parasternal end-systolic cine view (video clip 11 👁). (b) Peak dobutamine end-systolic cine view (video clip 12 👁). (c) RAO caudal: 70% proximal; LAD, 80% OM2, 60%, distal circumflex (video clip 13 👁). (d) 80% mid RCA (red arrow) (video clip 14 👁).

Example 5. Preoperative risk assessment with stress perfusion CMR

A 65-year-old man presented for a preoperative evaluation for elective right carotid endarterectomy. Dobutamine stress echo images were inadequate to determine

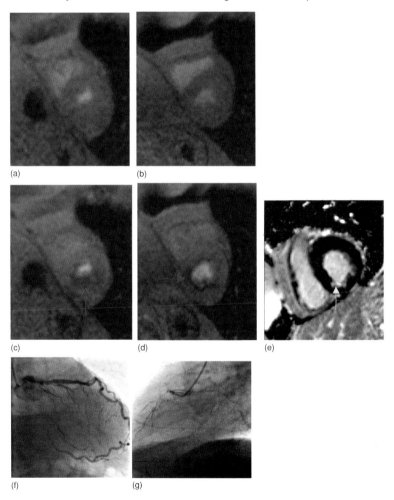

ischemia. The patient underwent adenosine CMR stress testing. (a,b) Resting images of apical and mid-short axes with no perfusion defects (video clips 15 and 16 👁). Adenosine CMR demonstrated (c,d) inferolateral and inferoseptal peri-infarct ischemia (red arrows) (video clips 17 and 18 👁) and (e) inferoseptal and inferior subendocardial infarcts (yellow arrow, delayed enhancement) (video clip 19 👁). The patient subsequently underwent a cardiac catheterization that showed (f) 100% occlusion of the proximal circumflex, 25% left main and LAD disease and (g) 100% occlusion of the RCA. A two-vessel off-pump CABG was performed successfully prior to the patient's right carotid endarterectomy.

References

1 Browner, W.S., Li, J., Mangano, D.T. (1992) In-hospital and long-term mortality in male veterans following non-cardiac surgery: the study of Perioperative Ischemia Research Group. *JAMA* **268**: 228–232.

2 Ashton, C.M., Petersen, N.J., Wray, N.P., *et al.* (1993) The incidence of perioperative myocardial infarction in men undergoing noncardiac surgery. *Ann Intern Med* **118**: 504–510.

3 Gilbert, K., Larocque, B.J., Patrick, L.T. (2000) Prospective evaluation of cardiac risk indices for patients undergoing noncardiac surgery. *Ann Intern Med* **133**: 356–359.

4 Khuri, S.F., Daley, J., Henderson, W., *et al.* (1995) The National Veterans for Administration Surgical Risk Study: risk adjustment for the comparative assessment of the quality of surgical care. *J Am Coll Surg* **180**: 519–531.

5 Shah, K.B., Kleinman, B.S., Rao, T.L., *et al.* (1990) Angina and other risk factors in patients with cardiac diseases undergoing noncardiac operations. *Anesth Analg* **70**: 240–247.

6 Badner, N.H., Knill, R.L., Brown, J.E., *et al.* (1998) Myocardial infarction after noncardiac surgery. *Anesthesiology* **88**: 572–578.

7 Mangano, D.T., Browner, W.S., Hollenberg, M., *et al.* (1992) Long-term prognosis following noncardiac surgery: the study of Perioperative Ischemia Research Group. *JAMA* **268**: 233–239.

8 Devereaux, P.J., Goldman, L., Cook, D.J,. *et al.* (2005) Perioperative cardiac events in patients undergoing noncardiac surgery: a review of the magnitude of the problem, the pathophysiology of the events and methods to estimate and communicate risk. *CMAJ* **173**(6): 627–634.

9 Mangano, D.T., Layug, E.L., Wallace, A., Tateo, I. (1996) Effect of atenolol on mortality and cardiovascular morbidity after noncardiac surgery: multicenter study of Perioperative Research Group. *N Engl J Med* **335**: 1713–1720.

10 Poldermans, D., Boersma, E., Bax, J.J., *et al.* (1999) The effect of bisoprolol on perioperative mortality and myocardial infarction in high-risk patients undergoing vascular surgery: Dutch Echocardiographic Cardiac Risk Evaluation Applying Stress Echocardiography Study Group. *N Engl J Med* **341**: 1789–1794.

11 Auerbach, A.D., Goldman, L. (2002) Beta blockers and reduction of cardiac events in noncardiac surgery. *JAMA* **287**: 1435–1444.

12 Fleisher, L.A., Beckman, J.A., Brown, K.A., *et al.* (2006) ACC/AHA 2006 guideline update on perioperative cardiovascular evaluation for noncardiac surgery: focused update on perioperative beta-blocker therapy. *J Am Coll Cardiol* **47**: 2343–2355.

13 Eagle, K.A., Berger, P.B., Calkins, H., *et al.* (2002) ACC/AHA guideline update for perioperative cardiovascular evaluation for noncardiac surgery—executive summary. *J Am Coll Cardiol* **39**(3): 542–553.

14 Fleischer, L.A., Bechman, J.A., Brown, K.A., *et al.* (2007) ACC/AHA 2007 Guidelines on preoperative cardiovascular evaluation and care for noncardiac surgery. *J Am Coll Cardiol* **50**: 1707–32.

15 Poldermans, P., Hoeks, S.E., Feringa, H.H. (2008) Pre-operative risk assessment and risk reduction before surgery. *J Am Coll Cardiol* **51**: 1913–1924.

16 Kertai, M.D., Boersma, E., Bax, J.J., *et al.* (2003) A meta-analysis comparing the prognostic accuracy of six diagnostic tests for predicting perioperative cardiac risk in patients undergoing major vascular surgery. *Heart* **89**: 1327–1334.

17 Lane, R.T., Sawada, S.G., Segar, D.S., *et al.* (1991) Dobutamine stress echocardiography as a predictor of perioperative cardiac events. *Am J Cardiol* **68**: 976.

18 Poldermans, D., Arnese, M., Fioretti, P.M., *et al.* (1995) Improved cardiac risk stratification in major vascular surgery with dobutamine-atropine stress echocardiography. *J Am Coll Cardiol* **26**: 648.

19 Shaw, L.J., Eagle, K.A., Gersh, B.J., *et al.* (1996) Meta-analysis of intravenous dipyridamole-thallium-201 imaging (1985–1994) and dobutamine echocardiography (1991–1994) for risk stratification before vascular surgery. *J Am Coll Cardiol* **27**: 787–798.

20 Eagle, K.A., Singer, D.E., Brewster, D.C., *et al.* (1987) Dipyridamole-thallium scanning in patients undergoing vascular surgery: optimizing preoperative evaluation of cardiac risk. *JAMA* **257**: 2185–2189.

21 Hsiah, A., Jollis, J.G., Kesler, K.L. (1996) Prognostic value of transthoracic echo in the Duke Cardiovascular Database. *Circulation* **94**: 1–27.

22 Kaul, S. (1997) Myocardial contrast echocardiography: 15 years of research and development. *Circulation* **96**: 3745–3760.

23 Vasan, R.S., Larson, M.G., Benjamin, E.J., *et al.* (1997) Left ventricular dilatation and the risk of congestive heart failure in people with myocardial infarction. *N Engl J Med* **335**: 1381–1382.

24 Ogden, C.L., Carroll, M.D., Curtin, L.R., *et al.* (2006) Prevalence of overweight and obesity in the United States, 1999–2004. *JAMA* **295**: 1549–1555.

25 Hansen, C.L., Woodhouse, S., Kramer, M. (2000) Effect of patient obesity on the accuracy of thallium-201 myocardial perfusion imaging. *Am J Cardiol* **85**: 749–754.

26 Freedman, N., Schechter, D., Klein, M., *et al.* (2000) SPECT attenuation artifacts in normal and overweight persons: insights from a retrospective comparison of Rb-82 positron emission tomography and TI-201 SPECT myocardial perfusion imaging. *Clin Nucl Med* **25**: 1019–1023.

27 Schuijf, J.D., Shaw, L.J., Wijns, W., *et al.* (2005) Cardiac imaging in coronary artery disease: differing modalities. *Heart* **91**: 1110–1117.

28 Dewey, M., Muller, M., Eddicks, S., *et al.* (2006) Evaluation of global and regional left ventricular function with 16-slice computed tomography, biplane cineventriculography and two-dimensional transthoracic echocardiography: comparison with magnetic resonance imaging. *J Am Coll Cardiol* **48**: 2034–2044.

29 Kazmers, A., Cerqeira, M.D., Zierler, R.E. (1988) The role of preoperative radionuclide ejection fraction in direct abdominal aortic aneurysm repair. *J Vasc Surg* **8**: 128.

30 Rose, E.L., Liu, X.J., Henley, M., *et al.* (1993) Prognostic value of noninvasive cardiac tests in the assessment of patients with peripheral vascular disease. *Am J Cardiol* **71**: 40.

31 Halm, E.A., Browner, W.S., Tubau, J.F., *et al.* (1996) Echocardiography for assessing cardiac risk in patients having noncardiac surgery. *Ann Intern Med* **125**: 433–441.

32 Smetana, G.W., Lawrence, V.A., Commell, J.E. (2006) Preoperative pulmonary risk stratification for non-cardiothoracic surgery. *Ann Intern Med* **144**: 581–595.

33 Hendel, R.C., Patel, M.R., Kramer, C.M., *et al.* (2006) Appropriateness criteria for cardiac computed tomography and cardiac magnetic resonance imaging. *J Am Coll Cardiol* **48**: 1475–1497.

34 Ntim, W.O., Hundley, W.G. (2007) Cardiac imaging in patients with chronic obstructive pulmonary disease and chronic heart failure. *J Am Coll Cardiol* **49**(18): 1900–1901.

35 Goldman, L., Caldera, D.L., Nussbaum, S.R., *et al.* (1977) Multifactorial index of cardiac risk in non-cardiac surgical procedures. *N Engl J Med* **297**: 845–850.

36 Detsky, A.S., Abrams, H.B., McLaughlin, J.R., *et al.* (1986) Predicting cardiac complications in patients undergoing noncardiac surgery. *J Gen Intern Med* **1**: 211.

37 Torsher, L.C., Shub, C., Rettke, S.R., *et al.* (1998) Risk of patients with severe aortic stenosis undergoing noncardiac surgery. *Am J Cardiol* **81**: 448–452.

38 Christ, M., Sharkova, Y., Geldner, G., *et al.* (2005) Preoperative and perioperative care for patients with suspected or established aortic stenosis facing noncardiac surgery. *Chest* **128**: 2944–2953.

39 Bonow, R.O., Carabello, B.A., Chatterjee, K., *et al.* (2006) ACC/AHA 2006 guidelines for the management of patients with valvular heart disease. *J Am Coll Cardiol* **48**: 1–148.

40 Oh, J.K., Seward, J.B., Tajik, A.J. (1999) *The Echo Manual*, 2nd ed. Lippincott, Williams & Wilkins, Philadelphia, 23–36.

41 Panza, J.A., Maron, B.J. (1988) Valvular aortic stenosis and asymmetric septal hypertrophy: diagnostic considerations and clinical therapeutic implications. *Eur Heart J* **9**(Suppl E): 71–76.

42 Susini, G., Zucchetti, M., Sisillo, E., *et al.* (1991) Diagnostic pitfalls with the combination of a hypertrophic cardiomyopathy and aortic valvular stenosis. *J Cardiothorac Vasc Anesth* **5**(1): 66–68.

43 Seward, J.B., Khandheria, B.K., Oh, J.K., *et al.* (1988) Transesophageal echocardiography: technique, anatomic correlations, implementation and clinical applications. *Mayo Clin Proc* **63**: 649–680.

44 Daniel, W.G., Erbel, R., Kasper, W., *et al.* (1991) Safety of transesophageal echocardiography: a multicenter survey of 10,419 examinations. *Circulation* **83**(3): 817–821.

45 Hundley, W.G., Li, H.F., Hillis, L.D., *et al.* (1995) Quantitation of cardiac output with velocity-encoded, phase difference magnetic resonance imaging. *Am J Cardiol* **75**: 1250–1255.

46 Sondergaard, L., Stahlberg, F., Thomsen, C. (1999) Magnetic resonance imaging of valvular heart disease. *J Magn Reson Imag* **10**: 627–638.

47 Caruthers, S.D., Lin, S.J., Brown, P., *et al.* (2003) Practical value of cardiac magnetic resonance imaging for clinical quantification of aortic valve stenosis: comparison with echocardiography. *Circulation* **108**: 2236–2243.

48 John, A.S., Dill, T., Brandt, R.R., *et al.* (2003) Magnetic resonance to assess the aortic valve area in aortic stenosis: how does it compare to current diagnostic studies? *J Am Coll Cardiol* **42**: 519–526.

49 Reant, P., Lederlin, M., Lafitte, S., *et al.* (2006) Absolute assessment of aortic valve stenosis by planimetry using cardiovascular magnetic resonance imaging:

comparison with transesophageal echocardiography, transthoracic echocardiography, and cardiac catheterization. *Eur J Radiol* **59**: 276–283.

50 Goldman, L., Caldera, D.L., Nussman, S.R., *et al.* (1977) Multifactorial index of cardiac risk in noncardiac surgical procedures. *N Engl J Med* **297**: 845–850.

51 Detsky, A.S., Abrams, H.B., McLauglin, J.R., *et al.* (1986) Predicting cardiac complications in patients undergoing non-cardiac surgery. *J Gen Intern Med* **1**: 211–219.

52 Lee, T.H., Marcantonio, E.R., Mangione, C.M., *et al.* (1999) Derivation and prospective validation of a simple index for prediction of cardiac risk of a major noncardiac surgery. *Circulation* **100**: 1043–1049.

53 Gilbert, K., Larocque, B.J., Patrick, L.T. (2000) Prospective evaluation of cardiac risk indices for patients undergoing noncardiac surgery. *Ann Intern Med* **133**: 356–359.

54 Warnes, C.A., Liberthson, R., Danielson, G.K., *et al.* (2001) Task Force 1: the changing profile of congenital heart disease in adult life. *J Am Coll Cardiol* **37**: 1170–1175.

55 Baum, V.C., Perloff, J.K. (1993) Anesthetic implications of adults with congenital heart disease. *Anesth Analg* **76**: 1342–1358.

56 Colman, J.M. (2003) Noncardiac surgery in adult congenital heart disease. In: Gatzoulis, M.A., Webb, G.D., Daubeney, P.E.F. (eds.), *Diagnosis and Management of Adult Congenital Heart Disease*. Churchill Livingstone, Philadelphia, 99–104.

57 Higgins, C.B., Byrd, B.F., III, Farmer, D.W., *et al.* (1984) Magnetic resonance imaging in patients with congential heart disease. *Circulation* **70**: 851–860.

58 Didier, D., Ratib, O., Beghetti, M., *et al.* (1999) Morphologic and functional evaluation of congenital heart disease by magnetic resonance imaging. *J Magn Reson Imag* **10**: 639–655.

59 Hirsch, R., Kilner, P.J., Connelly, M.S., *et al.* (1994) Diagnosis in adolescents and adults with congenital heart disease. Prospective assessment of individual and combined roles of magnetic resonance imaging and transesophageal echocardiography. *Circulation* **90**: 2937–2951.

60 Fogel, M.A. (2006) Editorial to special issue on congenital heart disease. *JCMR* **8**: 569–571.

61 Cranney, G.B., Lotan, C.S., Dean, L., *et al.* (1990) Left ventricular volume measurement using cardiac axis nuclear magnetic resonance imaging: validation by calibrated ventricular angiography. *Circulation* **82**: 154–163.

62 Deanfield, J., Thaulow, E., Warnes, C., *et al.* (2003) Management of the grown-up congenital heart disease. *Eur Heart J* **24**: 1035–1084.

63 Geva, T., Sandweiss, B.M., Gaureau, K., *et al.* (2004) Factors associated with impaired clinical status in long-term survivors of tetralogy of Fallot repair evaluated by magnetic resonance imaging. *J Am Coll Cardiol* **43**: 1068–1074.

64 Nielsen, J.C., Powell, A.J., Gauvreau, K., *et al.* (2005) Magnetic resonance imaging predictors of coarctation severity. *Circulation* **111**: 622–628.

65 Brenner, L.D., Caputo, G.R., Mostbeck, G., *et al.* (1992) Quantification of left to right atrial shunts with velocity-encoded cine nuclear magnetic resonance imaging. *J Am Coll Cardiol* **20**: 1246–1250.

66 Hundley, W.G., Li, H.F., Lange, R.A., *et al.* (1995) Assessment of left-to-right intracardiac shunting by velocity-encoded, phase difference magnetic resonance imaging: a comparison with oximetric and indicator dilution techniques. *Circulation* **91**: 2955–2960.

67 Campbell, R.M., Moreau, G.A., Johns, J.A., *et al.* (1987) Detection of caval obstruction by MRI after intra-atrial repair of transposition of great arteries. *Am J Cardiol* **60**: 688–691.

68 Chung, K.J., Simpson, I.A., Glass, R.F., *et al.* (1998) Cine MR after surgical repair of patients with transposition of great arteries. *Circulation* **77**: 104–109.

69 Didier, O., Ratib, O. (2003) *Dynamic Cardiovascular MRI: principles and Practical Examples*, 1st ed. Georg Thieme Verlag, Stuttgart, Germany, 31–73.

70 Jahnke, C., Nagel, E., Gebker, R., *et al.* (2007) Prognostic value of cardiac magnetic resonance stress test. *Circulation* **115**: 1769–1776.

71 Rerkpattanapipat, P., Morgan, T.M., Neagle, C.M., *et al.* (2002) Assessment of preoperative cardiac risk with magnetic resonance imaging. *Am J Cardiol* **90**: 416–419.

72 Eagle, K.A., Brundage, B.H., Chaitman, B.R., *et al.* (1996) Guidelines for perioperative cardiovascular evaluation for noncardiac surgery: report of the ACC/AHA Task Force on Practice Guidelines (Committee on Perioperative Cardiovascular Evaluation for Noncardiac Surgery). *J Am Coll Cardiol* **27**: 910–948.

73 Younis, L.T., Aguirre, F., Byers, S., *et al.* (1990) Perioperative and long-term prognostic value of intravenous dipyridamole thallium scintigraphy in patients with peripheral vascular disease. *Am Heart J* **119**: 1287.

74 L'Italien, G.J., Cambria, R.P., Cutler, B.S., *et al.* (1995) Comparative early and late cardiac morbidity among patients requiring different vascular surgery procedures. *J Vasc Surg* **21**: 935.

75 Stratmann, H.G., Younis, L.T., Wittry, M.D., *et al.* (1996) Dipyridamole technetium-99m sestamibi myocardial tomography in patients evaluated for elective vascular surgery: prognostic value for perioperative and late cardiac events. *Am Heart J* **131**: 923.

76 Schwitter, J., Nanz, D., Kneifel, S., *et al.* (2001) Assessment of myocardial perfusion in coronary artery disease by magnetic resonance: a comparison with positron emission tomography and coronary angiography. *Circulation* **103**: 2230–2235.

77 Ishida, N., Sakuma, H., Motoyasu, M., *et al.* (2003) Noninfarcted myocardium: correlation between dynamic first-pass contrast-enhanced myocardial MR imaging and quantitative coronary angiography. *Radiology* **229**: 209–216.

78 Klem, I., Heitner, J.F., Shah, D.J., *et al.* (2006) Improved detection of coronary artery disease by stress perfusion cardiovascular magnetic resonance with the use of delayed enhancement infarction imaging. *J Am Coll Cardiol* **47**: 1630–1638.

79 Ishida, M., Sakuma, H., Kato, N., *et al.* (2005) Contrast-enhanced MR imaging for evaluation of coronary artery disease before elective repair of aortic aneurysm. *Radiology* **237**: 458–464.

80 Assomull, R.G., Prasad, S.K., Lyne, J., *et al.* (2006) Cardiovascular magnetic resonance, fibrosis and prognosis in dilated cardiomyopathy. *J Am Coll Cardiol* **48**: 1977–1985.

81 Saeed, M., Weber, O., Lee, R., *et al.* (2006) Discrimination of myocardial acute and chronic (scar) infarctions on delayed contrast enhanced magnetic resonance imaging with intravascular magnetic resonance contrast media. *J Am Coll Cardiol* **48**: 1961–1968.

82 L'Italien, G.J., Cambria, R.P., Cutler, B.S., *et al.* (1995) Comparative early and late cardiac morbidity among patients requiring different vascular surgery procedures. *J Vasc Surg* **21**: 935–944.

83 Leppo, J.A., Dahlberg, S.T. (2005) *Clinical Nuclear Cardiology, State of the Art and Future Directions*. Mosby, Philadelphia, 323–337.

84 Ibrahim, T., Bulow, H.P., Hackl, T., *et al.* (2007) Diagnostic value of contrast-enhanced magnetic resonance imaging and single-photon emission computed tomography for detection of myocardial necrosis early after acute myocardial infarction. *J Am Coll Cardiol* **49**: 208–216.

85 Nieman, K., Cademartiri, F., Lemos, P.A., *et al.* (2002) Reliable noninvasive coronary angiography with fast submillimeter multislice spiral computer tomography. *Circulation* **106**: 2051–2054.

86 Mollet, N.R., Cademartiri, F., Krestin, G.P., *et al.* (2005) Improved diagnostic accuracy with 16-row multi-slice computed tomography coronary angiography. *J Am Coll Cardiol* **45**: 128–132.

87 Leschka, S., Alkadhi, H., Plass, A., *et al.* (2005) Accuracy of MSCT coronary angiography with 64-slice technology: first experience. *Eur Heart J* **26**: 1482–1487.

88 Achenbach, S. (2006) *Cardiac CT Imaging: Diagnosis of Cardiovascular Disease*. Springer, New York, 123–133.

89 Raff, G.L., Goldstein, J.A. (2007) Coronary angiography by computed tomography: coronary imaging evolves. *J Am Coll Cardiol* **49**: 1830–1833.

90 Schuijf, J.D., Bax, J.J., Shaw, L.T., *et al.* (2006) Meta-analysis of comparative diagnostic performance of magnetic resonance imaging and multislice computed tomography for noninvasive coronary angiography. *Am Heart J* **151**: 404–411.

91 Mohlenkamp, S., Lehmann, N., Schmermund, A., *et al.* (2003) Prognostic value of extensive coronary calcium quantities in symptomatic males—a 5-year follow-up study. *Eur Hear J* **24**: 845–854.

92 Budoff, M.J., Shaw, L.J., Liu, S.T., *et al.* (2007) Long-term prognosis associated with coronary calcification. *J Am Coll Cardiol* **49**: 1860–1870.

93 Wyman, R.M., Safian, R.D., Portway, V., *et al.* (1988) Current complications of diagnostic and therapeutic cardiac catheterization. *J Am Coll Cardiol* **12**: 1400.

94 McFalls, E.O., Ward, H.B., Moritz, T.E., *et al.* (2004) Coronary artery revascularization before elective major vascular surgery. *N Engl J Med* **351**: 2795–2804.

95 Poldermans, D., Schouten, O., Vidakovic, R., *et al.* (2007) A clinical randomized trial to evaluate the safety of a noninvasive approach in high-risk patients undergoing major vascular surgery. The DECREASE-V Pilot Study. *J Am Coll Cardiol* **49**: 1763–1769.

96 Gilard, M., Cornily, J., Pennec, P., *et al.* (2006) Accuracy of multislice computed tomography in the preoperative coronary disease in patients with aortic valve stenosis. *J Am Coll Cardiol* **47**: 2020–2024.

97 Manghat, N.E., Morgan-Hughes, G.J., Broadley, A.J., *et al.* (2006) 16-detector row computed tomography in patients undergoing evaluation for aortic valve replacement: comparison with catheter angiography. *Clin Radiol* **61**: 749–757.

98 Meijboom, W.B., Mollet, N.R., Van Mieghem, C.A.G., *et al.* (2006) Pre-operative computed tomography coronary angiography to detect significant coronary artery disease in patients referred for cardiac valve surgery. *J Am Coll Cardiol* **48**: 1658–1665.

99 Reant, P., Brunot, S., Lafitte, S., *et al.* (2006) Predictive value of noninvasive coronary angiography with multidetector computed tomography to detect significant coronary stenosis before valve surgery. *Am J Cardiol* **97**: 1506–1510.

100 Roth, B.J., Meyer, C.A. (1997) Coronary artery calcification at CT as a predictor of cardiac complications of thoracic surgery. *J Comput Assist Tomogr* **21**(4): 619–622.

Chapter 13

Evaluating the Patient before Interventional Electrophysiology

Riple J. Hansalia and Mario J. Garcia

The role of cardiac imaging in electrophysiology is ever expanding. Newer electrophysiology techniques such as catheter-based ablation procedures for atrial fibrillation and cardiac resynchronization therapy are both enhanced with an intimate knowledge of individual cardiac anatomy not attainable by fluoroscopy. Procedure duration and fluoroscopy time are significantly reduced with co-registered computerized tomography (CT) and fluoroscopic-guided ablation compared to fluoroscopic guidance alone [1]. Cardiac resynchronization is aided by pre-implantation venous delineation. This chapter will discuss the role of CT and cardiac magnetic resonance imaging (CMR) in atrial fibrillation ablation procedures and cardiac resynchronization therapy for heart failure.

Atrial Fibrillation

Atrial fibrillation is the most common sustained cardiac rhythm disturbance affecting nearly 5% of the population over 65 years of age [2]. Associated with significant morbidity and mortality, atrial fibrillation gives rise to two main complications: thromboembolism and hemodynamic instability. Thromboemboli, usually originating in the left atrial appendage, contribute to the large number of ischemic strokes seen in patients with atrial fibrillation and to the overall higher rates of systemic arterial emboli [3]. Hemodynamic instability results from heart rates that are either too fast or too slow to maintain adequate cardiac output, especially in those patients with structural heart disease.

The pathophysiology of atrial fibrillation is poorly understood. Multiple ectopic electrical atrial foci discharge independently of each other, delivering the

---

Novel Techniques for Imaging the Heart, 1st edition. Edited by M. Di Carli and R. Kwong.
© 2008 American Heart Association, ISBN: 9-781405-1-7533-3.

atrioventricular (AV) node up to 300 stimuli per minute, replacing P waves on the surface electrocardiogram (ECG) by irregular fibrillatory waves [4]. Ectopic foci have been found in the superior vena cava, the left and right atrium, the crista terminalis, coronary sinus ostium, interatrial septum, and the muscular sleeves of the distal pulmonary veins. The ventricular response, determined by the refractoriness of the AV node, sympathetic and vagal tone, and the presence of accessory pathways, can range anywhere between less than 30 to over 300 beats per minute. With the many limitations of anti-arrhythmic therapy, including a success rate of only about 63% in maintaining sinus rhythm, an ablation approach to atrial fibrillation is becoming more widespread [5]. Up to 88% of patients without structural heart disease are free of symptomatic atrial fibrillation after ablation [6].

There are currently two mainstream approaches to the ablation of atrial fibrillation: electric isolation of the pulmonary veins (PVI) and the mapping of high dominant-frequency areas and areas with complex fractionated atrial electrograms. Both techniques use radiofrequency to create scars that either electrically isolate an active area of discharge or inactivate it permanently. Initially, electrophysiologic mapping, a lengthy invasive procedure, was the only method available to identify foci responsible for the generation of extra stimuli. In the current paradigm, anatomical imaging using cardiac ultrasound, CMR, or CT angiography are all helpful in identifying these areas. CT or CMR evaluation prior to ablation is most applicable in PVI but can also be used with mapping ablation techniques.

The main goals of pre-ablation scanning are to delineate and display the left atrial volume contour and pulmonary venous anatomy in a three-dimensional model. Additionally, any variant anatomy or significant incidentals that might interfere with ablation such as anatomical relationships between the esophagus, atria, and pulmonary veins can be identified [3]. CT scanners with at least four slices and CMR can be used for this purpose.

Pulmonary Venous Anatomy

The pulmonary veins are divided into segments between branch points retrograde from the atriopulmonary junction, also know as the *ostium* [7]. An *ostial branch* is defined as a vein branch within 5 mm of the ostium. Therefore, by default any initial segment with an ostial branch is less than 5 mm in length. The *intravenous saddle* is the vein wall common to branches of a single pulmonary vein, whereas the *intervenous saddle* is the atrial wall separating distinct ostia of ipsilateral pulmonary veins. Common or *conjoined veins* arise when superior and inferior veins combine proximal to the left atrium, resulting in only one atriopulmonary junction on the affected side. Independent atriopulmonary junctions, aside from the left and right inferior and superior veins, give rise to accessory veins and are named for the pulmonary lobe or segment that they drain.

(a)

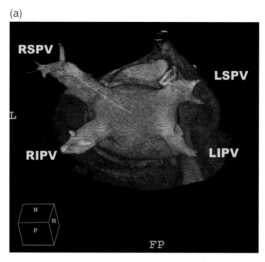

(b)

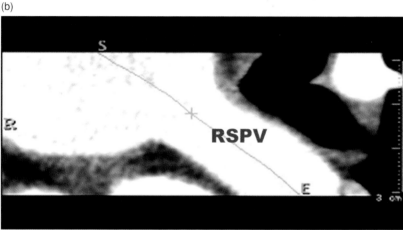

Fig. 13.1 (a) A 3D volume-rendered posterior view of the left atrium and pulmonary veins. (b) Longitudinal and (c) cross-sectional multiplanar 2D views of the left superior pulmonary vein. LIPV: left inferior pulmonary vein; LSPV: left superior pulmonary vein; RIPV: right inferior pulmonary vein; RSPV: right superior pulmonary vein. (d) A 3D volume-rendered view of the left atrium and pulmonary veins as seen by cardiac computed tomography.

A number of anatomic variants of left atrial pulmonary venous drainage have been described [8]. The moniker of "normal pulmonary venous anatomy" allows for a variety of scenarios, including not only the classic four-pattern of left/right superior and inferior veins with four distinct ostia but also common veins and accessory veins (Figure 13.1). A wide spectrum of normal configurations is seen

(c)

(d)

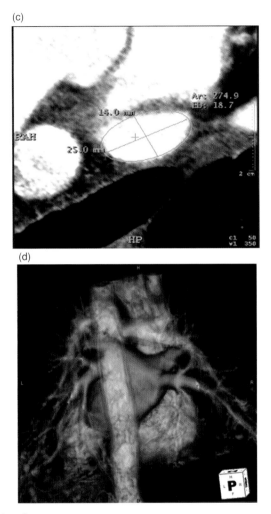

Fig. 13.1 (*continued*)

in case series: accessory veins, 30%; left common ostium, 83%; right common ostium, 39%; right ostial branching, 83%; and left ostial branching, 13% [7]. Most often, the right side will have accessory veins (usually draining the middle lobe) whereas the left side has a more regularly conjoined physiology (Figure 13.2) [9]. Atrial fibrillation is known to significantly increase pulmonary vein and left atrial dimensions compared to normal sinus rhythm controls. However, morphologic detail is not changed [10]. This variation in pulmonary vein anatomy was also confirmed by CMR in a series of 55 patients [11,12]. Because most PVI

(a)

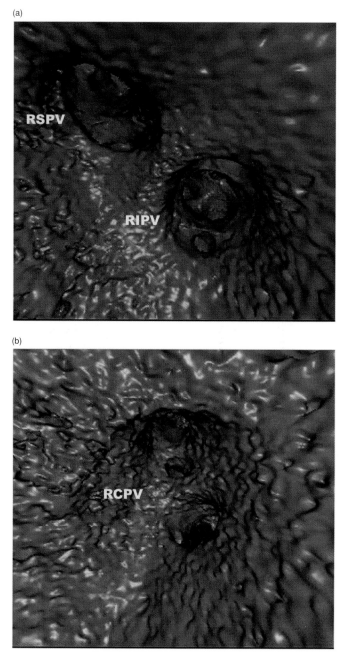

(b)

Fig. 13.2 3D internal projections of (a) separate right inferior (RIPV) and superior (RSPV) pulmonary vein configuration, and (b) common right pulmonary vein antrum (RCPV).

techniques rely on defined anatomical landmarks, pre-procedural imaging with CT or CMR with 3D reconstructions has become the standard of care.

Pulmonary Vein Stenosis

Pulmonary vein stenosis (PVS) is a recognized complication of atrial fibrillation ablation. The incidence of stenosis ranges anywhere between 3% and 42% depending on case series, the location of radiofrequency lesions, and energy applied [13,14]. In the largest study examining PVS, a total of 335 patients were screened by CT three months after ablation, or sooner if symptoms warranted. Eighteen patients were found to have a greater than 70% pulmonary vein stenosis in at least one of the ablated pulmonary veins. Symptoms of pulmonary stenosis varied widely: shortness of breath, 44%; cough, 39%; and hemoptysis, 28%. Astonishingly, PVS was not considered in the diagnostic workup of any symptomatic patient at the time of presentation. All follow-up CT scans were deemed interpretable [14]. Wongcharoen *et al.* calculated the incidence of pre-ablation PVS (defined as greater than 50%) at 2.8% in a series of 178 subjects referred for PVI, thus suggesting that postablation imaging should be performed to evaluate for PVS in those patients who are symptomatic (Figure 13.3) [15].

Multiple studies have also validated CMR as an accurate and sensitive modality in diagnosing PVS postablation [16,17]. In a group of 41 patients, 14% of the cohort was found to have moderate to severe stenosis postablation. Overall, 38% of the identified pulmonary veins had some detectable narrowing [18,19]. Predictors for stenosis included a larger pulmonary vein size and selective circumferential ablation around each pulmonary vein rather than a wide circumferential ablation around grouped ostia [18].

Left Atrial Appendage

The role of CT for the evaluation of the left atrial appendage (LAA) has been recently studied. The morphologic CT characteristics of the LAA, roof, and septum were characterized in one study of 47 enrollees [20]. Patients with atrial fibrillation had significantly greater LAA orifice size, neck size, and length of roofline compared to 49 controls. There have been several case reports of the detection of LAA thrombus by multidetector CT but only a few small series studying the diagnostic accuracy of this modality compared to transesophageal echocardiography (Figure 13.4) [21–25]. These preliminary series suggest that a normal contrast-enhanced CT virtually excludes the probability of thrombus, but without the use of contrast opacification, thrombus is not reliably detected by CT. Although CMR has the advantage of not needing ionizing radiation and nephrotoxic contrast agents, only limited preliminary data exists regarding the diagnostic utility of detecting LAA thrombus using current CMR techniques [25].

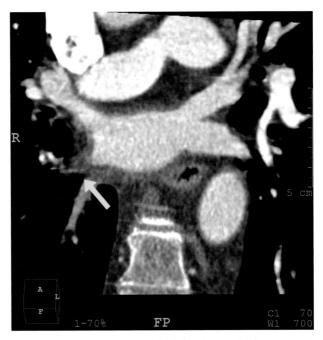

Fig. 13.3 Maximum intensity projection of the left atrium and pulmonary veins obtained from a patient with severe RIPV stenosis (arrow).

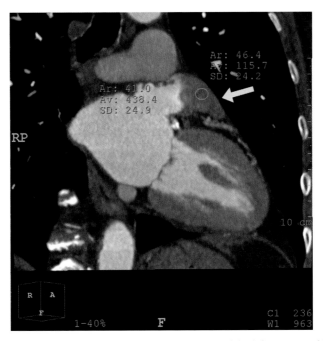

Fig. 13.4 An oblique maximum-intensity projection view of the left atrium and left ventricle. A thrombus (arrow) is seen in the left atrial appendage (average attenuation, 115 HU).

Anatomical Position of the Esophagus

Pappone *et al.* first described two cases of atrioesophageal fistulas (AEF) as a complication of percutaneous transcatheter ablation of atrial fibrillation [26]. With mortality rates of 50% or higher, AEF is a devastating complication. The course of the esophagus can easily be defined by CT scan or CMR and thus potentially reduce the risk of AEF. Tsao *et al.* proposed that there are two major types of esophageal routes based on a series of 80 patients [27]. Type 1 routes (42 patients) have the lower portion of the esophagus near the ostium of the left inferior pulmonary vein (LIPV). Type 2 routes (6 patients) have the lower portion of the esophagus near the ostium of the right inferior pulmonary vein (RIPV). Both Type 1 and Type 2 patients were further subdivided into three groups based on the distance to either the left superior pulmonary vein (LSPV) and left inferior pulmonary vein (for Type 1 routes) or the distance to the right superior pulmonary vein (RSPV) and right inferior pulmonary vein (for Type 2 routes). Type 1a classification ($n = 24$) encompasses a straight esophageal route less than 10 mm from the LSPV and LIPV. Type 1b classification ($n = 16$) encompasses an oblique esophageal route greater than 10 mm from the LSPV and less than 10 mm from the LIPV. Type 1c classification ($n = 2$) encompasses a straight esophageal route greater than 10 mm apart from both the LIPV and LSPV. Type 2a classification ($n = 3$) includes a straight esophageal course less than 10 mm from the RSPV and RIPV. Type 2b classification ($n = 2$) includes an oblique esophageal course less than 10 mm from the RIPV. Type 2c classification ($n = 1$) includes a straight esophageal course greater than 10 mm from both the RIPV and RSPV (Figure 13.5). Overall, only 54% of patients possessed a thin layer of fat between the adventitia of the esophagus and epicardium of the posterior left atrium; otherwise, the left atrium and esophagus were juxtaposed.

Procedure Guidance

Co-registering CT and CMR images with electroanatomic mapping at the time of ablation has been widely reported and now validated. Fluoroscopy alone does not provide enough anatomic detail to guide PVI — all operators also rely on an electroanatomic map of the left atrium generated at the time of ablation. The process of registration necessitates the alignment of anatomical features in one view of the object with the corresponding features in another view of that same object (Figure 13.6) [28]. Integrating software available in several electrophysiology mapping systems now automatically rotates, translates, and scales segmented CT or CMR images, accounting for table position and image detector configuration [1]. Accuracy between the two image datasets has been shown to be within 2.3 ± 0.4 mm in one study of 32 patients and within 3.05 ± 0.41 mm in another study of 16 patients [29,30]. Cardiac rhythm at the time of the study had no significant effect on total or regional surface registration accuracy [29].

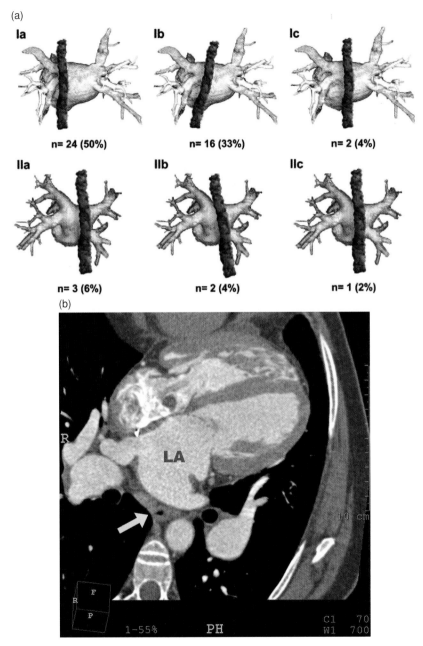

Fig. 13.5 (a) Common variants of anatomical relationships between the esophagus and the left atrium. Adapted from Tsao *et al.* (see text for details) [27]. (b) Oblique axial image demonstrating the anatomical relationship of the esophagus (arrow) and the left atrium in a patient referred for pulmonary vein isolation.

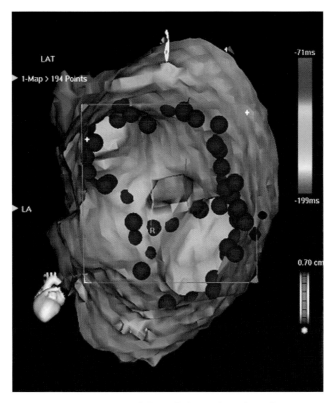

Fig. 13.6 Merged 3D volume-rendered CT and electrophysiological mapping images of the left atrium from a right projection. The right dots indicate the location of delivered radiofrequency ablation lesions.

Cardiac Resynchronization

Heart failure as an aggregate cost the United States' economy nearly $30 billion in 2006 and is the leading cause of admission in patients over 65 years of age [31]. Even with treatment advances, heart failure remains a progressive disease with nearly 40% of patients dying within the first year after diagnosis. Although many medical therapies are currently available for heart failure, there are also nonmedical interventions. One of these options, cardiac resynchronization or biventricular pacing, targets the aberrant pattern of ventricular activation, thereby reducing intra- and interventricular asynchrony. Three pacemaker leads (one in the right atrium, one in the right ventricle, and one in the coronary sinus posterior or lateral to the left ventricle) are placed in the heart, which then supplant the diseased natural conduction system. Currently, heart failure patients with New York Heart Association Class III or IV symptoms, a QRS duration greater than 120 ms, and an ejection fraction less than or equal to

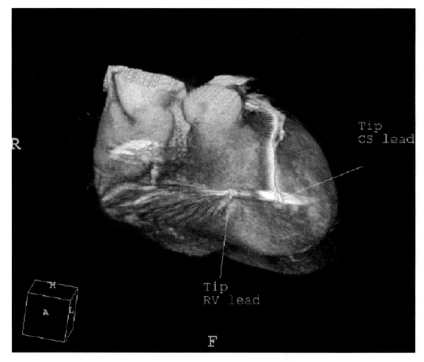

Fig. 13.7 A 3D volume-rendered image demonstrating the abnormal positioning of a left ventricular pacing lead in the anterior cardiac vein. Notice the close proximity between the tips of the right and left ventricular pacing leads.

35% qualify for cardiac resynchronization. A meta-analysis of cardiac resynchronization in patients with symptomatic heart failure revealed an improvement in ejection fraction, an improvement in quality of life, a reduction in heart failure mortality, and a reduction of heart failure hospitalizations [32]. However, up to 30% of patients are deemed "nonresponders" with little to no improvement in symptoms, exercise capacity, or left ventricular function [33].

Crucial to successful biventricular pacemaker implant is the cannulation of the coronary sinus for the left ventricular pacing lead (Figure 13.7). Clinically, the left ventricular lead must be located in the region of latest ventricular activation, usually identified by echocardiography with tissue Doppler imaging [34]. The patency and availability of nearby coronary venous vessels can be obtained by CT or CMR. Consequently, there has been renewed interest on coronary venous anatomy.

CMR enhancement late gadolinium (LGE) imaging is currently the best method of characterizing myocardial scar. Scar location and total scar burden have been preliminarily validated as markers of response after cardiac resynchronization therapy. Bleeker *et al.* found that posterolateral left ventricular transmural scar tissue (identified by CMR) resulted in clinical and echocardiographic nonresponse to CRT [35]. Using CMR and the LGE technique, a total scar burden of 15% or less predicted a response to biventricular pacing with a sensitivity and specificity of 85% and 90%, respectively [36].

Coronary Vein Anatomy

The interventricular sulcus gives rise to the *anterior interventricular vein* (also know as the great cardiac vein). After the anterior interventricular vein turns around the left aspect of the atrioventricular junction, it runs inferiorly in the atrioventricular groove, where it is also called the left coronary vein. The anterior interventricular vein drains into the coronary sinus at the level of the left atrioventricular sulcus, and the coronary sinus empties into the right atrium through the atrium's diaphragmatic left lateral wall. Occasionally, the origin of the coronary sinus is protected by a thin duplication fold of the endomyocardium (the Thebesian valve). The middle cardiac vein or the interventricular vein originates in the distal portion of the posterior interventricular sulcus and joins the coronary sinus proximal to its orifice in the right atrium. Also joining the coronary sinus near its origin in the right atrium is the small cardiac vein, which runs in the right atrioventricular sulcus. The posterior cardiac vein or posterior vein of the left ventricle derives from the diaphragmatic portion of the left ventricle and also drains directly into the coronary sinus. The most inferior vein at the obtuse angle of the heart draining into the terminal portion of the anterior interventricular vein is the left marginal vein. The coronary sinus, together with the great cardiac vein, forms a semicircular venous channel at the posterolateral aspect of the mitral valve annulus (Figure 13.8) [37,38].

In one series of 100 individuals using a 64-slice CT scanner, the coronary sinus and anterior interventricular vein were observed in nearly all patients studied (control patients, patients with significant coronary artery disease, and patients with a history of infarction) [39]. The coronary sinus entered the right atrium in a variety of positions compared to the inferior vena cava aperture: 41% above, 56% the same level, and 3% below. Only in those patients with significant coronary artery disease and a history of myocardial infarction did visualization of the left marginal vein decrease compared to controls. Patients with a history of either a lateral or anterolateral Q wave myocardial infarction did not have CT visualization of the left marginal vein in a study of 100 individuals [39]. The largest variability of the coronary venous system was seen in the number of branches between the posterior interventricular vein and the anterior interventricular vein. Sixty-three percent of patients had evidence of a posterior cardiac vein, and 73 to 88% of patients had evidence of a left marginal vein in

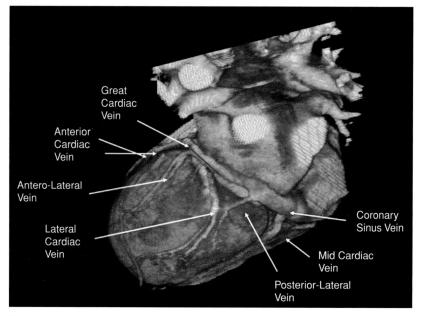

Fig. 13.8 A 3D volume-rendered image indicating the normal anatomy of the cardiac veins seen from a right projection.

both anatomic series [39,40]. On conventional angiography, the posterior cardiac vein was visualized in only 55% of cases and the left marginal vein in 83% of cases. In contrast, in a series of 231 patients undergoing cardiac CT, Mao *et al.* identified the coronary sinus in 100% of cases, the posterior interventricular vein in 78% of cases, and the left marginal vein in 81% of cases [41].

Relative Merits of CT and CMR

Both CT and CMR have their benefits and limitations. The advantages of CT are numerous: widely accessible, abbreviated scan time (less than 15 sec with 64-slice scanners), higher spatial resolution compared to CMR, and straightforward protocols. However, CT imaging is difficult in patients without rate-controlled atrial fibrillation as image quality may be compromised. Chronic renal insufficiency is a relative contraindication for contrast enhancement with either iodine agents or gadolinium. Magnetic resonance angiography can be performed without contrast, although with lower spatial and contrast resolution. Recent publications have highlighted that radiation doses from CT scanning are not inconsequential [42].

CMR has the advantage of higher temporal resolution and tissue contrast compared to CT. With higher temporal resolution (less than 50 ms) by standard cine steady state free precession (SSFP) technique, CMR can characterize atrial mechanical function, even in some patients with atrial fibrillation. With a good contrast-to-noise ratio, CMR may also be able to characterize myocardial scar in the ventricles and even in the atria. However, CMR scanning is currently precluded in those patients with pacemakers and defibrillators, and is challenging in a minority of patients with claustrophobia. Technical improvements in the latest generation of pacemaker and defibrillators and newer CMR scanner design may help overcome these limitations. CMR is usually the only option in those patients who cannot receive iodinated contrast.

Conclusions

CT, CMR, and invasive electrophysiology are currently intertwined with no foreseeable plans for separation. Future directions will most certainly include real-time tomography for resynchronization and ablation and perhaps even CT dyssynchrony assessment prior to resynchronization. Factors that currently limit this potential and will need to be overcome include radiation exposure to the operator and patient, hardware costs, and equipment maneuverability. Nonetheless, the integration of CT and CMR imaging with electrophysiology at all levels is ever increasing.

References

1 Sra, J., Narayan, G., Krum, D., *et al.* (2007) Computed tomography-fluoroscopy image integration-guided catheter ablation of atrial fibrillation. *J Cardiovasc Electrophysiol* **18**(4): 409–414.

2 Falk, R.H. (2001) Atrial fibrillation. *N Engl J Med* **344**(14): 1067–1078.

3 Lacomis, J.M., Goitein, O., Deible, C., Schwartzman, D. (2007) CT of the pulmonary veins. *J Thorac Imaging* **22**(1): 63–76.

4 Fishman, M., Hoffman, A., Klausner, R., *et al.* (1985) *Medicine.* J.B. Lippincott, Philadelphia.

5 Camm, J. (2006) Medical management of atrial fibrillation: state of the art. *J Cardiovasc Electrophysiol* **17**(Suppl 2): S2–6.

6 Oral, H., Scharf, C., Chugh, A., *et al.* (2003) Catheter ablation for paroxysmal atrial fibrillation: segmental pulmonary vein ostial ablation versus left atrial ablation. *Circulation* **108**(19): 2355–2360.

7 Lacomis, J.M., Wigginton, W., Fuhrman, C., *et al.* (2003) Multi-detector row CT of the left atrium and pulmonary veins before radio-frequency catheter ablation for atrial fibrillation. *Radiographics* Spec No. S35, **48**; disc. S48–50.

8 Jongbloed, M.R., Dirksen, M.S., Bax, J.J., *et al.* (2005) Atrial fibrillation: multi-detector row CT of pulmonary vein anatomy prior to radiofrequency catheter ablation—initial experience. *Radiology* **234**(3): 702–709.

9 Marom, E.M., Herndon, J.E., Kim, Y.H., McAdams, H.P. (2004) Variations in pulmonary venous drainage to the left atrium: implications for radiofrequency ablation. *Radiology* **230**(3): 824–829.

10 Schwartzman, D., Lacomis, J., Wigginton, W.G. (2003) Characterization of left atrium and distal pulmonary vein morphology using multidimensional computed tomography. *J Am Coll Cardiol* **41**(8): 1349–1357.

11 Kato, R., Lickfett, L., Meininger, G., *et al.* (2003) Pulmonary vein anatomy in patients undergoing catheter ablation of atrial fibrillation: lessons learned by use of magnetic resonance imaging. *Circulation* **107**(15): 2004–2010.

12 Takase, B., Nagata, M., Matsui, T., *et al.* (2004) Pulmonary vein dimensions and variation of branching pattern in patients with paroxysmal atrial fibrillation using magnetic resonance angiography. *Japanese Heart J* **45**(1): 81–92.

13 Kalusche, D., Arentz, T., Haissaguerre, M. (2000) Atrial fibrillation: healing by focal high frequency catheter ablation? *Z Kardiol* **89**(12): 1141–1145.

14 Saad, E.B., Marrouche, N.F., Saad, C.P., *et al.* (2003) Pulmonary vein stenosis after catheter ablation of atrial fibrillation: emergence of a new clinical syndrome. *Ann Intern Med* **138**(8): 634–638.

15 Wongcharoen, W., Tsao, H.M., Wu, M.H., *et al.* (2006) Preexisting pulmonary vein stenosis in patients undergoing atrial fibrillation ablation: a report of five cases. *J Cardiovasc Electrophysiol* **17**(4): 423–425.

16 Tamborero, D., Mont, L., Nava, S., *et al.* (2005) Incidence of pulmonary vein stenosis in patients submitted to atrial fibrillation ablation: a comparison of the selective segmental ostial ablation vs. the circumferential pulmonary veins ablation. *J Interv Card Electrophysiol* **14**(1): 21–25.

17 Tintera, J., Porod, V., Cihak, R., *et al.* (2006) Assessment of pulmonary venous stenosis after radiofrequency catheter ablation for atrial fibrillation by magnetic resonance angiography: a comparison of linear and cross-sectional area measurements. *Eur Radiol* **16**(12): 2757–2767.

18 Dong, J., Vasamreddy, C.R., Jayam, V., *et al.* (2005) Incidence and predictors of pulmonary vein stenosis following catheter ablation of atrial fibrillation using the anatomic pulmonary vein ablation approach: results from paired magnetic resonance imaging. *J Cardiovasc Electrophysiol* **16**(8): 845–852.

19 Anselme, F., Gahide, G., Savoure, A., *et al.* (2006) MR evaluation of pulmonary vein diameter reduction after radiofrequency catheter ablation of atrial fibrillation. *Eur Radiol* **16**(11): 2505–2511.

20 Wongcharoen, W., Tsao, H.M., Wu, M.H., *et al.* (2006) Morphologic characteristics of the left atrial appendage, roof, and septum: implications for the ablation of atrial fibrillation. *J Cardiovasc Electrophysiol* **17**(9): 951–956.

21 Alam, G., Addo, F., Malik, M., *et al.* (2003) Detection of left atrial appendage thrombus by spiral CT scan. *Echocardiography* **20**(1): 99–100.

22 Gottlieb, I., Pinheiro, A., Brinker, J.A., *et al.* (2007) Resolution of left atrial appendage thrombus by 64-detector CT scan. *J Cardiovasc Electrophysiol* Jul 26.

23 Achenbach, S., Sacher, D., Ropers, D., *et al.* (2004) Electron beam computed tomography for the detection of left atrial thrombi in patients with atrial fibrillation. *Heart* **90**(12): 1477–1478.

24 Jaber, W.A., White, R.D., Kuzmiak, S.A., *et al.* (2004) Comparison of ability to identify left atrial thrombus by three-dimensional tomography versus transesophageal echocardiography in patients with atrial fibrillation. *Am J Cardiol* **93**(4): 486–489.

25 Mohrs, O.K., Nowak, B., Petersen, S.E., *et al.* (2006) Thrombus detection in the left atrial appendage using contrast-enhanced MRI: a pilot study. *AJR* **186**(1): 198–205.

26 Pappone, C., Oral, H., Santinelli, V., *et al.* (2004) Atrio-esophageal fistula as a complication of percutaneous transcatheter ablation of atrial fibrillation. *Circulation* **109**(22): 2724–2726.

27 Tsao, H.M., Wu, M.H., Higa, S., *et al.* (2005) Anatomic relationship of the esophagus and left atrium: implication for catheter ablation of atrial fibrillation. *Chest* **128**(4): 2581–2587.

28 Sra, J., Narayan, G., Krum, D., Akhtar, M. (2006) Registration of 3D computed tomographic images with interventional systems: implications for catheter ablation of atrial fibrillation. *J Interv Card Electrophysiol* **16**(3): 141–148.

29 Kistler, P.M., Earley, M.J., Harris, S., *et al.* (2006) Validation of three-dimensional cardiac image integration: use of integrated CT image into electroanatomic mapping system to perform catheter ablation of atrial fibrillation. *J Cardiovasc Electrophysiol* **17**(4): 341–348.

30 Dong, J., Dickfeld, T., Dalal, D., *et al.* (2006) Initial experience in the use of integrated electroanatomic mapping with three-dimensional MR/CT images to guide catheter ablation of atrial fibrillation. *J Cardiovasc Electrophysiol* **17**(5): 459–466.

31 Thom, T., Haase, N., Rosamond, W., *et al.* (2006) Heart disease and stroke statistics—2006 update: a report from the American Heart Association Statistics Committee and Stroke Statistics Subcommittee. *Circulation* **113**: e85.

32 Bradley, D.J., Bradley, E.A., Baughman, K.L., *et al.* (2003) Cardiac resynchronization and death from progressive heart failure: a meta-analysis of randomized controlled trials. *JAMA* **289**(6): 730–740.

33 Bax, J.J., Ansalone, G., Breithardt, O.A., *et al.* (2004) Echocardiographic evaluation of cardiac resynchronization therapy: ready for routine clinical use? A critical appraisal. *J Am Coll Cardiol* **44**(1): 1–9.

34 Ansalone, G., Giannantoni, P., Ricci, R., *et al.* (2002) Doppler myocardial imaging to evaluate the effectiveness of pacing sites in patients receiving biventricular pacing. *J Am Coll Cardiol* **39**(3): 489–499.

35 Bleeker, G.B., Kaandorp, T.A., Lamb, H.J., *et al.* (2006) Effect of posterolateral scar tissue on clinical and echocardiographic improvement after cardiac resynchronization therapy. *Circulation* **113**(7): 969–976.

36 White, J.A., Yee, R., Yuan, X., *et al.* (2006) Delayed enhancement magnetic resonance imaging predicts response to cardiac resynchronization therapy in patients with intraventricular dyssynchrony. *J Am Coll Cardiol* **48**(10): 1953–1960.

37 El-Maasarany, S., Ferrett, C.G., Firth, A., *et al.* (2005) The coronary sinus conduit function: anatomical study (relationship to adjacent structures). *Europace* **7**(5): 475–481.

38 Schaffler, G.J., Groell, R., Peichel, K.H., Rienmuller, R. (2000) Imaging the coronary venous drainage system using electron-beam CT. *Surg Radiol Anat* **22**(1): 35–39.

39 Van de Veire, N.R., Schuijf, J.D., De Sutter, J., *et al.* (2006) Non-invasive visualization of the cardiac venous system in coronary artery disease patients using 64-slice computed tomography. *J Am Coll Cardiol* **48**(9): 1832–1838.

40 Muhlenbruch, G., Koos, R., Wildberger, J.E., *et al.* (2005) Imaging of the cardiac venous system: comparison of MDCT and conventional angiography. *AJR* **185**(5): 1252–1257.

41 Mao, S., Shinbane, J.S., Girsky, M.J., *et al.* (2005) Coronary venous imaging with electron beam computed tomographic angiography: three-dimensional mapping and relationship with coronary arteries. *Am Heart J* **150**(2): 315–322.

42 Einstein, A.J., Moser, K.W., Thompson, R.C., *et al.* (2007) Radiation dose to patients from cardiac diagnostic imaging. *Circulation* **116**(11): 1290–1305.

Chapter 14

Assessment of Blood Flow and Heart Valve Disease by CMR

Philip J. Kilner

Cardiovascular magnetic resonance (CMR) offers unrivalled versatility and comprehensiveness in the visualization and measurement of blood flow, without ionizing radiation or contrast agent. Although echocardiography is generally used for first-line assessment of heart valve disease, CMR can make several important contributions [1]:

- Depiction by cine imaging of valve movements and jet flow in planes of any orientation, with unrestricted access to the whole of the right as well as the left ventricular outflow tract.
- Measurement of right as well as left ventricular volumes by multislice cine imaging.
- Measurement of volume flow and regurgitation (pulmonary and aortic, at least) by phase contrast velocity mapping.
- Assessment of the context and consequences of heart valve disease using the wide fields of view, multiple image slices, and the versatility of tissue characterization available to CMR.

The Visibility of Flow in CMR Cine Images

Most breath-hold, bright-blood cine CMR acquisitions allow flow to be visualized by recovering signal from the blood with slightly different intensities in different flow regions. The signal is generally bright where there is coherent flow, contrasting with slightly darker regions where there is shear or turbulence. Exact appearances depend on the cine sequence used but most acquisitions give qualitative information on flow in the plane of the image, which can be aligned

Novel Techniques for Imaging the Heart, 1st edition. Edited by M. Di Carli and R. Kwong.
© 2008 American Heart Association, ISBN: 9-781-4051-7533-3.

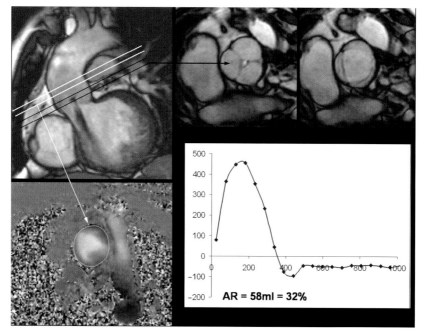

Fig. 14.1 Moderate aortic regurgitation shown by SSFP cine imaging (upper panels; see video clips 20 and 21) and phase contrast velocity mapping (lower panels). With respect to the oblique coronal LVOT image (above left), the black lines mark the plane chosen for imaging the valve leaflets, and the white lines the plane chosen for through-plane flow measurement. The flow curve shows systolic forward and diastolic reversed flow through the velocity mapping plane, recording a regurgitant fraction of 32% in this case. This value is likely to be an underestimate, probably by at least 5%, due to upward diastolic movement of the aortic root relative to the plane of velocity acquisition.

with flow through a valve, cavity, or vessel. In steady state free precession (SSFP) imaging, which is widely used for cine imaging at 1.5 T, the edges of a jet typically appear dark due to the de-phasing of signal in the shear layer where a range of velocities occur in single voxel. If appropriately aligned, the dark shear layer contrasts with bright signal from the coherent core of the jet (Figure 14.1), but this is only the case if there is a coherent core and if the image plane is aligned in a way that shows it. The same jet may appear dark, with no bright core, if the imaging plane is displaced slightly to one side, tangential to the shear layer. For this reason, the careful alignment of planes is crucial.

There are two useful strategies for achieving alignment that differ from the "sweep" used while scanning with 2D ultrasound. One approach is the sequential cross-cutting of one cine plane with a second and a third, each orthogonal to the previous, homing in on a narrow area of interest such as the core of the jet. The second approach is to acquire a contiguous or slightly overlapping stack of parallel slices that can afterward be viewed one after another. For attempted planimetry of the cross-sectional area of a jet through a stenotic or regurgitant orifice, such a stack should transect the jet core orthogonally, proceeding from upstream to a few millimeters downstream of the orifice. There may then be one slice in the stack suitable for planimetry that clearly depicts the cross-sectional area of the jet. However, if it is not clearly delineated it could be because the jet is splayed or fragmented, with peripheral jet regions deflected oblique to the image plane. Planimetry is then unlikely to be reliable. This situation is often the case for jets of mitral regurgitation. An alternative approach here is to acquire a stack of cines aligned with the left ventricular outflow tract, progressing from the more superior to the inferior mitral commissure without gaps so that no part of the line of mitral coaptation is overlooked.

In the assessment of a stenotic or regurgitant lesion of a heart valve, it is well worth acquiring enough cine views to assess the valve leaflets and jets fully, as indicated previously, before proceeding to measurements of flow and ventricular function, if appropriate. Each jet should be imaged in at least three planes — preferably six or more — before the operator can be confident that the size, shape, and functional significance of a jet have been adequately depicted.

A particular strength of CMR cine imaging is the visualization of subvalvar and supravalvar stenoses, distinguishing these from stenoses at the valve level. On the right ventricular side, a subinfundibular stenosis or double-chambered right ventricle, usually associated with a small ventricular septal defect, is an important lesion to recognize and distinguish from stenosis at an infundibular or valve level [2]. On the left ventricular side, subaortic stenosis due to the thickening of the basal septum combined with systolic anterior motion of the mitral valve can be recognized and distinguished from a subaortic ridge by appropriate cine imaging. Stenoses can be present at more than one level in either outflow tract.

Phase Contrast Velocity Mapping

For phase contrast velocity mapping, one or more of the directional components of velocity are encoded in the phase of the signal in each voxel of images throughout the cardiac cycle [3]. In the case of in-plane velocity measurements, velocity components in the x or y directions (or both, as in Figure 14.2) can be measured. However, velocity is usually encoded through the plane of the image in the direction of the slice select gradient, as in Figure 14.1. The principal direction of flow is then aligned with the elongated voxels that make up the slice.

As with Doppler flow measurement, velocity information is encoded in phase shifts and is subject to aliasing. To avoid aliasing, an appropriate

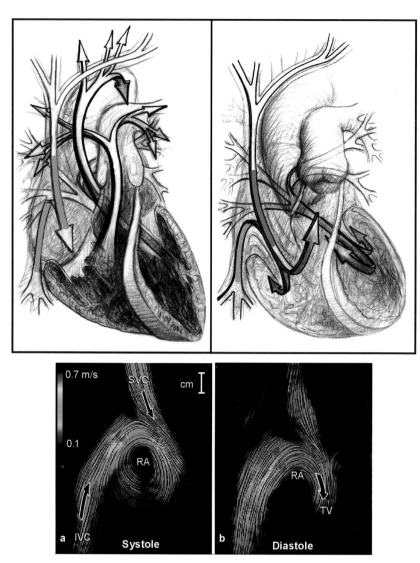

Fig. 14.2 Drawings of the principal paths of flow through the heart in systole and diastole (above) based on CMR cine and velocity acquisitions. Panels (a) and (b) below (see video clip 22 👁) show instantaneous streamlines in systole and diastole, color-coded for local speed, reconstructed from a 2D CMR velocity acquisition in an oblique sagittal plane through the right atrium of a healthy adult. Flows in other chambers and vessels were studied by velocity mapping in additional oblique planes. The momentum changes of flow through the looped curvatures of the heart are likely to take on a significant role during strenuous exertion. There will then be dynamic, directional exchanges of force between the alternately contracting atria and ventricles and the rapidly changing momentum of the passing blood. From Kilner, P.J., Yang, G.Z., Wilkes, A.J., Mohiaddin, R.H., Firmin, D.N., Yacoub, MH. Asymmetric redirection of flow through the heart. *Nature* 2000; **13**: 759–61.

velocity-encoding range (VENC) should be chosen before acquiring velocity data. An appropriate VENC exceeds the peak expected velocity by 10 to 50%. Too great a VENC reduces the sensitivity of velocity mapping by reducing the amount of velocity-related phase shifts relative to background noise or other artifact-related phase shifts.

The Multidirectional Nature of Flow through the Heart

Flow through the heart as a whole is not only distributed in 3D space, changing through the cardiac cycle, but is also multidirectional (Figure 14.2) [4]. The comprehensive measurement of flow through the whole heart requires the measurement of all three directional components of velocity (x, y, and z) for each point in space and time. In a sense, this is "seven-dimensional," but is more correctly described as three-dimensional, three-directional, time-resolved velocity data. With certain provisos, phase contrast magnetic resonance can achieve comprehensive flow measurement, whereas Doppler ultrasound measures only the components of velocity directed toward or away from the transducer [5]. Comprehensive CMR flow acquisition currently takes minutes rather than seconds, during which the fluctuations of unstable flow are averaged across many heart beats. Post-processing for visualization or measurement is challenging, and there can be blurring due to respiratory movements unless extra time is taken for diaphragm navigator acquisition.

The acquisition of comprehensive, multidirectional flow data is interesting in relation to the dynamics of flow through the normal curvatures of the heart and great vessels, and potentially in relation to congenital malformations (Figure 14.3) or an acquired pathology of the heart [6]. However, in clinical practice comprehensive acquisition is not usually needed. The measurement of one directional component through the plane of acquisition is usually adequate for clinical measurements of jet velocities, volume flows in the great vessels, and regurgitant fractions.

Jet Velocity Measurement by CMR

Measurements by CMR of jet velocity are subject to certain limitations. A key consideration is the shape, size, and orientation of voxels relative to those of the jet. The velocity of a jet can only be measured reliably by CMR if it has a coherent jet core (its central, high-velocity, low-shear region) large enough to contain entire voxels. The voxels are relatively long and thin, their length being the through-plane slice thickness, which is typically 5 to 8 mm. The cores of coherent jets are also long and thin, extending downstream from the orifice. Jet velocity is therefore best measured through a plane located carefully to transect the core of the jet, immediately downstream of the orifice. However, irregular or narrow jets, particularly those of regurgitant valves or a calcified and severely

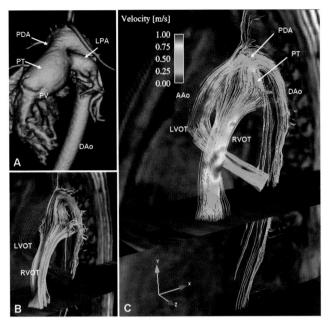

Fig. 14.3 An example of three-dimensional, three-directional, time-resolved CMR velocity mapping in a patient with a large patent ductus arteriosus (PDA). (a) Contrast enhanced magnetic resonance angiography. The volume-rendered images show the large PDA between the dilated pulmonary trunk (PT) and the aorta. PV, pulmonary valve; DAo, descending aorta; LPA, left pulmonary artery. (b) 3D streamlines originating from the left (LVOT, red) and from the right ventricular outflow tract (RVOT, blue). (c) Color-coded 3D streamlines demonstrating differences in flow velocities of the left and right outflow tract, with the right ventricle predominantly contributing to aortic filling (see video clip 23 👁) [5,6].

stenosed aortic valve, may be fragmented and unsuitable for accurate velocity measurement by CMR, although cine appearances of the valve, jet, and ventricle upstream usually make the severity obvious in such cases. Doppler ultrasound is not necessarily subject to the same limitations and is a more appropriate and reproducible method for measuring the velocity and time course of very narrow or fragmented jets.

Measurements of Volume Flow and Regurgitation

Measurements by phase contrast velocity mapping of volume flow through planes transecting the great arteries should provide the most accurate measurements available of cardiac output, shunt flow, aortic or pulmonary regurgitation (Figure 14.4), and, in combination with left ventricular volume or mitral inflow

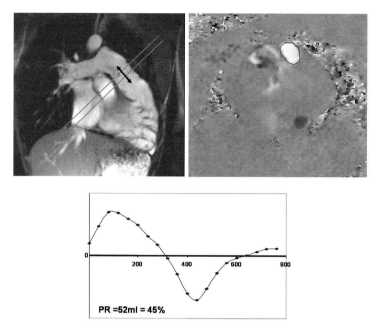

PR =52ml = 45%

Fig. 14.4 Free pulmonary regurgitation, late after repair of Fallot's tetralogy, shown using SSFP cine imaging (above left; see video clip 24 ⟨👁⟩) and through-plane velocity mapping (above right; see video clip 25 ⟨👁⟩). There was little or no effective valve action. The regurgitant fraction was 38%, which is typical of such cases. The flow curve (below) shows systolic forward flow, early diastolic reversal, and then late diastolic forward flow when the right ventricle is full and acts as a conduit, transmitting systemic venous return, boosted atrial systole, through to the pulmonary trunk.

measurements, of mitral regurgitation [7–13]. However, measurements of volume flow can be subject to errors [14]. Hardware, software, and acquisition protocols each must be optimized to achieve accurate results [15]. On some CMR systems, inaccuracies of flow measurement are caused by background phase errors due to eddy currents or uncorrected concomitant gradients. Measurements of regurgitant or shunt flow can be seriously affected by these errors, which should be minimized or corrected by appropriate hardware and software design. If they have not been, inaccuracies can be detected and corrected by repeating identical velocity acquisitions on a static phantom and subtracting the corresponding apparent phantom velocities from those of the clinical acquisition [14].

During a clinical study, planes of acquisition must be located appropriately with respect to the vessels in question. For reproducibility, and to avoid convergent, accelerating flow into a regurgitant orifice, a plane for aortic flow measurement is probably best located at or immediately above the sinotubular junction at end-diastole. This position keeps the plane clear of any convergent, accelerating diastolic flow in the vicinity of a regurgitant orifice, but it must be understood that coronary flow — which is typically about 5% of the cardiac output — does not reach this plane.

All four heart valves normally move with respect to the chest wall and the magnet during the cardiac cycle. Such movement may be reduced after previous surgery — for example, for tetralogy of Fallot — but otherwise the displacements of valve planes can affect attempted measurements of regurgitant flow. In diastole, when an aortic regurgitant jet is flowing back into the ventricle, the root moves up in the opposite direction, typically by about 6 to 12 mm. This movement tends to cause an underestimation of the regurgitant volume or regurgitant fraction. If the root is dilated and mobile, the underestimation of the regurgitant fraction could be as much as 10 or 15% of the forward flow volume — which, if unrecognized, could give misleading evidence regarding the need for surgical intervention.

A solution to this source of inaccuracy is the implementation of motion tracking and heart-motion adapted flow measurements as described by Kozerke and colleagues in 1999 and 2000 [16,17]. This technique has yet to be made available on most commercial CMR systems. The displacements of the aortic root or mitral annulus can be tracked by a modified tagging technique, and both the location of the velocity mapping slice and the through-plane velocity offsets are adjusted to take account of the annular movements through the phases of the cardiac cycle. In this way, velocities are measured relative to the valve annulus rather than relative to the magnet or the body. In their second paper, the authors showed how this procedure corrected significant underestimates of aortic regurgitant fractions in patients, and that the need for correction was even greater for accurate measurement of mitral flow. Although it may not be realistic to measure mitral regurgitant flow directly due to the shape of the valve and the narrow or splayed nature of jets, mitral regurgitant volume is calculable by subtracting systolic aortic outflow from diastolic mitral inflow, as long as both are measured accurately.

On the pulmonary side, the regurgitant orifice can be wide, and a complete absence of effective pulmonary valve function is relatively common after repair of tetralogy of Fallot or valvotomy for congenital pulmonary stenosis. A regurgitant fraction of about 40% is typical in patients with no effective pulmonary valve action, but it can vary considerably depending on upstream and downstream factors, not only on the incompetence of the valve itself [18].

Measures of the Severity of Valve Lesions

A guide to measures of the severity of stenotic and regurgitant valve lesions is offered in Table 14.1 (see page 347). Of course, measurements are dependent on appropriate methods of acquisition, and experience is needed both to optimize acquisitions and to recognize when image quality is not adequate for accurate measurement.

Other Velocity Mapping Applications

The through-plane velocity mapping technique can be used for the sizing of atrial septal defects, ventricular septal defects, and regurgitant orifices, particularly of the tricuspid and pulmonary valves. For these applications, the velocity mapping slice is located to transect the jet or stream passing through the orifice. Appropriately low VENCs are used for low-velocity jets — for example, 100 cm/s for an ASD stream and 250 cm/s for sizing the defect of a severely regurgitant tricuspid valve. Shunts due to a septal defect or patent arterial duct are quantified by the measurement of main pulmonary artery relative to ascending aortic flow [8,14]. With simultaneous catheter measurements of pressure, pulmonary arterial flow measurements probably allow the most accurate available calculations of pulmonary resistance, particularly when shunts complicate the use of indicator dilution techniques [18].

Conclusions

CMR offers unrivalled versatility and comprehensiveness in the visualization and measurement of flow. For investigating heart valve disease, important strengths lie in the visualization and quantification of regurgitation, the measurement of ventricular volumes, function and mass, and the investigation of associated congenital or acquired pathology. Freedom of access and the free orientation of planes make CMR a useful second-line approach for patients in whom ultrasonic access is limited, particularly for abnormalities of the right ventricular outflow tract. Measurements of volume flow and regurgitant fraction are a unique capability of CMR but can be subject to errors. To avoid these, concerted efforts toward optimization are needed from manufacturers and users to make appropriate use of phase contrast flow measurement techniques.

References

1 Bonow, R.O., *et al.* (2006) ACC/AHA Guidelines for the management of patients with valvular heart disease. *Circulation* **114**: e84–e231.
2 Kilner, P.J., Sievers, B., Meyer, G.P., Ho, S.Y. (2002) Double-chambered right ventricle or sub-infundibular stenosis assessed by cardiovascular magnetic resonance. *J Cardiovasc Magn Reson* **4**(3): 373–379.
3 Gatehouse, P.D., Keegan, J., Crowe, L.A., *et al.* (2005) Applications of phase-contrast flow and velocity imaging in cardiovascular MRI. *Eur Radiol* **15**(10): 2172–2184.
4 Kilner, P.J., Yang, G.Z., Wilkes, A.J., *et al.* (2000) Asymmetric redirection of flow through the heart. *Nature* **13**: 759–761.

5 Markl, M., Harloff, A., Bley, T.A., et al. (2007) Time-resolved 3D MR velocity mapping at 3T: improved navigator-gated assessment of vascular anatomy and blood flow. *J Magn Reson Imaging* **25**(4): 824–831.

6 Frydrychowicz, A., Bley, T.A., Dittrich, S., et al. (2007) Visualization of vascular hemodynamics in a case of a large patent ductus arteriosus using flow sensitive 3D CMR at 3T. *J Cardiovasc Magn Reson* **9**(3): 585–587.

7 Petersen, S.E., Voigtlander, T., Kreitner, K.F., et al. (2002) Quantification of shunt volumes in congenital heart diseases using a breath-hold MR phase contrast technique—comparison with oximetry. *Int J Cardiovasc Imaging* **18**: 53–60.

8 Colletti, P.M. (2005) Evaluation of intracardiac shunts with cardiac magnetic resonance. *Curr Cardiol Rep* **7**: 52–58.

9 Rebergen, S.A., Chin, J.G.L., Ottenkamp, J., et al. (1993) Pulmonary regurgitation in the late post-operative follow-up of tetralogy of Fallot: volumetric quantification by nuclear magnetic resonance velocity mapping. *Circulation* **88**: 2257–2266.

10 Gelfand, E.V., Hughes, S., Hauser, T.H., et al. (2006) Severity of mitral and aortic regurgitation as assessed by cardiovascular magnetic resonance: optimizing correlation with Doppler echocardiography. *J Cardiovasc Magn Reson* **8**(3): 503–507.

11 Hundley, W.G., Li, H.F., Willard, J.E., et al. (1995) Magnetic resonance imaging assessment of the severity of mitral regurgitation. *Circulation* **92**: 1151–1158.

12 Kon, M.W., Myerson, S.G., Moat, N.E., Pennell, D.J. (2004) Quantification of regurgitant fraction in mitral regurgitation by cardiovascular magnetic resonance: comparison of techniques. *J Heart Valve Dis* **13**(4): 600–607.

13 Chai, P., Mohiaddin, R. (2005) How we perform cardiovascular magnetic resonance flow assessment using phase-contrast velocity mapping. *J Cardiovasc Magn Reson* **7**(4): 705–716.

14 Chernobelsky, A., Shubayev, O., Comeau, C.R., Wolff, S.D. Baseline correction of phase contrast images improves quantification of blood flow in the great vessels. *J Cardiovas Magn Res* (in press).

15 Kilner, P.J., Gatehouse, P.D., Firmin, D.N. Flow measurement by magnetic resonance: a unique asset worth optimising. *J Cardiovas Magn Res* (in press).

16 Kozerke, S., Scheidegger, M.B., Pedersen, E.M., Boesiger, P. (1999) Heart motion adapted cine phase-contrast flow measurements through the aortic valve. *Magn Reson Med* **42**(5): 970–978.

17 Kozerke, S., Schwitter, J., Pedersen, E.M., Boesiger, P. (2001) Aortic and mitral regurgitation: quantification using moving slice velocity mapping. *J Magn Reson Imaging* **14**(2): 106–112.

18 Redington, A.N. (2006) Determinants and assessment of pulmonary regurgitation in tetralogy of Fallot: practice and pitfalls. *Cardiol Clin* **24**(4): 631–639.

19 Muthurangu, V., Taylor, A., Andriantsimiavona, R., et al. (2004) Novel method of quantifying pulmonary vascular resistance by use of simultaneous invasive pressure monitoring and phase-contrast magnetic resonance flow. *Circulation* **110**: 826–834.

Chapter 15

Relative Merits of CTA and MRA for Coronary Artery Imaging

Xin Liu, James C. Carr, and Debiao Li

Catheter-based, x-ray coronary angiography remains the gold standard for the detection of coronary stenosis due to its high spatial and temporal resolution (0.13 to 0.20 mm and 20 ms, respectively). However, it is an expensive procedure with a small risk of serious complications [1]. Furthermore, only one-third of these examinations are performed in conjunction with an interventional therapeutic procedure [2]. Thus, a noninvasive assessment of coronary arteries is highly desirable for the diagnosis of coronary artery disease (CAD).

Over the past decade, multislice computed tomography angiography (CTA) and magnetic resonance angiography (MRA) have evolved as potential noninvasive tools for the detection of significant CAD. The noninvasive imaging of coronary arteries is challenging because the coronary arteries are small in size, have tortuous courses and similar imaging characteristics to the surrounding tissues, and are in constant motion caused by heart beat and respiration. Although temporal and spatial resolutions of coronary CTA and MRA are still inferior to x-ray coronary angiography, both techniques have successfully addressed these challenges using various imaging strategies. In this chapter, we will briefly review CTA and MRA techniques for coronary artery imaging and discuss the relative merits of the two techniques.

Technologies of Coronary CTA and MRA

Spatial Resolution

The coronary arteries are generally less than 6 mm in diameter near the coronary ostia. Successful imaging of the small vessels requires a spatial resolution of

Novel Techniques for Imaging the Heart, 1st edition. Edited by M. Di Carli and R. Kwong.
© 2008 American Heart Association, ISBN: 9-781-4051-7533-3.

less than 1 mm, and a much higher spatial resolution of less than 0.5 mm is necessary for the identification of focal coronary stenoses [3,4]. In addition, isotropic resolution and whole-heart coverage are highly desirable for depicting coronary arteries in different planes.

For coronary CTA, high spatial resolution was achieved with the introduction of 64-detector scanners that use significant doses of radiation to generate isotropic voxel sizes approaching $0.4 \times 0.4 \times 0.4$ mm^3. For coronary MRA, the newly developed whole-heart imaging approach allows a spatial resolution of $1.1 \times 1.1 \times 1.3$ mm^3 by using the steady state free precession (SSFP) pulse sequence and parallel imaging techniques [5–9]. Further resolution improvements are expected at higher field (3.0 T) magnetic resonance systems [10–14].

Suppression of Motion Artifacts

To minimize the motion artifacts caused by cardiac motion, both coronary CTA and MRA use electrocardiographic (ECG) gating to acquire data during the period of minimal motion in each cardiac cycle. As discussed in Chapters 1 and 3, coronary CTA can collect data throughout the cardiac cycle using either retrospective or prospective ECG gating [15]. Although radiation exposure increases with the retrospective ECG gating acquisition, vessel-specific reconstruction with optimal image quality can be performed for each of the major coronary arteries [15,16]. Coronary MRA uses prospective ECG gating to synchronize data acquisition to the rest period in each cardiac cycle, identified by inspecting coronary artery motion on a cine scan. Because coronary artery motions in various vessel segments are different during the cardiac cycle, residual motion artifacts can occur, especially in patients with relatively high heart rates. A cardiac motion-resolved (4D) imaging approach has been developed to address this problem, which allows the retrospective selection of cardiac frames that best depict each major coronary artery [17].

The duration of the rest period in mid-to-end-diastole is typically 70 to 80 ms when the heart rate is greater than 65 beats per minute, and can extend to 150 ms or longer when the heart rate is less than 60 beats per minute [18]. For coronary CTA, the duration of data acquisition (reconstruction window) per slice is equal to half of the x-ray tube rotation time [19]. Reduction of the x-ray tube rotation time to around 330 ms now allows for the reconstruction window to be as short as 165 ms with 64-slice computed tomography (CT) scanners and 83 ms with dual source CT machines [20]. Thus, beta-blocker administration is still required for 64-slice CT in patients with heart rates greater than 65 beats per minute. The use of sublingual nitrates is also helpful to improve image quality. With the increased tube rotation speed and number of detectors, coronary CTA with 64-slice scanners can now be performed in less than 15 cardiac cycles to cover the normal heart with an average cranio-caudal size of 12 cm. In the future, it may be possible to perform a coronary CTA examination of the entire heart during a single heart beat by using volume CT (320 slices, or 16 cm axial coverage) [21]. With coronary MRA, the duration of data acquisition (acquisition window) varies from 50 to 150 ms, according to the patient's heart rate. Three hundred or more consecutive heart beats are typically required to obtain image data of the entire heart [22]. The exact number of heart beats is dependent on the spatial resolution and the duration of the acquisition window in each cardiac cycle. Because a regular rhythm and accurate ECG synchronization are required to achieve high image quality, the image quality of coronary MRA is more sensitive to arrhythmias than that of coronary CTA.

The suppression of respiratory motion artifacts for coronary CTA is accomplished with a single sustained breath-hold of less than 12 s. For coronary MRA, two methods have been used to compensate for respiratory motion. Breath-hold could eliminate respiratory motion more completely with cooperative patients, but the coverage and spatial resolution are limited by the short breath-hold time, and separate breath-holds are required for each of the major coronary arteries. A free-breathing approach using real-time gating and motion correction based on the diaphragmatic navigator echo allows greater resolution and larger coverage, but a significant limitation of the prolonged imaging time can result in poor image quality if heart beats or breathing patterns are inconsistent [23]. Further improvements in respiratory motion suppression techniques or very rapid single breath-hold acquisition using parallel imaging at high-field systems are required to increase the success rate of coronary MRA in patients [24,25].

Coronary Artery Contrast

Because blood in the coronary artery lumen has similar imaging characteristics to nearby fat, myocardium, and cardiac veins, coronary CTA requires the intravenous bolus injection of a large volume of highly iodinated contrast agents to provide sufficient contrast between blood and these surrounding structures. With magnetic resonance imaging (MRI), coronary artery contrast is generated by using specific imaging sequences and pre-pulses without the use of exogenous contrast agents. SSFP sequence is the preferred method for coronary lumen imaging at 1.5 T due to its intrinsically high blood-signal intensity and blood-myocardial contrast [26]. In addition, frequency-selective pre-pulses are applied to saturate signal from fat tissue, and T2-preparation pre-pulses are used to suppress myocardium and cardiac veins [27]. Exogenous magnetic resonance contrast agents, typically classified as extracellular (interstitial) and intravascular (blood pool) agents, have been used in coronary MRA to further improve the signal-to-noise ratio (SNR) and contrast-to-noise ratio (CNR) [28,29]. However, extravascular agents that diffuse to interstitial space quickly are not appropriate for free-breathing coronary MRA, which requires an imaging time of a few to more than 10 minutes. Recently, contrast-enhanced coronary MRA with the slow infusion of a high-relaxivity extravascular contrast agent showed promising results, with an improved SNR and reduced imaging time at 3.0 T [30]. Intravascular contrast agents allow much higher T1 relaxivity and longer half-lives in the blood pool, but they are not yet approved for clinical use in the United States [31].

Clinical Applications of Coronary CTA and MRA

Visualization of Normal Coronary Arteries

The introduction of 64-slice CT gave rise to major improvements in image quality and the robustness of coronary CTA. Recent studies showed that at experienced sites and with careful patient preparation, 88% to 100% of coronary arteries, including almost all major segments and larger side branches (greater than 1.5 mm in diameter), were assessable [32–36].

For coronary MRA, 3D techniques with SSFP at 1.5 T are the predominant methods. However, limited by SNR, spatial resolution, and imaging time, they are still difficult to depict distal coronary segments routinely and reliably. The rate of assessable coronary segments (greater than 2.0 mm in diameter) is typically 80 to 87% [9,37,38]. Recently, a multicenter study in 109 patients demonstrated that coronary MRA could reliably visualize proximal and middle segments of major coronary arteries [37].

Detection of Anomalous Coronary Arteries and Coronary Artery Aneurysm in Kawasaki's Disease

The ability of coronary MRA to reliably visualize major coronary arteries is ideally suited for the identification and characterization of anomalous coronary arteries. Anomalous coronary arteries are a well known but rare cause of myocardial ischemia and sudden death in children and young adults. Previous studies have demonstrated the high accuracy of coronary MRA for the detection and definition of anomalous coronary arteries in patients with suspected anomalous coronary arteries or congenital conditions associated with anomalous coronary arteries [39–41]. Coronary MRA has several advantages in the diagnosis of coronary artery anomalies. In addition to being noninvasive and not requiring ionizing radiation or iodinated contrast agents (likely to be an important consideration for adolescents and young adults), coronary MRA provides a 3D roadmap of anomalous coronary arteries that can be visualized in any orientation (Figure 15.1). Further, coronary MRA has shown to be very effective for both visualizing and measuring the dimensions of coronary aneurysms in pediatric patients with Kawasaki's disease (Figure 15.2) [42–44].

The presence of coronary artery anomalies and coronary artery aneurysms can be adequately assessed by coronary CTA [45,46]. However, the requirements for radiation exposure and potentially nephrotoxic contrast agents limit its routine application in young adults and children.

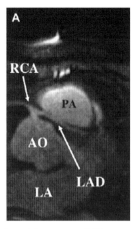
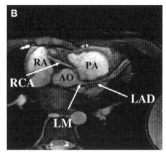

Fig. 15.1 Free-breathing targeted 3D coronary MRI using T2 pre-pulse navigator gating with real-time motion correction. (a) Transverse orientation depicting a malignant-type anomalous left anterior descending coronary artery originating from the right coronary artery (RCA). (b) Transverse image in another patient with a malignant-type anomalous origin of the RCA from the left coronary cusp. Ao, aorta; PA, pulmonary artery; LA, left atrium; RA, right atrium. From Manning *et al.*, used with permission. Reprinted with permission from Manning, W.J., Nezafat, R., Appelbaum, E., *et al.* (2007) *Cardiol Clin* **25**: 141–170.

Detection of Coronary Artery Stenoses

With the high spatial and temporal resolution of 64-slice CT, coronary CTA has achieved a high diagnostic accuracy for the detection of hemodynamically relevant coronary artery stenoses. A systematic analysis (15 studies in 1027 patients) showed that the pooled sensitivity, specificity, positive predictive value, and

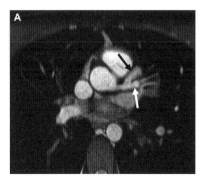
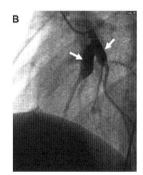

Fig. 15.2 (a) Transverse targeted 3D T2 pre-pulse coronary MRI of a subject with a left coronary artery aneurysm and (b) corresponding radiograph angiogram, demonstrating the good correlation of coronary MRI findings. From Manning *et al.*, used with permission. Reprinted with permission from Manning, W.J., Nezafat, R., Appelbaum, E., *et al.* (2007) *Cardiol Clin* **25**: 141–170.

negative predictive value of 64-slice CT for detecting significant coronary stenosis (greater than or equal to 50% diameter reduction) were 97, 88, 94, and 95% for patient-based assessment; 92, 92, 78, and 98% for vessel-based assessment; and 90, 96, 75, and 98% for segment-based assessment, respectively [47]. Although a relative high prevalence of CAD presented in these studies, the high negative predictive value indicates that 64-slice CT scanners can be clinically used to reliably rule out the presence of significant coronary artery stenoses.

However, coronary CTA has several limitations and should not be expected to widely replace x-ray angiography in the foreseeable future. First, the requirement of radiation exposure that is greater than conventional x-ray angiography (15.2 mSv for men and 21.4 mSv for women versus 6.0 mSv) limits its application for serial measurements (for example, during stress, at rest, and delayed scan) and follow-up examination (such as for plaque assessment), as well as its use in young patients [48,49]. However, as discussed in Chapter 3 prospective gating with either step-and-shoot acquisition techniques or the use of volume CT are expected to reduce radiation exposure significantly (to about 2 to 4 mSv). Second, spatial resolution limits the ability of coronary CTA to provide exact, quantitative measures of stenosis severity. Third, patients with atrial fibrillation or other arrhythmias as well as patients with contraindications to iodinated contrast media cannot be studied. Finally, the blooming artifacts from high-density materials such as coronary calcifications or stents can hamper the accurate assessment of the integrity of the coronary lumen.

Limited by relatively low spatial resolution, the diagnostic accuracy of current coronary MRA techniques is still inadequate for its clinical use for the identification of significant CAD. A meta-analysis (25 studies in 993 patients) demonstrated that the weighted average sensitivity and specificity of coronary MRA for the detection of significant coronary stenoses were 73 and 86%, respectively [5]. However, coronary MRA appears to be of clinical value for assessing coronary arteries in selected patients. A multicenter study with 109 patients demonstrated that 3D coronary MRA at 1.5 T is reliable for the assessment of left main coronary artery or three-vessel disease [37]. Recently, a new whole-heart MRA approach allowed greater diagnostic accuracy, with sensitivity, specificity, and positive and negative predictive values of 82, 90, 88, and 86%, respectively, based on patient analysis [9]. In addition, coronary MRA has been found to be especially valuable for determining the etiology of the cardiomyopathy by the combination with delayed enhancement MRI in patients who present with dilated cardiomyopathy in the absence of clinical infarction [3].

There are a few direct comparisons between coronary CTA and MRA for the detection of significant coronary artery stenosis. Recently, a comparison of 108 patients between 16-slice CT and 1.5-T MRI reported that coronary CTA outperformed MRA with higher sensitivity (92% versus 74%; $p = 0.013$), whereas specificity was comparable for the two techniques (79% versus 75%; $p = 0.643$) in the per-patient analysis [38]. Data from a meta-analysis also suggest that

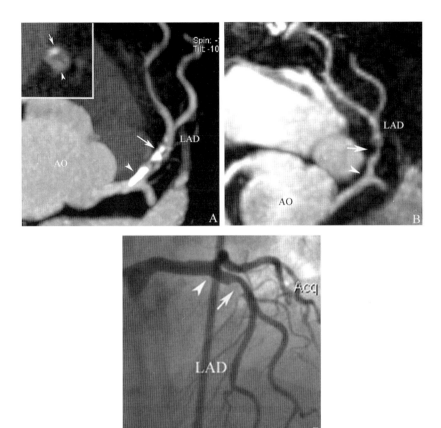

Fig. 15.3 A 60-year-old woman with chest pain. (a) A calcification in the left main coronary artery (arrowhead) and a mixed plaque in the proximal left anterior descending coronary artery (LAD) (arrow) seen on a CTA maximum intensity projection (MIP) image. The cross-sectional image (insert) shows noncalcified components within the plaque. (b) The MRA MIP image shows a significant stenosis in the proximal LAD (arrow) but a normal LM (arrowhead). (c) The findings from MRA are consistent with those from x-ray angiography (arrow and arrowhead, respectively). From Liu *et al.*, used with permission [51].

coronary CTA has a greater diagnostic accuracy than MRA for the detection of significant coronary stenosis [50]. However, a recent comparative study demonstrated that coronary MRA might be useful for the visualization of coronary artery lumen covered with severe calcification (Figure 15.3) [51].

Coronary Artery Bypass Grafts

The post-coronary artery bypass graft (CABG) follow-up using coronary CTA and MRA includes the assessment of venous and artery bypass grafts as well as the evaluation of native coronary arteries. The visualization of venous bypass grafts is relative easy because the motion of venous bypasses is limited and the size is relative large. The imaging of internal mammary artery grafts in some cases can be more difficult because of artifacts caused by metal clips placed alongside the bypass grafts. With coronary CTA, recent studies demonstrated that 64-slice CT allows the accurate exclusion of greater than 50% graft stenosis and the detection of vein graft disease at an early stage, but the assessment of distal anastomotic stenosis is limited [52,53]. The sensitivity, specificity, positive predictive value, and negative predictive value of 64-slice CT for the detection of greater than 50% graft stenoses were 85, 95, 80, and 96%, respectively [54]. With coronary MRA, 3D acquisition allows the assessment of venous graft patency and stenosis. A study reported that coronary MRA with free-breathing 3D gradient echo sequence has good diagnostic performance for assessing the severity of vein graft stenosis [54]. However, the imaging of arterial grafts is often more difficult for coronary MRA due to the metallic implants.

The assessment of native coronary arteries is challenging for both coronary CTA and MRA in patients after bypass surgery because they tend to calcify heavily and are frequently of small size. These characteristics limit the clinical usefulness of coronary CTA in patients who develop chest pain after bypass surgery because it is usually necessary to assess the status of both the bypass grafts and the native coronary arteries. As discussed in Chapters 9 and 10, stress myocardial perfusion imaging is a more effective approach to evaluate recurrent chest pain after coronary bypass surgery.

Coronary Artery Stents

Because of high-density artifacts caused by metal, visualization of the lumen within coronary artery stents by CT is more difficult than the assessment of native coronary arteries. Improved spatial resolution of 64-slice CT scanners allows a more accurate assessment of in-stent restenosis. A recent study reported that the sensitivity, specificity, and positive and negative predictive value of 64-slice CT for the detection of high-grade (greater than or equal to 50%) in-stent restenosis were 91, 93, 77, and 98%, respectively, when excluding unassessable coronary segments [55]. Another study reported that coronary CTA with 64-slice CT has a high accuracy rate of 98% for stents implanted in the left main coronary artery, and an intravascular ultrasound threshold value of greater than or equal to 1 mm was identified to reliably detect in-stent neointima hyperplasia [56]. In addition, the type of stent and stent diameter play a significant role in the assessment of in-stent restenosis by CT.

Coronary MRA should allow the potential assessment of in-stent restenosis without the blooming artifacts caused by the metallic stents. However, local field susceptibility changes may lead to signal voids at the site of the stent. The size of the signal void depends on both the stent material and the MRI sequence [57].

Coronary Atherosclerotic Plaque

As discussed in detail in Chapter 6, coronary CTA permits the depiction of atherosclerotic plaque [58,59]. Sensitivities for the detection of plaque, whether calcified or noncalcified, have been reported to be approximately 80 to 90% [59–61]. Coronary CTA with 64-slice CT allows the detection of atherosclerotic lesions with no significant stenosis and the measurement of plaque volume [61].

MRI allows the imaging of the arterial vessel wall with black-blood techniques that typically use a dual inversion pre-pulse for suppressing the blood signal. The techniques have been a great success in carotid arteries due to their superficial locations and relative absence of motion. Using spin density-, T1-, and T2-weighted acquisitions, magnetic resonance studies have demonstrated the characterization of normal and pathological arterial walls, the quantification of plaque size and therapeutic regression, and the detection of fibrous cap integrity, as well as disruption-related transient ischemic attack or stroke [62–64].

However, the imaging of the coronary artery wall is more challenging due to the small dimensions and the constant motions of the coronary arteries. Early studies of coronary vessel wall imaging used a 2D dual-inversion, fast spin echo technique with breath-hold or free-breathing [65,66]. Both coronary artery wall thickening and focal atherosclerotic plaque were assessed. More recently, 3D coronary vessel wall imaging with a near-isotropic, high-resolution, and larger coverage was reported (Figure 15.4) [67]. This approach has the potential to quantify subclinical plaques and measure the coronary plaque burden rapidly [68]. Magnetic resonance has the potential to monitor vessel wall thickness following interventions [69]. Future studies will include the use of contrast agents for plaque characterizations and greater field strength (3.0 T) imaging [70–73].

Conclusions

Coronary MRA allows the accurate assessment of anomalous coronary arteries, coronary aneurysms, and venous bypass graft patency. It has also demonstrated an initial clinical value for assessing native CAD in patients with suspected left main coronary artery or multivessel diseases. A normal coronary MRA strongly suggests the absence of severe multivessel disease. Compared to CTA, MRA does not require ionizing radiation or iodinated contrast media, and can assess coronary artery lumen in the presence of severe calcification. More importantly, coronary MRA can be combined with other cardiac magnetic resonance tests such as function, perfusion, hemodynamic, and tissue viability assessments for a comprehensive examination. However, the relatively low spatial resolution and long acquisition time limit its routine use for detecting significant coronary artery stenoses. Coronary MRA techniques are more complex and image quality is more variable, being somewhat dependent on the experience of the operator.

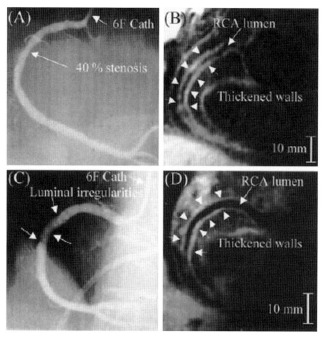

Fig. 15.4 X-ray angiography in two patients with (a) a focal 40% stenosis (white arrow) and (c) minor (about 10% stenosis) luminal irregularities (white arrows) of the proximal RCA. The corresponding black-blood 3D CMR vessel wall scans (b) and (d) demonstrate an irregularly thickened RCA wall (greater than 2 mm), indicative of an increased atherosclerotic plaque burden. The inner and outer RCA walls are indicated by the white dotted arrows. The catheter size for the x-ray was 6F. From Kim *et al.*, used with permission [67].

Further technical advances in motion suppression and faster imaging methods, improved multichannel radiofrequency coils, high field strength (such as 3.0 T) imaging, and novel magnetic resonance contrast agents will no doubt facilitate improved accuracy and widespread clinical use of coronary MRA.

As compared to coronary MRA, coronary CTA using 64-slice CT has been accepted as a clinical tool for the detection of significant CAD with its higher spatial resolution, diagnostic accuracy, and ease of use. However, the exclusive visualization of the coronary vessel wall cannot be obtained by CT, and the interpretation of coronary CTA is often impaired by severe coronary calcification. Furthermore, radiation and the use of nephrotoxic contrast media are a concern, especially for young patients and follow-up examinations. Coronary CTA should be carefully used for the detection of significant stenoses in symptomatic patients with a low pre-test probability of significant CAD.

References

1 Scanlon, P.J., Faxon, D.P., Audet, A.M., *et al.* (1999) ACC/AHA guidelines for coronary angiography: a report of the American College of Cardiology/American Heart Association Task Force on practice guidelines (Committee on Coronary Angiography). Developed in collaboration with the Society for Cardiac Angiography and Interventions. *J Am Coll Cardiol* **33**: 1756–1824.

2 American Heart Association, American Stroke Association. (2002) *Heart and Stroke Statistical Update.* American Heart Association, Dallas, TX.

3 Manning, W.J., Nezafat, R., Appelbaum, E., *et al.* (2007) Coronary magnetic resonance imaging (review). *Cardiol Clin* **25**: 141–170.

4 Schar, M., Kim, W., Stuber, M. (2001) The impact of spatial resolution and respiratory motion on MR imaging of atherosclerotic plaque. *J Magn Reson Imaging* **14**: 311–318.

5 Danias, P.G., Roussakis, A., Ioannidis, J.P.A. (2004) Diagnostic performance of coronary magnetic resonance angiography as compared against conventional X-ray angiography (a meta analysis). *J Am Coll Cardiol* **44**: 1867–1876.

6 Weber, O.M., Martin, A.J., Higgins, C.B. (2003) Whole-heart steady-state free processing coronary artery magnetic resonance angiography. *Magn Reson Med* **50**: 1223–1228.

7 Sakuma, H., Ichikawa, Y., Suzawa, N., *et al.* (2005) Assessment of coronary arteries with total study time of less than 30 minutes by using whole-heart coronary MR angiography. *Radiology* **237**: 316–321.

8 Bi, X., Deshpande, V., Carr, J., Li, D. (2006) Coronary MR angiography: a comparison between the whole-heart and volume-targeted methods using a T2-prepared SSFP sequence. *J Cardiovasc Magn Reson* **8**: 703–707.

9 Sakuma, H., Ichikawa, Y., Chino, S., *et al.* (2006) Detection of coronary artery stenosis with whole-heart coronary magnetic resonance angiography. *J Am Coll Cardiol* **48**: 1946–1950.

10 Stuber, M., Botnar, R.M., Fischer, S.E., *et al.* (2002) Preliminary report on in vivo coronary MRA at 3 Tesla in humans. *Magn Reson Med* **48**: 425–429.

11 Yang, P.C., Nguyen, P., Shimakawa, A., *et al.* (2004) Spiral magnetic resonance coronary angiography—direct comparison of 1.5 Tesla vs. 3 Tesla. *J Cardiovasc Magn Reson* **6**: 877–884.

12 Sommer T., Hackenbroch M., Hofer, U., *et al.* (2005) Coronary MR angiography at 3.0 T versus that at 1.5 T: initial results in patients suspected of having coronary artery disease. *Radiology* **234**: 718–725.

13 Bi, X., Li, D. (2005) Coronary arteries at 3.0 T: contrast-enhanced magnetization-prepared three-dimensional breathhold MR angiography. *J Magn Reson Imaging* **21**: 133–139.

14 Nezafat, R., Stuber, M., Ouwerkerk, R., *et al.* (2006) B_1-insensitive T_2 preparation for improved coronary magnetic resonance angiography at 3 T. *Magn Reson Med* **55**: 858–864.

15 Kopp, A.F., Schroeder, S., Kuettner, A., *et al.* (2001) Coronary arteries: retrospectively ECG-gated multi-detector row CT angiography with selective optimization of the image reconstruction window. *Radiology* **221**: 683–688.

16 Leschka, S., Husmann, L., Desbiolles, L.M., *et al.* (2006) Optimal image reconstruction intervals for non-invasive coronary angiography with 64-slice CT. *Eur Radiol* **16**: 1964–1972.

17 Park, J., Larson, A.C., Zhang, Q., *et al.* (2005) 4D radial coronary artery imaging within a single breath-hold: cine angiography with phase-sensitive fat suppression (CAPS). *Magn Reson Med* **54**: 833–840.

18 Wang, Y., Vidan, E., Bergman, G.W. (1999) Cardiac motion of coronary arteries: variability in the rest period and implications for coronary MR angiography. *Radiology* **213**: 751–758.

19 Flohr, T., Kuttner, A., Bruder, H., *et al.* (2003) Performance evaluation of a multi-slice CT system half rotation time with 16-slice detector and increased gantry rotation speed for isotropic submillimeter imaging of the heart. *Herz* **28**: 7–19.

20 Achenbach, S., Ropers, D., Kuettner, A., *et al.* (2006) Contrast-enhanced coronary artery visualization by dual-source computed tomography—initial experience. *Eur J Radiol* **57**: 331–335.

21 Mizuno, N., Funabashi, N., Imada, M., *et al.* (2007) Superiority of synchrony of 256-slice cone beam computed tomography for acquiring pulsating objects. Comparison with conventional multislice computed tomography. *Int J Cardiol* **118**: 400–405.

22 Stuber, M., Weiss, R.G. (2007) Coronary magnetic resonance angiography (review). *J Magn Reson Imaging* **26**: 219–2134.

23 Manning, W.J., Botnar, R.M., Kissinger, K.V., Stuber, M. (2002) Impact of navigator timing on free-breathing submillimeter 3D coronary magnetic resonance angiography. *Magn Reson Med* **47**: 196–201.

24 Santos, J.M., Cunningham, C.H., Lustig, M., *et al.* (2006) Single breath-hold whole-heart MRA using variable-density spirals at 3 T. *Magn Reson Med* **55**: 371–379.

25 Niendorf, T., Hardy, C.J., Giaquinto, R.O., *et al.* (2006) Toward single breath-hold whole-heart coverage coronary MR angiography using highly accelerated parallel imaging with a 32-channel MR system. *Magn Reson Med* **56**: 167–176.

26 Deshpande, V.S., Wielopolski, P.A., Shea, S.M., *et al.* (2001) 3D magnetization-prepared true-FISP: a new technique for imaging coronary arteries. *Magn Reson Med* **46**: 494–502.

27 Shea, S.M., Deshpande, V.S., Chung, Y.C., Li, D. (2002) Three-dimensional true-FISP imaging of the coronary arteries: improved contrast with T2-preparation. *J Magn Reson Imaging* **15**: 597–602.

28 Stuber, M., Botnar, R.M., Danias, P.G., *et al.* (1999) Contrast agent-enhanced, free-breathing, three-dimensional coronary magnetic resonance angiography. *J Magn Reson Imaging* **10**: 790–799.

29 Li, D., Carr, J.C., Shea, S.M., *et al.* (2001) Coronary arteries: magnetization-prepared contrast-enhanced three-dimensional volume-targeted breath-hold MR angiography. *Radiology* **219**: 270–277.

30 Bi, X., Carr, J., Li, D. (2007) Whole-heart coronary magnetic resonance angiography at 3 Tesla in 5 minutes with slow infusion of Gd-BOPTA, a high relaxivity clinical contrast agent. *Magn Reson Med* **58**: 1–7.

31 Paetsch, I., Jahnke, C., Barkhausen, J., *et al.* (2006) Detection of coronary stenoses with contrast enhanced, three-dimensional free breathing coronary MR angiography using the gadolinium-based intravascular contrast agent gadocoletic acid (B-22956). *J Cardiovasc Magn Reson* **8**: 509–516.

32 Leschka, S., Alkadhi, H., Plass, A., *et al.* (2005) Accuracy of MSCT coronary angiography with 64-slice technology: first experience. *Eur Heart J* **26**: 1482–1487.

33 Leber, A.W., Knez, A., von Ziegler, F., *et al.* (2005) Quantification of obstructive and nonobstructive coronary lesions by 64-slice computed tomography: a comparative study with quantitative coronary angiography and intravascular ultrasound. *J Am Coll Cardiol* **46**: 147–154.

34 Raff, G.L., Gallagher, M.J., O'Neill, W.W., Goldstein, J.A. (2005) Diagnostic accuracy of noninvasive coronary angiography using 64-slice spiral computed tomography. *J Am Coll Cardiol* **46**: 552–557.

35 Mollet, N.R., Cademartiri, F., van Mieghem, C.A., *et al.* (2005) High-resolution spiral computed tomography coronary angiography in patients referred for diagnostic conventional coronary angiography. *Circulation* **112**: 2318–2323.

36 Schuijf, J.D., Pundziute, G., Jukema, J.W., *et al.* (2006) Diagnostic accuracy of 64-slice multislice computed tomography in the noninvasive evaluation of significant coronary artery disease. *Am J Cardiol* **98**: 145–148.

37 Kim, W.Y., Danias, P.G., Stuber, M., *et al.* (2001) Coronary magnetic resonance angiography for the detection of coronary stenoses. *N Engl J Med* **345**: 1863–1869.

38 Dewey, M., Teige, F., Schnapauff, D., *et al.* (2006) Noninvasive detection of coronary artery stenoses with multislice computed tomography or magnetic resonance imaging. *Ann Intern Med* **145**: 407–415.

39 Taylor, A.M., Thorne, S.A., Rubens, M.B., *et al.* (2000) Coronary artery imaging in grown-up congenital heart disease: complementary role of magnetic resonance and x-ray coronary angiography. *Circulation* **101**: 1670–1678.

40 McConnell, M.V., Stuber, M., Manning, W.J. (2000) Clinical role of coronary magnetic resonance angiography in the diagnosis of anomalous coronary arteries (review). *J Cardiovasc Magn Reson* **2**: 217–224.

41 Bunce, N.H., Lorenz, C.H., Keegan, J., *et al.* (2003) Coronary artery anomalies: assessment with free-breathing three-dimensional coronary MR angiography. *Radiology* **227**: 201–208.

42 Duerinckx, A.J., Troutman, B., Allada, V., Kim, D. (1997) Coronary MR angiography in Kawasaki disease. *AJR* **168**: 114–116.

43 Mavrogeni, S., Papadopoulos, G., Douskou, M., *et al.* (2002) Coronary magnetic resonance angiography in adolescents and young adults with Kawasaki disease. *Circulation* **105**: 908–911.

44 Mavrogeni, S., Papadopoulos, G., Douskou, M., *et al.* (2004) Magnetic resonance angiography is equivalent to x-ray coronary angiography for the evaluation of coronary arteries in Kawasaki disease. *J Am Coll Cardiol* **43**: 649–652.

45 Datta, J., White, C.S., Gilkeson, R.C., *et al.* (2005) Anomalous coronary arteries in adults: depiction at multi-detector row CT angiography. *Radiology* **235**: 812–818.

46 Goo, H.W., Park, I.S., Ko, J.K., Kim, Y.H. (2006) Coronary CT angiography and MR angiography of Kawasaki disease. *Pediatr Radiol* **36**: 697–705.

47 Sun, Z., Lin, C., Davidson, R., *et al.* (2008) Diagnostic value of 64-slice CT angiography in coronary artery disease: a systematic review. *Eur J Radiol* **67**: 78–84.

48 Jakobs, T.F., Becker, C.R., Ohnesorge, B., *et al.* (2002) Multislice helical CT of the heart with retrospective ECG gating: reduction of radiation exposure by ECG-controlled tube current modulation. *Eur Radiol* **12**: 1081–1086.

49 Brenner, D.J., Hall, E.J. (2007) Computed tomography—an increasing source of radiation exposure (review). *N Engl J Med* **357**: 2277–2284.

50 Schuijf, J.D., Bax, J.J., Shaw, L.J., *et al.* (2006) Meta-analysis of comparative diagnostic performance of magnetic resonance imaging and multislice computed tomography for noninvasive coronary angiography. *Am Heart J* **151**: 404–411.

51 Liu, X., Zhao, X., Huang, J., *et al.* (2007) Comparison of 3D free-breathing coronary MR angiography and 64-MDCT angiography for detection of coronary stenosis in patients with high calcium scores. *AJR* **189**: 1326–1332.

52 Pache, G., Saueressig, U., Frydrychowicz, A., *et al.* (2006) Initial experience with 64-slice cardiac CT: non-invasive visualization of coronary artery bypass grafts. *Eur Heart J* **27**: 976–980.

53 Feuchtner, G.M., Schachner, T., Bonatti, J., *et al.* (2007) Diagnostic performance of 64-slice computed tomography in evaluation of coronary artery bypass grafts. *AJR* **189**: 574–580.

54 Langerak, S.E., Vliegen, H.W., de Roos, A., *et al.* (2002) Detection of vein graft disease using high-resolution magnetic resonance angiography. *Circulation* **105**: 328–333.

55 Ehara, M., Kawai, M., Surmely, J.F., *et al.* (2007) Diagnostic accuracy of coronary in-stent restenosis using 64-slice computed tomography: comparison with invasive coronary angiography. *J Am Coll Cardiol* **49**: 951–959.

56 Van Mieghem, C.A., Cademartiri, F., Mollet, N.R., *et al.* (2006) Multislice spiral computed tomography for the evaluation of stent patency after left main coronary artery stenting: a comparison with conventional coronary angiography and intravascular ultrasound. *Circulation* **114**: 645–653.

57 Maintz, D., Botnar, R.M., Fischbach, R., *et al.* (2002) Coronary magnetic resonance angiography for assessment of the stent lumen: a phantom study. *J Cardiovasc Magn Reson* **4**: 359–367.

58 Becker, C.R., Nikolaou, K., Muders, M., *et al.* (2003) Ex vivo coronary atherosclerotic plaque characterization with multi-detector-row CT. *Eur Radiol* **13**: 2094–2098.

59 Leber, A.W., Knez, A., Becker, A., *et al.* (2004) Accuracy of multidetector spiral computed tomography in identifying and differentiating the composition of coronary atherosclerotic plaques, A comparative study with intracoronary ultrasound. *J Am Coll Cardiol* **43**: 1241–1247.

60 Achenbach, S., Moselewski, F., Ropers, D., *et al.* (2004) Detection of calcified, submillimeter multidetector spiral computed tomography: a segment-based comparison with intravascular ultrasound. *Circulation* **109**: 14–17.

61 Leber, A.W., Becker, A., Knez, A., *et al.* (2006) Accuracy of 64-slice computed tomography to classify and quantify plaque volumes in the proximal coronary system: a comparative study using intravascular ultrasound. *J Am Coll Cardiol* **47**: 672–677.

62 Yuan, C., Mitsumori, L.M., Ferguson, M.S., *et al.* (2001) In vivo accuracy of multispectral magnetic resonance imaging for identifying lipid-rich necrotic cores and intraplaque hemorrhage in advanced human carotid plaques. *Circulation* **104**: 2051–2056.

63 Corti, R., Fuster, V., Fayad, Z.A., *et al.* (2002) Lipid lowering by simvastatin induces regression of human atherosclerotic lesions: two years' follow-up by high-resolution noninvasive magnetic resonance imaging. *Circulation* **106**: 2884–2887.

64 Yuan, C., Zhang, S.H., Polissar, N.L., *et al.* (2002) Identification of fibrous cap rupture with magnetic resonance imaging is highly associated with recent transient ischemic attack or stroke. *Circulation* **105**: 181–185.

65 Fayad, Z.A., Fuster, V., Fallon, J.T., *et al.* (2000) Noninvasive in vivo human coronary artery lumen and wall imaging using black-blood magnetic resonance imaging. *Circulation* **102**: 506–510.

66 Botnar, R.M., Stuber, M., Kissinger, K.V., *et al.* (2000) Noninvasive coronary vessel wall and plaque imaging with magnetic resonance imaging. *Circulation* **102**: 2582–2587.

67 Kim, W.Y., Stuber, M., Bornert, P., *et al.* (2002) Three-dimensional black-blood cardiac magnetic resonance coronary vessel wall imaging detects positive arterial remodeling in patients with nonsignificant coronary artery disease. *Circulation* **106**: 296–299.

68 Kim, W.Y., Astrup, A.S., Stuber, M., *et al.* (2007) Subclinical coronary and aortic atherosclerosis detected by magnetic resonance imaging in type 1 diabetes with and without diabetic nephropathy. *Circulation* **115**: 228–235.

69 Nissen, S.E., Tsunoda, T., Tuzcu, E.M., *et al.* (2003) Effect of recombinant ApoA-I Milano on coronary atherosclerosis in patients with acute coronary syndromes: a randomized controlled trial. *JAMA* **290**: 2292–2300.

70 Sirol, M., Itskovich, V.V., Mani, V., *et al.* (2004) Lipid-rich atherosclerotic plaques detected by gadofluorine-enhanced in vivo magnetic resonance imaging. *Circulation* **109**: 2890–2896.

71 Yeon, S.B., Sabir, A., Clouse, M., *et al.* (2007) Delay-enhancement cardiovascular magnetic resonance coronary artery wall imaging: comparison with multislice computed tomography and quantitative coronary angiography. *J Am Coll Cardiol* **50**: 441–447.

72 Koktzoglou, I., Simonetti, O., Li, D. (2005) Coronary artery wall imaging: initial experience at 3 Tesla. *J Magn Reson Imaging* **21**: 128–132.

73 Bansmann, P.M., Priest, A.N., Muellerleile, K., *et al.* (2007) MRI of the coronary vessel wall at 3 T: comparison of radial and Cartesian k-space sampling. *AJR* **188**: 70–74.

Chapter 16

Can Atherosclerosis Imaging Improve Patient Management?

Allen J. Taylor and Robert O. Bonow

Detection of latent cardiovascular risk has traditionally focused on demographic factors such as age and gender, coupled with the measurement of risk factors such as blood pressure and blood levels of cholesterol and glucose. This approach, whether through simplified risk factor counting algorithms or using prospectively derived logistic equations, provides a moderately accurate initial assessment of cardiovascular risk across modest time horizons of up to 10 years [1–4]. The practicality of this approach includes its reliance on simple and largely treatable factors. However, the practicality of this population-derived risk estimation tool is diminished when applied to individual patients versus groups of patients. Furthermore, this method leads to the grouping of risk into broad ranges (e.g., low, intermediate, and high) and among middle-aged individuals yields a large "intermediate" risk group that, because of its large size, accounts for a large proportion of the "population attributable risk" [5]. Lastly, the risk algorithms do not account for family history, for new factors that contribute to cardiovascular risk (e.g., C-reactive protein), nor for the exposure duration of individual risk factors [6]. All together, risk factor assessments lead to a practical and valuable but limited initial estimate of cardiovascular risk. To extend beyond these limitations, the imaging of atherosclerosis is evolving into a central method in cardiovascular medicine to refine the clinical risk prediction of coronary heart disease (CHD).

Atherosclerosis imaging provides a more individualized case identification method for use in asymptomatic patients in need of presymptomatic coronary risk estimation. Over the past decade, pivotal publications on methods such as carotid ultrasonography for the detection of intima-media thickness and cardiac

Novel Techniques for Imaging the Heart, 1st edition. Edited by M. Di Carli and R. Kwong.
© 2008 American Heart Association, ISBN: 9-781-4051-7533-3.

computed tomography (CT) for the detection of coronary artery calcium (CAC) have convincingly shown that these tests independently predict incident CHD events [7,8]. Subsequently, expert recommendations have endorsed the use of these tests as reasonable methods to refine clinical risk prediction with the aim of improved discrimination of coronary disease risk and the guidance of therapeutic selections (Table 16.1) [1,8–11]. Similarly, the development of magnetic resonance angiography has led to its initial application for atherosclerosis imaging, with preliminary data supporting its accuracy and emerging potential as a clinical surrogate [12–16].

Despite this wealth of information on the predictive value of atherosclerosis imaging, it remains to be established whether presymptomatic atherosclerosis imaging improves clinical outcomes. As solely diagnostic tests, the pathway to improved outcomes following imaging is entirely dependent on the subsequent management impact of the information obtained. In this regard, atherosclerosis imaging is postulated to lead to favorable changes in patient coronary risk behaviors and to more effective patient management decisions.

Atherosclerosis Imaging as a Behavioral Modification Tool

Evidence supporting the primacy of healthy cardiovascular behaviors in the optimization of cardiovascular risk is undeniable. Suboptimal coronary risk behaviors and modifiable factors may account for the majority — up to 80 or 90% — of coronary events, and medication adherence and persistence is often poor in both primary and secondary prevention [17–20]. Thus, a method that improves the patient's motivation for change, and moreover leads to measurable behavioral change, could have important benefits on coronary outcomes. Atherosclerosis imaging has been postulated to motivate patient behavior but is there evidence to support such a claim, or are we simply asking too much of an imaging test? Despite anecdotal and logical plausibility, the evidence to date fails to suggest a long-term, durable effect of atherosclerosis imaging on patient motivation. Several survey studies among primarily referred populations using either cardiac CT for the detection of coronary calcium or carotid ultrasonography for the detection of intima-media thickness or plaque have suggested that survey respondents report being motivated to healthy behavioral change presumably through an increased perception of risk [21–23]. In contrast, studies of measured behavioral change have yielded conflicting results. A study of 153 smokers showed a six-fold greater cessation rate of smoking at six months (22.2%) among smokers with evidence of carotid plaque who were shown their plaque on carotid ultrasonography (Figure 16.1). However, in general biomedical aids to enhance smoking cessation have not been shown to be effective [24,25]. Two randomized trials of coronary calcium have also shown imaging to be ineffective in motivating behavioral change. In studies of coronary calcium screening among healthy middle-aged military personnel (Prospective Army

Table 16.1 Recent Medical Society Statements on Atherosclerosis Imaging in Asymptomatic Individuals to Refine Patient Risk Stratification and Management

Source	Publication Year	Statement
American Heart Association, Prevention V [11]	2000	"In asymptomatic individuals older than 45 years of age, carefully performed carotid ultrasound examination with IMT measurement can add incremental information to traditional risk factor assessment. In experienced laboratories, this test can now be considered for further clarification of CHD risk assessment at the request of a physician."
NCEP ATP 3 [2, 30]	2001, 2004	"High coronary calcium scores signify and confirm increased risk for CHD when persons have multiple risk factors. Therefore, measurement of coronary calcium is an option for advanced risk assessment in appropriately selected persons, provided the test is ordered by a physician who is familiar with the strengths and weaknesses of noninvasive testing. In persons with multiple risk factors, high coronary calcium scores (e.g., $\geq 75^{th}$ percentile for age and sex) denotes advanced coronary atherosclerosis and provides a rationale for intensified LDL-lowering therapy. Moreover, measurement of coronary calcium is promising for older persons in whom the traditional risk factors lose some of their predictive power. For example, a high coronary calcium score could be used to tip the balance in favor of a decision to introduce LDL-lowering drugs for primary prevention in older persons. "Coronary calcium scores above the 75th percentile "denote advanced atherosclerosis and as such provide a rationale for intensified lipid lowering therapy."
ACC Bethesda Conference 34 [10]	2003	"Selecting intermediate-risk patients for screening with plaque burden assessment has potential theoretical advantages within a Bayesian approach to screening."
American Heart Association [9]	2006	"In clinically selected, intermediate-risk patients, it may be reasonable to measure the atherosclerosis burden using EBCT or MDCT to refine clinical risk prediction and to select patients for more aggressive target values for lipid-lowering therapies."
American College of Cardiology [8]	2007	"The Committee judged that it may be reasonable to consider use of CAC measurement in asymptomatic patients with intermediate CHD risk (between 10% and 20% 10-year risk of estimated coronary events based on available evidence that demonstrates incremental risk prediction information in this selected (intermediate risk) patient group. This conclusion is based on the possibility that such patients might be reclassified to a higher risk status based on high CAC score, and subsequent patient management may be modified."

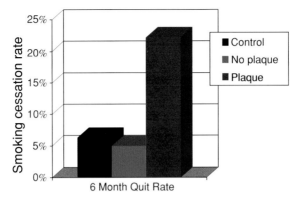

Fig. 16.1 A randomized study of carotid ultrasound in smokers found a six-fold higher cessation rate among smokers shown evidence of carotid plaque than controls or smokers without carotid plaque. The cessation rate at six months in smokers shown plaque was 22.2%. Data from Bovet, P., Peret F., Cornuz, J., Quilindo, J., Paccaud, F. (2002) Improved smoking cessation in smokers given ultrasound photographs of their own atherosclerotic plaques. *Prev Med* **34**(2): 215–20.

Coronary Calcium Study, or PACC) and of postmenopausal women, there was no relationship between imaging and behavioral change or motivation after one year [26,27]. These findings are hardly surprising given the limited motivational impact that even definite cardiac events such as myocardial infarction have on long-term patient behavior. Notably, within the factorial design of the PACC Project randomized trial, a randomization arm of a nurse case management approach to behavioral change was successful in stabilizing coronary risk (Figure 16.2), reducing the incidence of metabolic syndrome, and increasing patient motivation for change [26,28]. Thus, although images could not enable durable behavioral change, a recurring relationship between a health care provider and a patient could match a paradigm seen in other health states such as nurse case management programs in heart failure [29].

Atherosclerosis Imaging as an Aide to Patient Management

Asymptomatic Individuals: Provision of Medications

The use and persistence of evidence-based cardiovascular preventive medications is low, and this underutilization represents a barrier to optimizing opportunities for cardiovascular risk reduction [20]. Atherosclerosis imaging represents an opportunity to ensure not only that patients needing guideline-based therapies are properly identified, it also provides a rational basis to treat beyond present guidelines. As an example, the statement of the National Cholesterol Education Program (NCEP) suggested that coronary calcium scores above the 75th percentile "denote advanced atherosclerosis and as such provide a rationale for intensified lipid lowering therapy" [30].

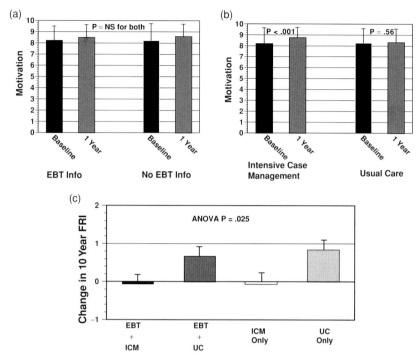

Fig. 16.2 Observed effects on motivation and coronary risk levels after one year in the randomized controlled trial of the PACC Project: motivation for healthy behavioral change with or without coronary calcium information (Panel A) and with or without nurse-based case management (Panel B). A significant increase in motivation behavioral change was observed only in goal-setting through a nurse-based case management program. At the conclusion of the one-year trial, the primary endpoint, a change in coronary risk levels, was met only in the case management group who showed stabilized cardiovascular risk (Panel C). EBT, electron beam tomography; ICM, intensive case management (nurse case management); UC, usual care (community-based provision of standard risk management). Data from O'Malley, P.G., Feuerstein, I.M., Taylor, A.J. (2003) Impact of electron beam tomography, with or without case management, on motivation, behavioral change, and cardiovascular risk profile: a randomized controlled trial. *JAMA* 7; **289**(17): 2215–23.

Is there evidence to support an effect of atherosclerosis imaging on the provision of risk-reducing medications? It is important to note that there are no completed randomized controlled trials, but several reports provide promise. Prospective observational data from the PACC Project in 1620 men followed for six years showed a 3.5- to 7-fold increase of the odds of community-based provision of statin or aspirin [31] (Figure 16.3). Furthermore, in this study there was a significantly more appropriate use of statins as indicated by NCEP guidelines, and a greater likelihood of beyond-guideline care when not indicated by NCEP guidelines.

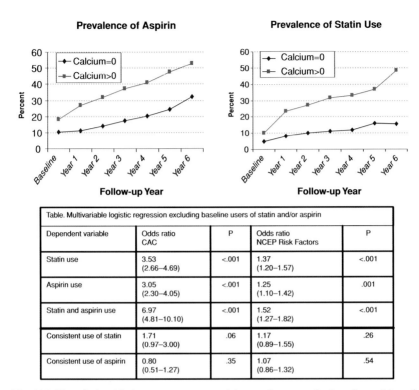

Fig. 16.3 The relationship between coronary calcium and community-based provision of aspirin and statin over six years. There was a strong, significant relationship between preventive medication usage and subclinical calcified coronary atherosclerosis that was incremental to standard risk factors and NCEP guidelines. Reprinted with permission from Taylor, A.J., Bindeman, J., Bauer, K., *et al.* (2007) *Circulation* **114**, 11–823. 2007.

Beyond the provision of medications, patient adherence is also critical to the success of pharmacotherapies. There are numerous barriers to medication adherence, many of which are rooted in behavioral patterns, such that isolated approaches are less effective than broad-based programs to improve adherence and promote persistence of use. To date, there are no convincing data that atherosclerosis imaging improves medication adherence, with negative findings from the PACC Project, but a suggestion of more prevalent statin usage (but not exercise or smoking cessation) on self report in a study by Budoff and colleagues [31,32]. Ultimately, only a properly designed clinical trial can separate the influence of the scan image from that of the interaction (and typically recurring interaction) with the health care provider.

Asymptomatic Patients: Selection for Further Testing

Although a relationship exists between increasing extent and multivessel CAC and obstructive coronary artery disease on coronary angiography, there is no evidence or sound rationale for invasive testing following presymptomatic atherosclerosis imaging. This result is particularly supported in light of clinical trial results showing optimal clinical outcomes with moderately intensive medical therapy versus an approach focused on coronary revascularization. However, recommendations from the American Society of Nuclear Cardiology do suggest it is appropriate to perform stress myocardial perfusion imaging at very high coronary calcium scores (Agatston scores greater than 400) to further refine the risk assessment among this high-risk group [33]. Recent data suggest that individuals with normal myocardial perfusion despite high coronary calcium scores have an excellent prognosis (Figure 16.4), providing a negative modifier for the adverse prognosis suggested by high coronary calcium scores alone [34].

Asymptomatic Patients: Preoperative Testing

Consistent with the general concept of low atherosclerosis burden correlating overall with a lower likelihood of obstructive coronary artery disease, atherosclerosis imaging has been tested as a preoperative risk-screening method to identify either risk for perioperative events during noncardiac surgery or the need for invasive coronary evaluation prior to valvular heart surgery [35,36]. Although generally successful in these applications, there is little interest in use of atherosclerosis imaging for these purposes given the availability of alternative screening mechanisms supported by more robust data and guidelines.

Symptomatic Patients: Use in the Emergency Room

Several studies have shown that patients presenting to the emergency department with chest pain represent a low-risk group for discharge when the coronary calcium score is low [37–39]. However, one important caveat is that solely noncalcified plaques can lead to acute coronary syndromes in younger patients. Furthermore, calcium scores have low specificity in older patients with prevalent coronary calcium. For these reasons, coronary calcium testing is not recommended for patient management in the emergency department. As discussed in Chapter 5, coronary CT angiography (CTA) appears to be superior to coronary calcium testing as it allows the identification of both calcified and noncalcified coronary plaques. Prospective studies are ongoing to evaluate the clinical utility of coronary CTA in the emergency department.

Areas of Controversy

Cost Effectiveness

A source of moderation within scientific statements on the clinical use of atherosclerosis imaging has been the uncertainty regarding cost-effectiveness. Notably, effectiveness has less to do with the test (beyond the incremental identification of risk) than with subsequent clinical decision making, therapeutic

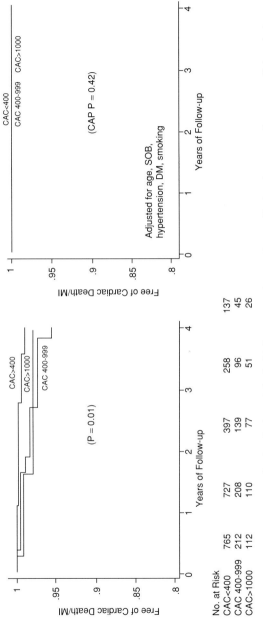

Fig. 16.4 Excellent prognosis of individuals with high CAC scores, and no evidence of ischemia on exercise myocardial perfusion scintigraphy. From Rozanski *et al.*, with permission [34].

relative risk reduction, and adherence to therapeutic selections. For example, in a study modeling the cost-effectiveness of coronary calcium testing, the procedure's cost-effectiveness was approximately $37,000 per quality adjusted life-year saved using a range of moderate assumptions [40]. However, cost-effectiveness was highly sensitive to the underlying assumptions, such that the marginal cost per quality adjusted life-year saved ranged from $10,000 to $1,700,000 for a range of relative risk reductions from 50 to 25%. Thus, once risk is accurately identified, the cost-effectiveness is highly dependent on external factors more related to clinical decision making. For these reasons, close coupling of the imaging procedure and clinical therapeutic decision making is needed.

Limiting the Application of Atherosclerosis Imaging to Intermediate-Risk Patients Only

Bayesian principles suggest that an intermediate-risk group is most likely to experience a shift in management following atherosclerosis imaging. However, this result adopts a focus on ten-year coronary risk rather than lifetime risk. In the Framingham Heart Study, the lifetime risk at age 50 of a low-risk man (44.2%) or woman (23.1%) was nearly that of those high-risk at age 50 (54.4 and 34.8% for men and women, respectively) [5]. Thus, recent trends are focusing on lifetime coronary risk as a more longitudinal approach to coronary disease risk. Under this rationale, presymptomatic testing even of low-risk individuals might hold value under a longer time horizon. Accurate lifetime risk calculators are needed, along with a focus on pre-emergent cardiovascular risk factors (such as obesity as a premonitory marker of diabetes mellitus).

Noncalcified Plaque as an Additional Imaging Target to Guide Patient Management

The imaging of noncalcified coronary arterial plaque requires multidetector CT with the administration of intravenous contrast and, presently, exposure to greater levels of radiation exposure than coronary calcium imaging. Theoretically, combining contrast and noncontrast cardiac CT will lead to a more comprehensive plaque burden assessment, as the relationship between plaque burden and calcium score varies between patients [41,42]. For asymptomatic patients without coronary calcium in whom the near-term prognosis is excellent, it is unlikely that the detection of solely noncalcified plaque will meaningfully refine cardiovascular prognosis or guide management. As such, the management of patients with calcium scores of zero should adhere to published risk factor-based recommendations. However, the potential exists for a clinical application for noncalcified plaque imaging among patients with intermediate coronary calcium scores for age, ethnicity, and gender with modestly elevated relative risk for CHD [43]. Before the routine detection of noncalcified coronary arterial plaque can be considered clinically appropriate, standardized and reproducible methods are needed for the quantification of noncalcified plaque, and studies must validate its independent prognostic value and potential for improving clinical management decision making.

Conclusions

Through an improved identification of risk, atherosclerosis imaging has the potential to shift clinical management decisions and thereby improve patient outcomes. Although the available data do not demonstrate a large attributable effect of atherosclerosis imaging on patient motivation, incorporating these data into a recurring clinical patient/physician relationship could lead to behavioral modification such as improved adherence to medical therapies. The provision of medications does appear to be strongly influenced by the detection of calcified coronary atherosclerosis, which is an important step in potentially translating imaging to improved CHD outcomes. Ultimately, with guidelines progressively endorsing the use of atherosclerosis imaging to refine the clinical risk assessment, it is incumbent upon those who perform and use these technologies to ensure that the test results enhance therapeutic decision making for the selection of well-evidenced treatments that reduce cardiovascular risk.

References

1 Grundy, S.M., Cleeman, J.I., Merz, C.N., *et al.* (2004) Implications of recent clinical trials for the National Cholesterol Education Program Adult Treatment Panel III Guidelines. *J Am Coll Cardiol* **44**(3): 720–372.

2 NCEP Writing Group. (2001) Executive summary of the third report of the National Cholesterol Education Program (NCEP) Expert Panel on Detection, Evaluation, and Treatment of High Blood Cholesterol in Adults (Adult Treatment Panel III). *JAMA* **285**(19): 2486–2497.

3 Wilson, P.W., D'Agostino, R.B., Levy, D., *et al.* (1998) Prediction of coronary heart disease using risk factor categories. *Circulation* **97**(18): 1837–1847 (see comments).

4 Grover, S.A., Coupal, L., Hu, X.P. (1995) Identifying adults at increased risk of coronary disease: how well do the current cholesterol guidelines work? *JAMA* **274**(10): 801–806.

5 Lloyd-Jones, D.M., Leip, E.P., Larson, M.G., *et al.* (2006) Prediction of lifetime risk for cardiovascular disease by risk factor burden at 50 years of age. *Circulation* **113**(6): 791–798.

6 Hemann, B.A., Bimson, W.F., Taylor, A.J. (2007) The Framingham Risk Score: an appraisal of its benefits and limitations. *Am Heart Hosp J* **5**(2):91–96.

7 Lorenz, M.W., Markus, H.S., Bots, M.L., *et al.* (2007) Prediction of clinical cardiovascular events with carotid intima-media thickness: a systematic review and meta-analysis. *Circulation* **115**(4): 459–467.

8 Greenland, P., Bonow, R.O., Brundage, B.H., *et al.* (2007) ACCF/AHA 2007 clinical expert consensus document on coronary artery calcium scoring by computed tomography in global cardiovascular risk assessment and in evaluation of patients with chest pain: a report of the American College of Cardiology Foundation Clinical Expert

Consensus Task Force (ACCF/AHA writing committee to update the 2000 expert consensus document on electron beam computed tomography) developed in collaboration with the Society of Atherosclerosis Imaging and Prevention and the Society of Cardiovascular Computed Tomography. *J Am Coll Cardiol* **49**(3): 378–402.

9 Budoff, M.J., Achenbach, S., Blumenthal, R.S., *et al.* (2006) Assessment of coronary artery disease by cardiac computed tomography: a scientific statement from the American Heart Association Committee on Cardiovascular Imaging and Intervention, Council on Cardiovascular Radiology and Intervention, and Committee on Cardiac Imaging, Council on Clinical Cardiology. *Circulation* **114**(16): 1761–1791.

10 Taylor, A.J., Merz, C.N., Udelson, J.E. (2003) 34th Bethesda Conference: executive summary — can atherosclerosis imaging techniques improve the detection of patients at risk for ischemic heart disease? *J Am Coll Cardiol* **41**(11): 1860–1862.

11 Greenland, P., Abrams, J., Aurigemma, G.P., *et al.* (2000) Prevention Conference V: beyond secondary prevention: identifying the high-risk patient for primary prevention: noninvasive tests of atherosclerotic burden: Writing Group III. *Circulation* **101**(1): E16–E22.

12 Kathiresan, S., Larson, M.G., Keyes, M.J., *et al.* (2007) Assessment by cardiovascular magnetic resonance, electron beam computed tomography, and carotid ultrasonography of the distribution of subclinical atherosclerosis across Framingham risk strata. *Am J Cardiol* **99**(3): 310–314.

13 Chan, S.K., Jaffer, F.A., Botnar, R.M., *et al.* (2001) Scan reproducibility of magnetic resonance imaging assessment of aortic atherosclerosis burden. *J Cardiovasc Magn Reson* **3**(4): 331–338.

14 Corti, R., Fayad, Z.A., Fuster, V., *et al.* (2001) Effects of lipid-lowering by simvastatin on human atherosclerotic lesions: a longitudinal study by high-resolution, noninvasive magnetic resonance imaging. *Circulation* **104**(3): 249–252.

15 Jaffer, F.A., O'Donnell, C.J., Larson, M.G., *et al.* (2002) Age and sex distribution of subclinical aortic atherosclerosis: a magnetic resonance imaging examination of the Framingham Heart Study. *Arterioscler Thromb Vasc Biol* **22**(5): 849–854.

16 Kathiresan, S., Larson, M.G., Keyes, M.J., *et al.* (2007) Assessment by cardiovascular magnetic resonance, electron beam computed tomography, and carotid ultrasonography of the distribution of subclinical atherosclerosis across Framingham risk strata. *Am J Cardiol* **99**(3): 310–314.

17 Yusuf, S., Hawken, S., Ounpuu, S., *et al.* (2004) Effect of potentially modifiable risk factors associated with myocardial infarction in 52 countries (the INTERHEART study): case-control study. *Lancet* **364**(9438): 937–952.

18 Stampfer, M.J., Hu, F.B., Manson, J.E., *et al.* (2000) Primary prevention of coronary heart disease in women through diet and lifestyle. *N Engl J Med* **343**(1): 16–22.

19 Ellis, J.J., Erickson, S.R., Stevenson, J.G., *et al.* (2004) Suboptimal statin adherence and discontinuation in primary and secondary prevention populations. *J Gen Intern Med* **19**(6): 638–645.

20 Newby, L.K., LaPointe, N.M., Chen, A.Y., *et al.* (2006) Long-term adherence to evidence-based secondary prevention therapies in coronary artery disease. *Circulation* **113**(2): 203–212.

21 Rupard, E.J., O'Malley, P.G., Jones, D.L., *et al.* Knowledge of preclinical coronary artery disease: the effect on motivation to change smoking behavior. *West J Med* (in press).

22 Wong, N.D., Detrano, R.C., Diamond, G., *et al.* (1996) Does coronary artery screening by electron beam computed tomography motivate potentially beneficial lifestyle behaviors? *Am J Cardiol* **78**(11): 1220–1223.

23 Shahab, L., Hall, S., Marteau, T. (2007) Showing smokers with vascular disease images of their arteries to motivate cessation: a pilot study. *Br J Health Psychol* **12**(Pt 2): 275–283.

24 Bovet, P., Perret, F., Cornuz, J., *et al.* (2002) Improved smoking cessation in smokers given ultrasound photographs of their own atherosclerotic plaques. *Prev Med* **34**(2): 215–220.

25 Bize, R., Burnand, B., Mueller, Y., Cornuz, J. (2005) Biomedical risk assessment as an aid for smoking cessation. *Cochrane Database Syst Rev* (**4**): CD004705.

26 O'Malley, P.G., Feuerstein, I.M., Taylor, A.J. (2003) Impact of electron beam tomography, with or without case management, on motivation, behavioral change, and cardiovascular risk profile: a randomized controlled trial. *JAMA* **289**(17): 2215–2223.

27 Lederman, J., Ballard, J., Njike, V.Y., *et al.* (2007) Information given to postmenopausal women on coronary computed tomography may influence cardiac risk reduction efforts. *J Clin Epidemiol* **60**(4): 389–396.

28 O'Malley, P.G., Kowalczyk, C., Bindeman, J., Taylor, A.J. (2006) A randomized trial assessing the impact of cardiovascular risk factor case-management on the metabolic syndrome. *J Cardiometabolic Syndrome* **1**(1): 6–12.

29 Vale, M.J., Jelinek, M.V., Best, J.D., *et al.* (2003) Coaching Patients on Achieving Cardiovascular Health (COACH): a multicenter randomized trial in patients with coronary heart disease. *Arch Intern Med* **163**(22): 2775–2783.

30 Grundy, S.M., Cleeman, J.I., Merz, C.N., *et al.* (2004) Implications of recent clinical trials for the National Cholesterol Education Program Adult Treatment Panel III guidelines. *Circulation* **110**(2): 227–239.

31 Taylor, A.J., Bindeman, J., Bauer, K., *et al.* (2007) Does the detection of coronary artery calcium lead to increased use of statin and aspirin in primary prevention? *Circulation* 114, II-823. Ref Type: Abstract.

32 Kalia, N.K., Miller, L.G., Nasir, K., *et al.* (2006) Visualizing coronary calcium is associated with improvements in adherence to statin therapy. *Atherosclerosis* **185**(2): 394–399.

33 Shaw, L.J., Berman, D.S., Bax, J.J., *et al.* (2005) Computed tomographic imaging within nuclear cardiology. *J Nucl Cardiol* **12**(1): 131–142.

34 Rozanski, A., Gransar, H., Wong, N.D., *et al.* (2007) Clinical outcomes after both coronary calcium scanning and exercise myocardial perfusion scintigraphy. *J Am Coll Cardiol* **49**(12): 1352–1361.

35 Caravalho, J., Jr., O'Donnell, S.D., Feuerstein, I.M., *et al.* (2002) Preoperative risk stratification using electron beam computed tomography in elective vascular surgery: relationship to clinical risk prediction and postoperative complications. *Ann Vasc Surg* **16**(5): 639–643.

36 Belhassen, L., Carville, C., Pelle, G., *et al.* (2002) Evaluation of carotid artery and aortic intima-media thickness measurements for exclusion of significant coronary atherosclerosis in patients scheduled for heart valve surgery. *J Am Coll Cardiol* **39**(7): 1139–1144.

37 Georgiou, D., Budoff, M.J., Kaufer, E., *et al.* (2001) Screening patients with chest pain in the emergency department using electron beam tomography: a follow-up study. *J Am Coll Cardiol* **38**(1): 105–10.

38 Laudon, D.A., Vukov, L.F., Breen, J.F., *et al.* (1999) Use of electron-beam computed tomography in the evaluation of chest pain patients in the emergency department. *Ann Emerg Med* **33**(1): 15–21.

39 McLaughlin, V.V., Balogh, T., Rich, S. (1999) Utility of electron beam computed tomography to stratify patients presenting to the emergency room with chest pain. *Am J Cardiol* **84**(3): 327–328, A8.

40 O'Malley, P.G., Greenberg, B.A., Taylor, A.J. (2004) Cost-effectiveness of using electron beam computed tomography to identify patients at risk for clinical coronary artery disease. *Am Heart J* **148**(1): 106–113.

41 Hausleiter, J., Meyer, T., Hadamitzky, M., *et al.* (2006) Prevalence of noncalcified coronary plaques by 64-slice computed tomography in patients with an intermediate risk for significant coronary artery disease. *J Am Coll Cardiol* **48**(2): 312–318.

42 Schmermund, A., Baumgart, D., Adamzik, M., *et al.* (1998) Comparison of electron-beam computed tomography and intracoronary ultrasound in detecting calcified and noncalcified plaques in patients with acute coronary syndromes and no or minimal to moderate angiographic coronary artery disease. *Am J Cardiol* **81**(2): 141–146.

43 Hausleiter, J., Meyer, T., Hadamitzky, M., *et al.* (2006) Prevalence of noncalcified coronary plaques by 64-slice computed tomography in patients with an intermediate risk for significant coronary artery disease. *J Am Coll Cardiol* **48**(2): 312–318.

PART III

Advanced Applications of CT and CMR Imaging

Chapter 17

Atherosclerosis Imaging: A Biological and Clinical Perspective

Peter Libby

We are currently witnessing an era of rapid evolution of cardiovascular imaging technologies. Much attention has focused on the potential of emerging imaging technologies to improve the noninvasive evaluation of atherosclerosis, a growing worldwide challenge to health and useful-life years. Given this expanding interest and realm of possibilities applicable to atherosclerosis imaging, a number of issues regarding the biology of this disease and its clinical expression require consideration. Indeed, concomitant with the rapid evolution in imaging technologies, the vascular biology of atherosclerosis and understanding of the clinical biology of this disease has changed considerably over the last decade [1–3]. Focusing imaging technologies on the biologically and medically most important questions requires an acquaintance with current concepts of the basic and clinical biology of this disease. This chapter aims to furnish a foundation for understanding the basic vascular biology of atherosclerosis from a clinical perspective. The union of clinical and basic biology with emerging imaging modalities promises to offer new options for the noninvasive evaluation of atherosclerosis, and to hasten the evaluation of novel therapies to lessen the clinical consequences of atherosclerotic cardiovascular disease.

Atherosclerotic Plaque Burden and Arterial Stenosis versus Clinical Events

For decades, the imaging of atherosclerosis has focused on assessing the degree of arterial stenosis at specific locations in the arterial tree. Angiographic techniques have provided a useful way of ascertaining information regarding the

Novel Techniques for Imaging the Heart, 1st edition. Edited by M. Di Carli and R. Kwong.
© 2008 American Heart Association, ISBN: 9-781-4051-7533-3.

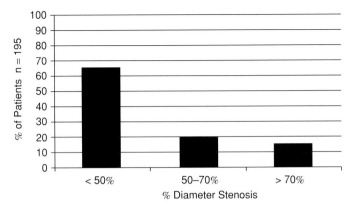

Smith, S.C.Circulation 1996; 93:2205-2211

Fig. 17.1 This graphic shows the degree of coronary artery stenosis on angiograms recorded before acute myocardial infarction. The 195 patients were from four studies: (1) Ambrose *et al., J Am Coll Cardiol* 1988; **12**: 56–62; (2) Giroud *et al., Am J Cardiol* 1992; **69**: 729–732; (3) Little *et al., Circulation* 1988; **78**: 1157–1166; and (4) Nobuyoshi *et al., J Am Coll Cardiol* 1991; **18**: 904–910.

localization and severity of arterial stenoses over the last half century. Many of our traditional treatment modalities aimed at combating atherosclerotic disease focus on stenoses. Revascularization by surgical or percutaneous techniques require a precise definition of the anatomy of arterial stenoses. The diagnostic information provided by traditional imaging techniques that identify stenoses goes hand-in-hand with revascularization therapies. Such imaging-directed revascularization strategies have proven highly effective in reducing ischemia due to arterial stenoses in the coronary, carotid, and peripheral beds.

Surprisingly, successful revascularization — although effective at relieving ischemia — has failed to forestall many morbid coronary events. We now recognize that most acute coronary syndromes derive from occlusions produced by thrombi rather than by the bulk of the atherosclerotic plaque itself [4,5]. This dawning recognition that acute thrombotic complications of atherosclerosis do not always correlate well with stenoses emerged from several lines of clinical evidence [4–6]. For example, serial angiographic studies performed independently in a number of centers yielded the surprising finding that the sites of culprit lesions that caused acute myocardial infarction on antecedent angiograms often had stenoses that would not cause flow limitation (Figure 17.1). Indeed, these serial studies showed that fewer than 20% of acute myocardial infarctions occurred at sites in the coronary arterial bed that had the angiographic appearance of stenoses greater than 60% on angiograms that had been recorded in the months preceding the acute coronary event. Serial angiographic findings in Europe and Japan show that the progression of coronary arterial stenoses did not occur in a linear monotonic fashion but appeared episodic, with periods of relative quiescence in growth punctuated by periods of more rapid progression of angiographic stenosis [7,8]. Angiographic studies performed on patients receiving thrombolytic therapy also proved revealing in this regard. After lysis of the culprit thrombus due to administration of lytic therapy, angiographic interrogation revealed an underlying stenosis of less than 60% in almost half of individuals undergoing a first myocardial infarction [9]. These convergent lines of angiographic evidence support the counterintuitive finding that many myocardial infarctions arise from lesions that do not produce critical coronary artery stenosis.

Observations performed by pathologists help us understand this disparity between angiographically determined stenoses and the propensity of plaque to produce an acute myocardial infarction. A number of independent studies of lesions that caused fatal acute myocardial infarction support the notion that a physical disruption of the atherosclerotic plaque rather than a critical stenosis causes fatal coronary events. Among several mechanisms of atherosclerotic plaque disruption that can provoke acute thrombosis, the rupture of the plaque's fibrous cap and superficial erosion of the endothelial lining cause most fatal thrombi [10,11]. Thus, an atherosclerotic plaque can rupture despite not causing a critical stenosis and provoking a fatal coronary event. The wall tension, a physical force that can promote plaque disruption, actually increases inversely with the degree of stenosis according to the Laplace relationship [12]. Clearly, highly stenotic coronary arterial plaques do cause acute myocardial infarctions. However, as nonocclusive atheromata far outnumber the relatively few critical stenoses, the majority of fatal coronary thrombi arise from plaques that by angiographic criteria we have traditionally considered "nonsignificant."

We have learned a great deal about the vascular biology of the types of plaque that appear particularly prone to provoking fatal coronary thrombosis (Figure 17.2). Basic scientific studies have established mechanisms that link inflammation to impaired ability of the arterial smooth muscle cell to elaborate the interstitial collagen needed to reinforce the plaque's fibrous skeleton that renders it resistant to rupture [13,14]. Inflammatory cells such as macrophages that accumulate in atheromatous plaques when exposed to pro-inflammatory cytokines can elaborate proteolytic enzymes that attack the macromolecules of the plaque's extracellular matrix that lend strength to the plaque's protective fibrous cap (Figure 17.3) [15–22]. Among several classes of collagen- and elastin-degrading enzymes, the matrix metalloproteinases and elastolytic cathepsins have received wide attention in this regard. Human atherosclerotic plaques that display markers of inflammation contain elevated levels of these extracellular matrix-degrading enzymes. Studies in genetically altered mice have shown the importance of proteolysis in regulating the collagen content and structure of experimental atherosclerotic plaques [23,24]. This conjunction of observations on human plaques and in vitro and in vivo laboratory experiments have

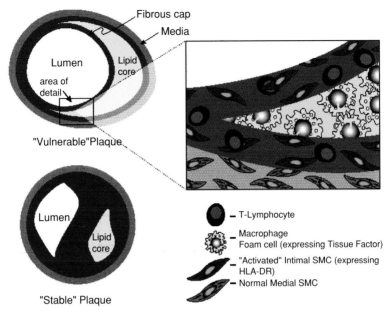

Fibrous cap
Media
Lumen
Lipid core
area of detail
"Vulnerable" Plaque
Lumen
Lipid core
"Stable" Plaque

— T-Lymphocyte
— Macrophage
  Foam cell (expressing Tissue Factor)
— "Activated" Intimal SMC (expressing HLA-DR)
— Normal Medial SMC

Fig. 17.2 A comparison of the characteristics attributed to "vulnerable" and "stable" plaques. The so-called "vulnerable" plaques often have a well-preserved lumen because plaques grow outward initially. The "vulnerable" plaque typically has a substantial lipid core and a thin fibrous cap separating the blood compartment from the lipid-rich core filled with macrophages bearing the potent pro-coagulant tissue factor. At sites of lesion disruption, smooth muscle cells (SMC) often display markers of an activated phenotype as detected by their expression of the transplantation antigen HLA-DR. In contrast, the stable plaque has a relatively thick fibrous cap protecting the lipid core from contact with the blood. Clinical data suggest that stable plaques more often show luminal narrowing detectable by angiography than do vulnerable plaques.

provided a strong link between inflammation and the integrity of the plaque's extracellular matrix, a critical determinant of the propensity to rupture. Moreover, when exposed to certain pro-inflammatory stimuli macrophages heighten their production of the potent pro-coagulant tissue factor [25]. Overexpression of tissue factor pro-coagulant documented in human atherosclerotic plaques can aggravate the thrombotic risk when a particular plaque disrupts. In this manner, inflammation not only controls the integrity of the plaque's extracellular matrix but also its thrombogenic potential.

The concept of arterial remodeling during atherogenesis has a major influence on our thinking about the distinction between the burden of disease, stenosis, and clinical events. Initial studies performed in experimental animals such as the nonhuman primates, and ultimately observations on atherosclerotic human arteries performed postmortem, pointed to a process of compensatory

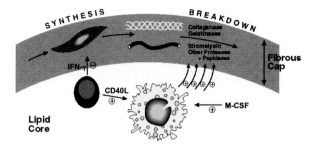

Fig. 17.3 Metabolism of collagen and elastin in the plaque's fibrous cap. The vascular smooth muscle cell synthesizes the extracellular matrix proteins collagen and elastin from amino acids. In the unstable plaque, interferon (IFN) -gamma secreted by activated T cells may inhibit collagen synthesis, interfering with the maintenance and repair of the collagenous framework of the plaque's fibrous cap. The activated macrophage secretes proteinases that can break down both collagen and elastin to peptides and eventually amino acids. This breakdown can weaken the fibrous cap, rendering it particularly susceptible to rupture and precipitation of acute coronary syndromes. IFN-gamma secreted by the T lymphocytes can also activate the macrophage. Plaques also contain other activators of macrophages, including tumor necrosis factor-alpha (TNFα), macrophage colony-stimulating factor (M-CSF), and macrophage chemoattractant protein-1 (MCP-1), among others.

enlargement during atherogenesis that preserves the lumen as the plaque enlarges due to "positive remodeling" or "compensatory enlargement" [26–28]. These experimental and human postmortem studies indicated that plaques grow initially in an outward abluminal direction, preserving a lumen until late in the stage of the disease. Invasive imaging studies using intravascular ultrasound have corroborated in living human patients the ubiquity of compensatory enlargement that preserves the lumen as the plaque enlarged outward [28]. This phenomenon of compensatory enlargement has major implications for the interpretation of lumenographic techniques such as coronary arteriography. Considerable plaque burden can accumulate in the coronary tree, which is invisible on the angiogram. These concealed or hidden plaques can be quite large and often harbor high degrees of inflammation. As noted previously, inflamed plaques tend to have impaired integrity of the protective fibrous cap and higher thrombogenicity than more fibrous or sclerotic plaques. Thus, the angiogram severely misleads the diagnostician regarding the actual burden of plaque, including many that share characteristics of those that have disrupted and provoked fatal thrombi.

The distinction between plaque burden, stenoses, and correlation of clinical events requires careful consideration when evaluating the information obtained from various imaging modalities. Traditional radiographic contrast angiography defines the lumen with high temporal and spatial resolution, but only indirectly discloses information regarding the arterial plaque. Angiographically apparent ulcers, filling defects, and certain patterns of irregularity can correlate with plaques that have produced thrombi or that have a high likelihood of doing so. Yet because of arterial remodeling, the angiogram cannot directly estimate plaque burden, nor can arteriography reliably disclose many characteristics of plaque related to thrombosis.

We have known for many years that the degree of coronary artery involvement as visualized on the arteriogram correlates with future clinical events. While serving as a marker of future coronary events, the very plaques that cause the events might not produce stenoses visible on the coronary arteriogram. By providing an index of the overall burden of coronary arterial atherosclerosis, the coronary arteriogram appears to serve as a marker of the nonstenotic plaques that "keep company" with the stenoses and on a lesion-per-lesion basis actually cause more acute myocardial infarction than the angiographically detected stenoses themselves.

The intima-media thickness of the carotid arteries detected ultrasonographically can visualize both actual atherosclerotic plaques and diffuse intimal thickening that can provide a fertile "soil" for atheroma growth or indicate a burden of atherosclerotic risk factors such as hypertension or dyslipidemia [29]. Certainly, considerable evidence supports the correlation of intima-media thickness with clinical events. Thus, when properly measured the carotid intima-media thickness serves as a validated biomarker of clinical cardiovascular complications [30]. However, this imaging modality does not visualize directly the culprit plaques that cause the vast majority of these events.

The measurement of coronary arterial calcium, first by electron beam computed tomography (EBCT) and more recently by successively more sophisticated multidetector computed tomographic (CT) scanners, has great appeal as a marker for coronary atherosclerotic disease burden [31–34]. As discussed in Chapter 15, a number of studies have shown positive correlations between the coronary calcium score and future cardiovascular events [35,36]. Issues regarding the selection of individuals entered into clinical cohorts to evaluate coronary calcium as a prognostic marker have given rise to some controversy. Others have argued that the information conveyed by the coronary calcium score might not add to the prognostic information already available from the application of classical coronary risk factors to individual patients.

However, recent studies affirm the ability of the calcium score to independently predict cardiovascular events. Curiously, calcified coronary plaques can themselves be less prone to provoking coronary thromboses, and hence acute coronary syndromes, than less calcified lipid-rich plaques. In one study, coronary calcium in individual lesions was assessed by acoustic shadowing as detected by intravascular ultrasound in a series of patients with stable angina pectoris or acute coronary syndromes [37]. The stenotic plaques responsible for the ischemia in the patients with stable angina tended to have more calcium than the plaques responsible for unstable angina. From the perspective of vascular biology, the lipid-rich plaque with many inflammatory cells may more likely rupture and cause coronary thrombosis than sclerotic calcified plaques that have a dense extracellular matrix component. Several postmortem studies have shown that culprit plaques of acute coronary syndromes have thinner fibrous caps than nonthrombosed plaques. As both lipid-rich plaques filled with inflammatory cells and atheromatous gruel coexist in the same coronary circulation with sclerotic calcified plaques, the correlation between calcium score and cardiovascular events might once again reflect the ability of the calcium score to indicate the overall burden of disease, although the very lesions that cause calcification may have less tendency on a per-plaque basis to cause thrombotic complications than the noncalcified plaques.

The distinction between lipid-rich atheromatous plaques and sclerotic calcified plaques has gained considerable currency in the field of computed tomographic angiographic (CTA) examination of the coronary arteries. Imaging specialists commonly refer to calcified plaques as "hard plaques" and to noncalcified plaques as "soft plaques." As opposed to EBCT, the CT angiogram promises to provide views not just of the lumen as in coronary arteriography, or of the amount of calcification as EBCT, but of both the lumen and the arterial wall. As the technology improves, greater degrees of resolution and shorter examination times increase the power of CTA techniques. From the perspective of the vascular biologist, the commonly employed terms "hard plaque" and "soft plaque" seem oversimplified. As CTA makes no biomechanical measurements, using terms that imply biomaterial properties seems inappropriate. Indeed, calcium within lesions can provide inhomogeneities in biomaterial properties that could increase stresses within the plaque and precipitate disruption [38]. However, recent bioengineering modeling has shown that microscopic collections of calcium within arterial plaques can dramatically alter the calculated local stress in the plaque [39]. Such microcalcifications on the order of 10 μm could evade the resolution of even the latest generation of CT scanners. Thus, plaques with clinically important calcium collections might appear "soft" by CTA, and lesions that contain considerable calcium could cause stenoses but might have less propensity to rupture and cause thrombotic events. Once again, as with the modalities discussed previously, CT visualization of atherosclerotic plaques — and in particular, their calcium content — may provide a biomarker of the burden of disease but not necessarily identify individual plaques at a high risk of rupture.

In sum, each anatomical imaging modality discussed here has promise as a biomarker of disease burden. Yet given the dissociation between the degree of stenosis, calcium content, and actual likelihood of precipitating a clinical event, these anatomical imaging modalities fall short of the ability to characterize an individual plaque in this regard, both with respect to theoretical considerations or convincing prospective clinical studies. Although these anatomical imaging modalities provide a foundation for the contemporary practice of cardiovascular medicine and surgery, future developments should strive to reach beyond anatomy and harness advances in vascular biology to gain more specific information about individual plaques and their clinical import beyond causing ischemia.

Toward Functional or Molecular Imaging of Atherosclerotic Plaques

The vascular biology of atherosclerosis promises to provide a myriad of molecular processes that could serve as targets for novel imaging technologies. These targets include endothelial activation; the recruitment, accumulation, and activation of inflammatory leukocytes; smooth muscle cell accumulation and activation; visualization of effector molecules of inflammation implicated in complications of atherosclerosis, or of metabolic activity of cells within the atherosclerotic plaque; procoagulant properties; proteinases; and reactive oxygen species, among others [40]. The next section will briefly introduce each of these biological processes and illustrate how molecular imaging might harness them.

Endothelial Activation

Even before atherosclerotic lesions form, risk factors associated with atherogenesis alter the function of the luminal endothelial cells in arteries. The endothelial monolayer in healthy arteries resists prolonged contact with blood leukocytes, elaborated endogenous vasodilator molecules, and displays a number of properties that combat thrombosis, favor fibrinolysis, and express antioxidant enzymes such as superoxide dismutase that can inactivate reactive oxygen species. Laminar sheer stress characteristic of normal arteries tends to promote these homeostatic endothelial functions [41–43]. However, when exposed to disturbed flow rather than laminar sheer stress, and in the presence of pro-atherogenic mediators such as modified lipoprotein or pro-inflammatory cytokines, endothelial cells become "dysfunctional." This laboratory jargon refers to a state of the endothelium in which production of endogenous vasodilators climbs, the elaboration of reactive oxygen species increases, adhesion molecules that promote the recruitment of leukocytes increase, and inhibitors of fibrinolysis increase, promoting the stability of thrombi.

Among these properties associated with endothelial dysfunction, the expression of leukocyte adhesion molecules has incited considerable interest as a target for molecular imaging. Of the leukocyte adhesion molecules expressed by endothelial cells in atherosclerotic lesions, vascular cell adhesion molecule-1 (VCAM-1) has gained wide acceptance as a marker of endothelial activation. Decreased function of VCAM-1 achieved by genetic manipulation limits experimental atherosclerosis in mice [44]. Thus, the plausibility of VCAM-1 as a direct marker of activated or dysfunctional endothelial cells has broad biological support. Unfortunately, the thin monolayer of endothelial cells that lines blood vessels provides a poor target for imaging, though in human atherosclerotic lesions the plexus of microvessels within plaques express much of the VCAM-1 [45]. There is considerable controversy regarding the ability of antibodies directed against VCAM-1 and coupled to various imaging indicators to serve as effective imaging agents. Evidence is increasing that under certain circumstances, VCAM-1 can internalize ligands and thus cause them to accumulate in activated endothelial and perhaps smooth muscle cells. In preliminary experimental work, magneto-optical agents internalized by VCAM-1 have demonstrated the feasibility for imaging atherosclerotic plaques, not based on anatomy but on the degree of endothelial activation [46]. The example of VCAM-1 illustrates how a well-defined molecular target with considerable biological and clinical validation may provide a molecular window on atherogenesis beyond anatomy.

In addition to leukocyte adhesion molecules, certain markers associated with an angiogenic phenotype of endothelial cells have undergone exploration as potential targets for molecular imaging. In particular, certain integrins expressed by microvessels in atherosclerotic arteries (notably $alpha_v beta_3$) may provide a functional window on angiogenesis in plaques, a process implicated in their complication [47].

Macrophage Accumulation and Activation

Once bound by endothelial leukocyte adhesion molecules such as VCAM-1, blood leukocytes can penetrate into the intima in response to chemoattractant mediators overexpressed in plaque. Mononuclear phagocytes, the most numerous of blood leukocytes recruited to atheromata, enter the arterial wall as monocytes and mature into macrophages. These cells express a number of functions that could provide targets for molecular imaging. For example, one could track the accumulation of these cells within lesions. As macrophages bear various markers on their surface, like many leukocytic subtypes, detection of the number of macrophages might provide a window on the accumulation of these inflammatory cells in plaque. Recent work has highlighted the heterogeneity of monocytes recruited to experimental atheromata [48]. In particular, subtypes of monocytes that bear markers of an inflammatory subset (high levels of an antigen known as Ly6c in mice) appear to accumulate preferentially in plaques and give rise to inflammatory macrophages. The extension of these observations in mice to human beings might reveal markers of particular monocyte/macrophage subsets that could provide targets for molecular imaging in the future.

Among the functions of macrophages, phagocytosis provides an enticing target for molecular imaging because it involves the uptake and intracellular accumulation of the phagocytic target, enhancing potential signals. A number of groups have explored the use of ultrasmall particulate iron oxide particles (USPIO) as potential markers of macrophage accumulation. Under T2-weighted imaging conditions, USPIO cause an attenuation of signal. Promising small-scale clinical imaging studies have established the possibility of imaging phagocytosis by macrophages within plaques, by macrophages, and perhaps other cells as a target for molecular imaging [49–51]. These preliminary observations certainly warrant follow-up in larger scale rigorous clinical investigations, correlated with histopathologic examination, and ultimately clinical event prediction.

Activated macrophages may have greater reliance on glycolytic pathways than other cells within plaques. There is currently great interest in the use of metabolic markers such as fluorodeoxyglucose (FDG) as a marker of glucose uptake, and hence the metabolic activity of cells within plaques, presumably activated macrophages. Although the detection of deoxyglucose tagged with ^{18}F provides ready external detection, CT or magnetic resonance techniques afford higher resolution. Hybrid positron emission tomographic (PET)-CT techniques promise to colocalize anatomical features with the PET signal, providing a complementary anatomicofunctional approach to imaging atherosclerosis. A number of preclinical and clinical studies have established the ability of PET scanning to localize FDG signals in the regions of diseased arteries [52,53].

Correlations with the number of macrophages provide a promising indicator of colocalization of FDG signal with the accumulation of inflammatory cells, though they do not themselves establish that the macrophages are the source of the signal [54]. Indeed, in mice brown fat surrounding arteries appears to provide a confounding source of FDG uptake in the region of mouse atherosclerotic vessels [55]. Although FDG uptake requires more rigorous validation as a marker of inflammation in atherosclerosis, its feasibility and ready clinical applicability has proven enticing. Validation of the use of this modality will require rigorous study of the regulation of glucose uptake in cells found in plaques and in the ability of FDG signals to predict clinical atherosclerotic events.

One of the principal properties of phagocytic cells within plaques is the elaboration of proteinases. The pathophysiologic role of matrix-degrading proteinases in weakening the fibrous skeleton of plaques discussed previously provides a firm pathophysiologic foundation for proteases as a target for molecular imaging in plaques. Moreover, the catalytic power of enzymes provides an amplifier of signals that should increase signal-to-background ratio. Based on strong clinical and histopathological observations on human atheromata, certain matrix metalloproteinases and elastolytic cathepsins provide promising targets for molecular imaging. Near-infrared fluorescent probes for matrix metalloproteinases can localize proteolytic activity within mouse atherosclerotic plaques. Cathepsin B, the matrix metalloproteinases, and the potent elastase cathepsin K provide plausible targets for molecular imaging [56,57]. Preclinical studies have established the feasibility of imaging these proteases implicated in plaque "destabilization," and thus clinical events. As pro-inflammatory cytokines augment the expression of these matrix-degrading proteinases in cells found in atheromata, including monocyte/macrophages, imaging these proteinases can provide a window not only on a specific pathobiological process (protein catabolism) but also a basic biological process strongly implicated in the biology of plaque complication.

Activated macrophages, smooth muscle cells, and endothelial cells can elaborate reactive oxygen species that contribute to oxidative stress within atheromata, promote cellular damage or death, and thus serve as both a marker of inflammatory activation and a mediator of pathogenic processes in atheromata. Among the generators of oxidative stress, NADPH oxidases that produce superoxide anions and myeloperoxidase that generates hypochlorous acid (HOCl) have generated considerable interest in the realm of atherosclerosis research [58–60]. These two reactive oxygen species provide plausible targets for molecular imaging. In preliminary work, the product of myeloperoxidase, hypochlorous acid, has undergone preliminary evaluation as a target for molecular imaging. Sensors for hypochlorite anion (OCl^-) exist. The optimization of hypochlorite probes might provide a detector for oxidative stress in atherosclerosis and other conditions [61]. While very preliminary, these initial investigations indicate the feasibility of monitoring oxidative stress in atheromata, providing yet another window on cellular functions that can add to anatomical features in determining the clinical significance of individual plaques.

The clinical application of such molecular imaging technologies will require considerable technological advance and rigorous validation. Yet we are inevitably approaching an era when we will fruitfully harness advances in the biology of atherosclerosis to evolving imaging technologies to go beyond structure and enhance our ability to determine clinically important characteristics of atheromata.

A Clinician's Perspective on the Integration of Atherosclerosis Imaging into Practice

From the clinician's perspective, the burgeoning of novel imaging approaches to atherosclerosis offers a number of exciting practical applications. The concluding segment of this chapter provides a highly personal viewpoint regarding the practical clinical application of these emerging modalities. I consider the use of imaging tools as aids to cardiovascular investigation and development and evaluation of therapies, as well as the use in risk stratification in apparently well individuals ("primary prevention") and in patients with established atherosclerotic cardiovascular disease ("secondary prevention").

Cardiovascular Imaging in Investigation and Therapeutic Development and Evaluation

Researchers have arrived at a very gratifying point in an understanding of the vascular biology of atherosclerosis. In vitro studies have revealed a great deal about the fundamental molecular mechanisms of processes that lead to atheroma formation and complication. In vivo experiments, most recently using genetically modified mice, have accelerated our ability to test the causality of various hypotheses regarding the pathobiology of atherosclerosis in vivo. Much of our clinical extension of this exciting vascular biology relies on the sampling of peripheral blood, a distant window indeed on the atherosclerotic plaque [2]. We have also learned a great deal from the histopathologic, biochemical, and molecular analysis of specimens retrieved at endarterectomy, atherectomy, or postmortem examination. However, these opportunities to examine human tissues represent merely one "slice in time" in the life history of an atheroma that can evolve over many decades. Molecular imaging technologies that report on specific pathobiological processes promise to provide a tool for the in vivo validation of our mechanistic hypotheses in intact human subjects. From this perspective, I view the development of molecular imaging of atherosclerosis as imperative to the clinical extension of the rich fabric of vascular biology woven by investigations over the last several decades.

We have reached an excruciatingly difficult point in the evaluation of novel therapeutic approaches to modifying atherosclerosis. Heartened by the success of statins and other proven modalities in preventing cardiovascular events, and by the identification of novel therapeutic targets such as those discussed here, we are equipped to develop novel therapeutics to address the unacceptable residual burden of morbidity and mortality due to atherosclerosis. Yet the very success of our therapies frustrates our ability to perform clinical evaluations that assess "hard" clinical endpoints such as myocardial infarction or cardiovascular death. The efficacy of standard therapies has lowered event rates to the extent that clinical trials powered to show benefits of novel therapeutics over and above currently accepted standard of care require large numbers of enrollees and longer periods of time than previously.

Even the best-funded entities, public or private, can finance only a limited number of such "hard endpoint" clinical trials in the cardiovascular arena. Therefore, we have an urgent need to develop biomarkers of efficacy of novel therapeutics to provide a way station on the road to their ultimate validation in studies that evaluate clinical endpoints. Eventually, some of the emerging imaging modalities discussed in this volume may achieve the status of surrogate endpoints for regulatory approval and clinical adoption of novel therapeutics [62]. However, in the current environment it appears that the use of imaging modalities as surrogate endpoints for these purposes will require a great deal of further validation. However, there is no obstacle in principle to adopting molecular imaging strategies that report on specific pathobiological processes to provide early clinical signals regarding the ability of novel therapeutics to influence the targeted process in vivo. Clinical studies of a relatively modest scale might provide assurance that a novel agent actually affects the target in vivo. Imaging reporters might provide a way of choosing doses of new drugs to be subsequently tested in more lengthy clinical trials on greater numbers of individuals monitored by clinical endpoints. Thus, molecular imaging modalities have the potential to expedite the development and evaluation of novel therapies and their clinical introduction.

Currently available anatomical imaging modalities have had variable success in aiding drug development. Intravascular ultrasound reports reliably on plaque volume but lacks the resolution required to determine the thickness of a plaque's fibrous cap. Radiofrequency information available from ultrasound examinations may provide information regarding tissue characterization [63]. However, to date methodologies such as palpography and virtual histology require further validation to serve as biomarkers for future clinical events. Although an indicator of disease burden and cardiovascular events, coronary calcium has not proven to indicate efficacy of therapeutics. For example, in the BELLES trial, a statin treatment regimen known to reduce events did not alter coronary calcium content as detected by EBCT [64].

The Role of Atherosclerosis Imaging in Primary Prevention

The screening of low-risk populations according to current guidelines requires the evaluation of certain readily obtainable features of the clinical history and well-established and validated biomarkers such as blood pressure, glucose measurements, and the lipid profile. These widely adopted and well-validated tools provide a great deal of information regarding the risk for first-ever cardiovascular events. Risk assessment tools such as the Framingham algorithm illustrate the utility of inexpensive and readily available biomarkers of cardiovascular risk in apparently well populations.

A number of emerging biomarkers may help sharpen risk prediction over and above the well-validated and accepted variables such as those used in the Framingham algorithm. Among these emerging biomarkers, C-reactive protein (CRP) measured by a high sensitivity assay (hsCRP) by many metrics adds to the predictive power of the Framingham covariates in risk prediction in both women and men [65]. Even an inexpensive and readily measured blood biomarker such as hsCRP has engendered considerable controversy as to its "added value" over the Framingham algorithm and its cost effectiveness in clinical practice as a screening tool for low-risk populations. Many other blood biomarkers, buttressed by less abundant data, vie for addition to the traditional Framingham covariates.

It is highly unlikely that an imaging modality will prove cost-effective or of "added value" in screening low-risk populations. This controversial personal viewpoint rests on two principles. First, emerging imaging modalities involve technological platforms that entail considerable expense. Although cost will inevitably drop as a function of scale and evolving technologies, it is highly unlikely that imaging modalities will supplant traditional risk factors and simple blood biomarkers as a first-level screening tool, even if they could add to their predictive power.

A second major limitation of imaging modalities in screening I have categorized as the "incidentaloma problem." Just as body surveys with CT can reveal unsuspected lesions that often precipitate further diagnostic follow-up in asymptomatic individuals, one must be concerned that identifying "silent" atherosclerotic disease may lead to further diagnostic and therapeutic interventions that entrain considerable expense and risk without promising clinical benefit. One cannot make an asymptomatic individual feel better. Scant evidence supports the ability of any revascularization intervention to prevent events or prolong life in broad categories of asymptomatic individuals, particularly when pitted against intensive medical management. Existing risk-prediction engines can stratify well populations for "preventive" therapies in a cost-effective fashion. I have great concern that using any imaging technology for atherosclerosis in apparently well populations may open Pandora's box and expose individuals to needless worry, expense, and risk without promising benefit. Future findings might assuage these concerns regarding the application of imaging to screening low-risk populations. The adoption of imaging to screen unselected low-risk individuals for atherosclerosis should await the rigorous evaluation of clinical efficacy and cost-effectiveness.

The Use of Imaging Modalities in Secondary Prevention

Individuals who have established atherosclerosis have a high risk of recurrent events. They warrant aggressive secondary prevention therapies according to established guidelines today. Given the unacceptable residual burden of events in individuals with established atherosclerosis, the implementation of imaging strategies for further risk stratification appears attractive. However, the use of imaging strategies even in secondary prevention scenarios requires careful consideration. Certainly, methods that rely on the detection of stenoses may not reveal potentially dangerous plaques that do not cause arterial stenosis. Moreover, most patients with established atherosclerotic disease will receive contemporary therapies that modify the biology of the plaque. For example, statins likely exert direct anti-inflammatory actions in addition to their LDL-lowering effects, and by both of these mechanisms may alter features of the plaque that render them less likely to rupture and cause thrombotic events. Despite these qualitative changes in plaques, the degree of stenosis may not decrease significantly with statin treatment. Thus, anatomical imaging modalities may not reliably report on cardiovascular risk in patients with atherosclerosis. Even if we had molecular imaging technologies in hand ready for clinical application, they would require considerable rigorous validation to warrant adoption in clinical practice. Patients with established atherosclerosis most often have widespread arterial involvement.

Recent studies have indicated that revascularization strategies may not provide a clinical benefit in a number of categories of individuals with established coronary disease. In the recent Open Artery Trial (OAT), revascularization in patients with acute myocardial infarction did not confer a survival benefit unless performed within the first days [66]. In patients with chronic stable angina, even those with considerable angiographic stenotic disease, revascularization strategies did not add benefit beyond intensive medical management [67]. Thus, we must not assume that interventions that target stenoses will improve clinical outcomes, despite their potential for complications and their expense and, in the case of drug-eluting stents, their commitment to long-term antiplatelet therapy.

Conclusions

We are entering an exciting era of accelerated application of emerging imaging modalities to patients with or at risk for atherosclerosis. No doubt many of these modalities will enter routine clinical practice in the future. The optimum adoption of emerging imaging modalities in cardiovascular practice will require consideration of some of the biological and clinical concerns discussed here. Certainly, imaging modalities will provide important investigative tools and new biomarkers for drug development and the evaluation of therapy. The use of imaging strategies in addition to established risk algorithms in patients with or without established atherosclerotic disease will require rigorous validation. It is likely that the cost-beneficial application of emerging imaging modalities for atherosclerosis will employ a tiered approach. Established clinical and laboratory biomarkers, and a few emerging biomarkers, will provide a first step in risk stratification. Those in whom a combination of traditional and emerging blood or genetic biomarkers of disease suggest heightened cardiovascular risk may prove appropriate subjects for the cost-beneficial application of imaging modalities. Carefully deployed, there is little doubt that new cardiovascular imaging techniques will add enormously to the practice of clinical cardiovascular medicine in years to come, and will help us tailor and personalize our management strategies for individual patients.

References

1 Tsimikas, S., *et al.* (2005) Oxidized phospholipids, Lp(a) lipoprotein, and coronary artery disease. *N Engl J Med* **353**(1): 46–57.
2 Libby, P., Ridker, P.M. (2006) Inflammation and atherothrombosis: from population biology and bench research to clinical practice. *J Am Coll Cardiol* **48**: A33–46.
3 Hansson, G.K., Libby, P. (2006) The immune response in atherosclerosis: a double-edged sword. *Nat Rev Immunol* **6**(7): 508–519.
4 Corti, R., Fuster, V., Badimon, J.J. (2003) Pathogenetic concepts of acute coronary syndromes. *J Am Coll Cardiol* **41**(4 Suppl S): 7S–14S.

5 Libby, P., Theroux, P. (2005) Pathophysiology of coronary artery disease. *Circulation* **111**: 3481–3488.

6 Smith, S., Jr., (1996) Risk-reduction therapy: the challenge to change. *Circulation* **93**(12): 2205–2211.

7 Bruschke, A.V., *et al.* (1989) The dynamics of progression of coronary atherosclerosis studied in 168 medically treated patients who underwent coronary arteriography three times. *Am Heart J* **117**(2): 296–305.

8 Yokoya, K., *et al.* (1999) Process of progression of coronary artery lesions from mild or moderate stenosis to moderate or severe stenosis: a study based on four serial coronary arteriograms per year. *Circulation* **100**(9): 903–909.

9 Hackett, D., Davies, G., Maseri, A. (1988) Pre-existing coronary stenoses in patients with first myocardial infarction are not necessarily severe. *Eur Heart J* **9**(12): 1317–1323.

10 Loree, H.M., *et al.* (1992) Effects of fibrous cap thickness on peak circumferential stress in model atherosclerotic vessels. *Circ Res* **71**(4): 850–858.

11 Virmani, R., *et al.* (2006) Pathology of the vulnerable plaque. *J Am Coll Cardiol* **47**(8 Suppl): C13–18.

12 Loree, H.M., *et al.* (1994) Static circumferential tangential modulus of human atherosclerotic tissue. *J Biomech* **27**(2): 195–204.

13 Amento, E.P., *et al.* (1991) Cytokines and growth factors positively and negatively regulate interstitial collagen gene expression in human vascular smooth muscle cells. *Arterioscler Thromb Vasc Biol* **11**: 1223–1230.

14 Rekhter, M., *et al.* (1993) Type I collagen gene expression in human atherosclerosis. Localization to specific plaque regions. *Am J Pathol* **143**: 1634–1648.

15 Henney, A.M., *et al.* (1991) Localization of stromelysin gene expression in atherosclerotic plaques by in situ hybridization. *Proc Natl Acad Sci USA* **88**(18): 8154–8158.

16 Galis, Z., *et al.* (1994) Increased expression of matrix metalloproteinases and matrix degrading activity in vulnerable regions of human atherosclerotic plaques. *J Clin Invest* **94**: 2493–2503.

17 Sukhova, G.K., *et al.* (1999) Evidence for increased collagenolysis by interstitial collagenases-1 and -3 in vulnerable human atheromatous plaques. *Circulation* **99**(19): 2503–2509.

18 Sukhova, G.K., *et al.* (1998) Expression of the elastolytic cathepsins S and K in human atheroma and regulation of their production in smooth muscle cells. *J Clin Invest* **102**(3): 576–583.

19 Herman, M.P., *et al.* (2001) Expression of neutrophil collagenase (matrix metalloproteinase-8) in human atheroma: a novel collagenolytic pathway suggested by transcriptional profiling. *Circulation* **104**(16): 1899–1904.

20 Dollery, C.M., Libby, P. (2006) Atherosclerosis and proteinase activation. *Cardiovasc Res* **69**(3): 625–635.

21 Nikkari, S.T., *et al.* (1995) Interstitial collagenase (MMP-1) expression in human carotid atherosclerosis. *Circulation* **92**(6): 1393–1398.

22 Liu, J., *et al.* (2004) Lysosomal cysteine proteases in atherosclerosis. *Arterioscler Thromb Vasc Biol* **24**(8): 1359–1366.

23 Fukumoto, Y., *et al.* (2004) Genetically determined resistance to collagenase action augments interstitial collagen accumulation in atherosclerotic plaques. *Circulation* **110**(14): 1953–1959.

24 Deguchi, J.O., *et al.* (2005) Matrix metalloproteinase-13/collagenase-3 deletion promotes collagen accumulation and organization in mouse atherosclerotic plaques. *Circulation* **112**(17): 2708–2715.

25 Mach, F., *et al.* (1997) Activation of monocyte/macrophage functions related to acute atheroma complication by ligation of CD40: induction of collagenase, stromelysin, and tissue factor. *Circulation* **96**: 396–399.

26 Clarkson, T.B., *et al.* (1994) Remodeling of coronary arteries in human and nonhuman primates. *JAMA* **271**(4): 289–294.

27 Glagov, S., *et al.* (1987) Compensatory enlargement of human atherosclerotic coronary arteries. *N Engl J Med* **316**: 371–375.

28 Schoenhagen, P., *et al.* (2000) Extent and direction of arterial remodeling in stable versus unstable coronary syndromes: an intravascular ultrasound study. *Circulation* **101**(6): 598–603.

29 Schwartz, S.M. (1999) The intima: a new soil. *Circ Res* **85**(10): 877–879.

30 Taylor, A.J. (2002) Atherosclerosis imaging to detect and monitor cardiovascular risk. *Am J Cardiol* **90**(10C): 8L–11L.

31 Greenland, P., *et al.* (2007) ACCF/AHA 2007 clinical expert consensus document on coronary artery calcium scoring by computed tomography in global cardiovascular risk assessment and in evaluation of patients with chest pain: a report of the American College of Cardiology Foundation Clinical Expert Consensus Task Force (ACCF/AHA writing committee to update the 2000 expert consensus document on electron beam computed tomography). *Circulation* **115**(3): 402–426.

32 Kronmal, R.A., *et al.* (2007) Risk factors for the progression of coronary artery calcification in asymptomatic subjects: results from the Multi-ethnic Study of Atherosclerosis (MESA). *Circulation* **115**(21): 2722–2730.

33 Cordeiro, M.A., Lima, J.A. (2006) Atherosclerotic plaque characterization by multidetector row computed tomography angiography. *J Am Coll Cardiol* **47**(8 Suppl): C40–47.

34 Fayad, Z.A., *et al.* (2002) Computed tomography and magnetic resonance imaging for noninvasive coronary angiography and plaque imaging: current and potential future concepts. *Circulation* **106**(15): 2026–2034.

35 Greenland, P., *et al.* (2004) Coronary artery calcium score combined with Framingham score for risk prediction in asymptomatic individuals. *JAMA* **291**(2): 210–215.

36 Budoff, M.J., *et al.* (2007) Long-term prognosis associated with coronary calcification: observations from a registry of 25,253 patients. *J Am Coll Cardiol* **49**(18): 1860–1870.

37 Beckman, J.A., *et al.* (2001) Relationship of clinical presentation and calcification of culprit coronary artery stenoses. *Arterioscler Thromb Vasc Biol* **21**(10): 1618–1622.

38 Loree, H.M., *et al.* (1994) Static circumferential tangential modulus of human atherosclerotic tissue. *J Biomech* **27**(2): 195–204.

39 Vengrenyuk, Y., *et al.* (2006) A hypothesis for vulnerable plaque rupture due to stress-induced debonding around cellular microcalcifications in thin fibrous caps. *Proc Natl Acad Sci USA* **103**(40): 14678–14683.

40 Jaffer, F.A., Libby, P., Weissleder, R. (2007) Molecular imaging of cardiovascular disease. *Circulation* **116**(9): 1052–1061.

41 Gimbrone, M.A., Jr., *et al.* (2000) Endothelial dysfunction, hemodynamic forces, and atherogenesis. *Ann NY Acad Sci* **902**: 230–239; disc. 239–240.

42 Libby, P., Aikawa, M., Jain, M.K. (2006) Vascular endothelium and atherosclerosis. *Handb Exp Pharmacol* **176**(Pt 2): 285–306.

43 Dai, G., *et al.* (2007) Biomechanical forces in atherosclerosis-resistant vascular regions regulate endothelial redox balance via phosphoinositol 3-kinase/Akt-dependent activation of Nrf2. *Circ Res* **101**(7): 723–733.

44 Cybulsky, M.I., *et al.* (2001) A major role for VCAM-1, but not ICAM-1, in early atherosclerosis. *J Clin Invest* **107**(10): 1255–1262.

45 O'Brien, K., *et al.* (1993) Vascular cell adhesion molecule-1 is expressed in human coronary atherosclerotic plaques: implications for the mode of progression of advanced coronary atherosclerosis. *J Clin Invest* **92**: 945–951.

46 Nahrendorf, M., *et al.* (2006) Noninvasive vascular cell adhesion molecule-1 imaging identifies inflammatory activation of cells in atherosclerosis. *Circulation* **114**(14): 1504–1511.

47 Winter, P.M., *et al.* (2003) Molecular imaging of angiogenesis in early-stage atherosclerosis with alpha(v)beta3-integrin-targeted nanoparticles. *Circulation* **108**(18): 2270–2274.

48 Tacke, F., *et al.* (2007) Monocyte subsets differentially employ CCR2, CCR5, and CX3CR1 to accumulate within atherosclerotic plaques. *J Clin Invest* **117**(1): 185–194.

49 Kooi, M.E., *et al.* (2003) Accumulation of ultrasmall superparamagnetic particles of iron oxide in human atherosclerotic plaques can be detected by in vivo magnetic resonance imaging. *Circulation* **107**(19): 2453–2458.

50 Durand, E., *et al.* (2007) Magnetic resonance imaging of ruptured plaques in the rabbit with ultrasmall superparamagnetic particles of iron oxide. *J Vasc Res* **44**(2): 119–128.

51 von Zur Muhlen, C., *et al.* (2007) Superparamagnetic iron oxide binding and uptake as imaged by magnetic resonance is mediated by the integrin receptor Mac-1 (CD11b/CD18): implications on imaging of atherosclerotic plaques. *Atherosclerosis* **193**(1): 102–111.

52 Rudd, J.H., *et al.* (2007) (18)Fluorodeoxyglucose positron emission tomography imaging of atherosclerotic plaque inflammation is highly reproducible: implications for atherosclerosis therapy trials. *J Am Coll Cardiol* **50**(9): 892–86.

53 Tawakol, A., *et al.* (2005) Noninvasive in vivo measurement of vascular inflammation with F-18 fluorodeoxyglucose positron emission tomography. *J Nucl Cardiol* **12**(3): 294–301.

54 Tawakol, A., *et al.* (2006) In vivo 18F-fluorodeoxyglucose positron emission tomography imaging provides a noninvasive measure of carotid plaque inflammation in patients. *J Am Coll Cardiol* **48**(9): 1818–1824.

55 Laurberg, J.M., *et al.* (2007) Imaging of vulnerable atherosclerotic plaques with FDG-microPET: no FDG accumulation. *Atherosclerosis* **192**(2): 275–282.

56 Chen, J., *et al.* (2002) In vivo imaging of proteolytic activity in atherosclerosis. *Circulation* **105**(23): 2766–2771.

57 Jaffer, F.A., *et al.* (2007) Optical visualization of cathepsin K activity in atherosclerosis with a novel, protease-activatable fluorescence sensor. *Circulation* **115**(17): 2292–2298.

58 Heinecke, J.W. (2003) Oxidative stress: new approaches to diagnosis and prognosis in atherosclerosis. *Am J Cardiol* **91**(3A): 12A–16A.

59 Seshiah, P.N., *et al.* (2002) Angiotensin II stimulation of NAD(P)H oxidase activity: upstream mediators. *Circ Res* **91**(5): 406–413.

60 Hazen, S.L. (2004) Myeloperoxidase and plaque vulnerability. *Arterioscler Thromb Vasc Biol* **24**(7): 1143–1146.

61 Shepherd, J., *et al.* (2007) A fluorescent probe for the detection of myeloperoxidase activity in atherosclerosis-associated macrophages. *Chem Biol* **14**(11): 1221–1231.

62 Tardif, J.C., *et al.* (2006) Vascular biomarkers and surrogates in cardiovascular disease. *Circulation* **113**(25): 2936–2942.

63 Schaar, J.A., *et al.* (2003) Characterizing vulnerable plaque features with intravascular elastography. *Circulation* **108**(21): 2636–2641.

64 Raggi, P., *et al.* (2005) Aggressive versus moderate lipid-lowering therapy in hypercholesterolemic postmenopausal women: Beyond Endorsed Lipid Lowering with EBT Scanning (BELLES). *Circulation* **112**(4): 563–571.

65 Ridker, P.M., *et al.* (2007) Development and validation of improved algorithms for the assessment of global cardiovascular risk in women: the Reynolds Risk Score. *JAMA* **297**(6): 611–619.

66 Hochman, J.S., *et al.* (2006) Coronary intervention for persistent occlusion after myocardial infarction. *N Engl J Med* **355**(23): 2395–2407.

67 Boden, W.E., *et al.* (2007) Optimal medical therapy with or without PCI for stable coronary disease. *N Engl J Med* **356**(15): 1503–1516.

Chapter 18

Stem Cell Imaging

Dara L. Kraitchman

The introduction of new gene, protein, and cellular therapies to treat cardiovascular disease has created new challenges for noninvasive imaging. In particular, the ability to image stem cells can be used to direct cellular delivery to specific anatomical locations, determine cell engraftment, and potentially to determine the fate of stem cells in vivo. The frequency with which routine magnetic resonance imaging (MRI) or computed tomography (CT) examinations are used to determine global and regional function as a surrogate for evaluating stem cell efficacy is on the rise. Furthermore, the high spatial resolution of MRI and CT is perfectly suited for detecting cellular therapies and examining cardiovascular anatomy. The potential to also track stem cells with these imaging modalities should lend insights into the development of optimized cellular therapies for the treatment of acute myocardial ischemia as well as congestive heart failure.

Stem Cell Labeling Strategies

Cellular labeling has been used extensively for fluorescence microscopy. A typical example is the use of 4′,6-diamidino-2-phenylindole (DAPI) in mounting medium that leads to strong nuclear binding, which appears blue when excited by ultraviolet light. Antibodies labeled with quantum dots have been targeted to donor cells in the heart to determine the cardiomyogenic fate of these cells [1]. The primary advantage of this technique is the narrow emission wavelength that is less likely to be confused with tissue autofluorescence, which is commonly present after ischemia and hemorrhage. Because tissue must be biopsied for histopathological analysis, the translation of these techniques to a noninvasive

Novel Techniques for Imaging the Heart, 1st edition. Edited by M. Di Carli and R. Kwong.
© 2008 American Heart Association, ISBN: 9-781-4051-7533-3.

imaging platform is unlikely. In addition, quantum dots contain heavy metals (e.g., cadmium) that are highly toxic, further limiting clinical translation.

Thus, cellular labeling strategies for noninvasive imaging have more stringent requirements than histological labels. Ideally, the label remains strongly bound or internalized within the cell. Furthermore, it is anticipated that stem cell therapies will lead to the production of daughter cells that will assume a cardiac myogenic fate or angiogenic phenotype. Thus, the label must not be diluted by cell division. Finally, the cell label must be biocompatible and not alter cell viability and differentiation.

At present, strategies for labeling stem cells for noninvasive imaging have been based on direct labeling and monoclonal antibody techniques that have been used for immunofluorescent histology and radionuclide imaging, respectively. For molecular imaging, magnetic labels bound to monoclonal antibodies have been used to detect immunoglobins produced during inflammation, atherosclerotic plaques, or neoplastic cells [2–4]. Because stem cells lack specific, distinct targets that are expressed in significantly great quantities and remain with cellular differentiation, monoclonal antibody techniques have not been used for stem cell imaging in the heart. Due to the high toxicity of iodinated contrast agents, whether bound to cells or internalized, labeling of stem cells with x-ray visible agents has been limited. Alternatively, one class of MRI contrast agents, superparamagnetic iron oxides (SPIO), was specifically developed for clinical use due to their avid uptake by Kupffer cells, a specialized macrophage, in the liver [5]. Neoplastic cells in the liver fail to take up the SPIOs and can be differentiated from normal liver parenchymal on MRI. However, stem cells are usually nonphagocytic. Thus, the direct labeling of stem cells requires approaches to encourage stem cells to bind or uptake magnetic labels.

An alternate approach is *reporter gene imaging*. In reporter gene imaging, cells are transduced with genetic material that results in production (or overproduction) of a receptor, transporter, protein, or enzyme [6–8]. The transduced cell is then interrogated with a reporter probe that is either bound to the receptor or internalized inside the cell (either due to the presence of the transporter or enzymatic degradation that traps the probe within the cell.) For example, expression of the human transferrin receptor in engineered glioma cells could be imaged after injection of an iron oxide nanoparticle linked to transferrin on T2-weighted MRI [7]. Alternatively, using magnetic resonance spectroscopy, one can look for shifts in spectral peaks in kinetic reactions due to the overproduction of a specific enzyme, such as creatine kinase in transfected mice, or the production of a nonmammalian enzyme, arginine kinase [9–11]. One of the primary advantages of reporter gene imaging is that cell viability must be maintained for gene expression. Despite 10 to 15 years of development of magnetic resonance reporter genes, the translation to the clinical realm remains more elusive than radiotracer reporter gene methods. The lack of adoption of MRI reporter gene imaging is in part due to the low sensitivity for MRI reporter gene products.

Furthermore, there are difficulties in creating sufficient contrast of the reporter probe from the background anatomical image. Lastly, difficulties in interpretation exist due to the accumulation of substances, such as iron oxides from receptor overexpression, which may persist even after cell death [12].

A new method for cell labeling has recently been reported that is a hybrid of tissue engineering and direct cell labeling. Several reports suggest that stem cells in patients with cardiovascular disease are impaired, and therefore healthy young donors may be preferable [13,14]. Many stem cells are exceedingly rare such that ex vivo expansion, which typically requires 10 to 20 days, will be required to obtain therapeutic quantities of stem cells [15]. Due to the acute nature of myocardial ischemia, expansion of stem cell products from autologous sources may not possible. Microencapsulation of cells can provide a protective coating to circumvent the need for immunosuppressive regimes, which often are cytotoxic on naive progenitor and stem cells. Microencapsulation's porous barrier allows the free flow of small molecules — such as cytokines, glucose, oxygen, and waste products — while restricting larger molecules, such as immunoglobulins. One microencapsulation scheme developed by Lim and Sun uses alginate, a biocompatible product of seaweed [16]. Alginate has been used as a cellular matrix or sponge for stem cell seeding that can then be used as a cardiovascular patch [17]. A logical extension of microencapsulation was to incorporate contrast agents into the alginate coating for both MRI and CT imaging of cells [18,19]. Because the contrast agent is moved further outside the cell, radiopaque agents can be employed with diminished issues of toxicity to enable the first method to track cells with an x-ray imaging modality. But direct labeling methods for MRI are currently the most advanced and have already been used clinically for cell tracking in noncardiovascular applications [20,21].

MRI Contrast Agents for Direct Cellular Labeling

There are three major classes of MRI contrast agents that can be used for direct cellular imaging. *Paramagnetic contrast agents*, including gadolinium-based agents, are the first class of agents. Typically, these agents are used for first-pass perfusion and viability imaging. The unpaired electrons in gadolinium alter the local magnetic field and reduce relaxation rates, resulting in hyperintensities on T1-weighted images. Because free gadolinium is highly toxic, these agents are chelated to substances such as DTPA and DOTA. Thus, direct labeling with gadolinium-based contrast agents poses the additional toxicity concern of de-chelation should the cell die. Another problem is that the ability of contrast agents to relax protons is diminished once restricted to the intracellular space [22]. Therefore, the concentration of paramagnetic agents required to directly detect labeled cells with clinically approved agents would be quite high. Further complicating this scenario are the concerns about nephrogenic systemic fibrosis/nephrogenic fibrosing dermopathy when these agents are used at high doses in renally compromised patients [23]. Recently, several investigators have successfully used new gadolinium formations with higher relaxivities to directly label cells [24,25].

The second class of agents is the *superparamagnetic agents*, which include SPIOs, monocrystalline iron oxides (MION), and micrometer-sized SPIOs (MPIO) [26,27]. These agents cause large field disruptions that lead to proton dephasing far from the particle. Thus, micromolar concentrations of these agents can be used to detect a small number of labeled cells. On T2*-weighted images, superparamagnetic labeled cells lead to susceptibility artifacts that appear as hypointensities (Figure 18.1). Toxicity concerns using iron oxide agents are minimal at the concentrations used to label cells because the free iron can be recycled using the normal iron pool turnover mechanisms. In fact, two reports of SPIO-labeled cells in patients suggest that these agents for cellular imaging will have an acceptable safety profile for cardiovascular stem cell delivery and tracking [20,21].

The third class of agents is agents the so-called *"hot spot" imaging agents*. Rather than using traditional proton MRI, multinuclear spectroscopy is combined with anatomical images from proton MRI for localization. One of the best known and perhaps earliest MRI contrast agent in this class is fluorine [28]. The absence of fluorine in the body results in a high sensitivity to the presence of the particles in ^{19}F MRI, similar to detecting radiotracers with radionuclide imaging. Indeed, preliminary images of in vivo labeling of stem cells with perfluoropolyether nanoparticles have been obtained [29]. As a relative newcomer to stem cell imaging, the toxicity profile of these agents has not been extensively studied. Moreover, the requirement of specialized hardware/software for multinuclear spectroscopy and the need for greater clinical field strengths to obtain adequate signal-to-noise ratios creates a hurdle for the rapid expansion of these techniques. Nonetheless, the potential to quantify stem cell numbers similar to counting emissions of radiotracers using "hot spot" imaging could be very powerful.

Direct Cell Labeling MRI Methods

Because stem cells are nonphagocytic, methods to encourage the efficient uptake of contrast agent for direct cellular labeling have been developed. Initial methods involved linking iron oxides to lectins or the HIV Tat peptide [30,31]. Another novel technique was to use magnetic cell sorting beads to label progenitor cells [32]. Encapsulation in liposomes has also been explored [33]. A chief disadvantage of these techniques is that they were often species-specific. To overcome that problem, compounds coated with dedrimers, which are highly charged polymers that bind to the cell membrane and induce endocytosis of the

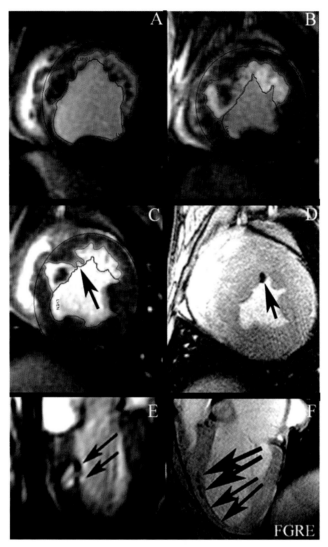

Fig. 18.1 Inversion recovery, delayed contrast enhanced MRI in the short-axis view in a reperfused canine myocardial infarction demonstrates a decreased area of hyperenhancement (red outlined area) consistent with remodeling of the myocardial infarction (MI) from (a) 72 hours post-MI, (b) one week post-MI, and (c) two weeks post-MI. (d) On fast-gradient echo MRI, an area of hypointensities is seen due to injection of SPIO-labeled mesenchymal stem cells (MSC). The area of stem cell injections corresponds to an area that was originally infarcted at 72 hours post-MI but appears viable at two weeks post-MI. Tracking the changes in the appearance of the hypointensities from delivery at (e) 72 hours and (f) eight weeks post-MI in long-axis images, one can appreciate the fading and spreading of the injection sites (arrows). From Bulte and Kraitchman, used with permission [47].

contrast agent, were developed [34,35]. Because all these agents were entirely new contrast agent formulations, rapid clinical adoption is unlikely.

A more convenient magnetic labeling method has been developed using commercially available SPIOs and gadolinium-based contrast agents in combination with transfection agents (TA), such as poly-L-lysine or protamine sulfate. For cell labeling, TAs are ideal in that the contrast agent-TA complex encourages endocytosis and stable incorporate into the cytoplasm or a perinuclear location; thus, toxicity is minimized. Magnetic labeling using TAs or "magnetofection" has become the most widely used method for cell labeling with MRI [36–40]. Typically, the contrast agent is incubated with the TA to coat the contrast agent with the TA. The contrast agent-TA mixture is then added to cell culture media and the cells are cultured for 24 to 48 hours, after which the cells are washed to remove any unincorporated contrast agent. Careful titration of the TA and contrast agent concentrations are required to prevent precipitates or agglomeration of the complexes, which may be cytotoxic. When using SPIOs, magnetofection typically results in each cell containing 10 to 30 pg of iron [36,41]. Overall, magnetofection is a simple, inexpensive method using clinical-grade pharmaceutical products to label cells. Additionally, the technique works well in a variety of species and cell lines.

For cardiovascular cellular therapy, the long incubation times required by magnetofection could present a problem for acute therapy. Electroporation, a well-established technique for transfecting cells with proteins and DNA, was proposed as a method for the rapid incorporation of contrast agents into cells. However, initial attempts resulted in markedly reduced viability, requiring the postlabeling incubation of 24 hours duration [42]. Recently, modifications to the voltage peaks and time duration of the pulses of "magnetoporation" allows for cells to be labeled instantly without loss of viability and, thus, the need for a recovery period [43]. Because no transfection agent is required, regulatory hurdles for adoption of this labeling method for clinical use should be reduced.

Stem Cell Delivery and Tracking Using MRI and X-ray Imaging

There are several routes for the delivery of stem cells for cardiovascular applications. Intravenous delivery provides the least invasive route. Systemic administration also may yield the smallest uptake of cells to the heart because cells are distributed to many organs other than the heart. Additionally, if the cells are large, trapping in the capillaries may occur [44–46]. Limited preclinical studies with magnetically labeled cells administered intravenously have now been performed in both murine and larger animal models [29,44,47]. Like many studies with histologically labeled cells, only a small number of cells could be detected in the heart at days to weeks postadministration [44,48]. Nonetheless, a phase I double-blind, placebo-controlled trial in patients using intravenously administered unlabeled allogeneic mesenchymal stem cells has been performed with preliminary evidence of efficacy and safety [49].

Intracoronary administration of labeled stem cells, while more invasive than intravenous administration, is an attractive route because it can be combined with primary percutaneous coronary interventions. A large number of clinical trials have been performed using intracoronary administration [50–55]. But the only studies to date that have been performed with labeled cells have used radiotracer labeling [56,57].

Intramyocardial administration of magnetic resonance-labeled stem cells has been performed in many preclinical models [38,58–70]. In murine models, the labeled cells are typically delivered using a standard needle and syringe under direct visualization during an open-chest procedure [58–61]. These hypointensities are readily visible over many weeks and months in the heart wall (Figure 18.2) but sometimes obscure the cardiac anatomy, making MRI tracking difficult. Nonetheless, fading of the hypointense signal over time is common. In large animals, transendocardial administration of stem cells has been performed under x-ray or electromechanical guidance using devices designed for patients with follow-up T2*-weighted MRI on clinical scanners (Figure 18.3) [38,62–67]. Because the magnetic resonance label cannot be visualized on x-ray, injection failures — which can be as high as 30% of the injections — cannot be determined. Alternatively, interventional MRI (iMRI) offers the ability to immediately visualize injection success as well as target the stem cells based on myocardial viability from delayed enhancement MRI (Figure 18.1), albeit at a lower temporal resolution than x-ray fluoroscopy. Specialized devices are required that are magnetic resonance-compatible and steerable for iMRI cellular delivery [71,72]. Frequently, electronics are included within these devices to make them active or "magnetic resonance-visible" (Figure 18.3). Interactive scan plan acquisitions with graphical interfaces that allow three-plane reconstruction, colorization of the injection device, and tracking of the catheter tip are becoming more common for these iMRI procedures to enhance delivery [73]. Even in the setting of x-ray fluoroscopic delivery, serial MRI of transmyocardially injected iron oxide-labeled stem cells has shown that the long-term engraftment of stem cells may be different depending on the myocardial viability status.

Hybrid x-ray fluoroscopic and MRI suites offer another means to harness the advantages of each imaging modality [74]. X-ray fusion with MRI (XFM) may become an increasingly common platform for stem cell delivery and imaging (Figure 18.4) [75]. In this scenario, MRI provides the anatomical detail to determine cardiac viability for targeting to peri-infarction zones and to avoid areas of wall thinning so that off-the-shelf devices and interactivity of x-ray fluoroscopy can be exploited. With the introduction of x-ray visible stem cells, these XFM platforms could provide a means of limiting ionizing radiation exposure and enhancing targeting on a platform more familiar to the cardiac interventionalist.

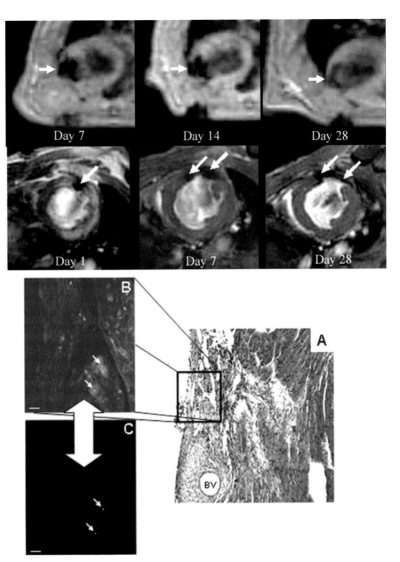

Fig. 18.2 Serial short-axis MRIs of intramyocardial injections of SPIO-labeled mesenchymal stem cells at 7, 14, and 28 days after coronary artery ligation in the female mouse. Hypointensities seen at 28 days on MRI were shown to be unrelated to the presence of donor male cells on polymerase chain reaction (from Amsalem *et al.*, used with permission) [61]. Short-axis MRIs in a reperfused mouse myocardial infarction at 1, 7, and 28 days postinjection of MPIO-labeled cardiac differentiated embryonic stem cells show hypointensities in the left ventricular wall (middle row). Hematoxylin and eosin (A) of the infarcted mouse ventricle with magnified fluorescent images processed at different exposure periods (B,C) show the presence of the MPIOs in the infarction indicative of the exogenous cells at 28 days (BV, blood vessel; scale bar = 10 μm; from Ebert *et al.*, used with permission) [59]. These studies indicate that the presence of hypointensities at several weeks postinjection of iron oxide-labeled stem cells may not be related to the engraftment of donor cells. However, this discrepancy may be related to cell type or perfusion status after myocardial infarction.

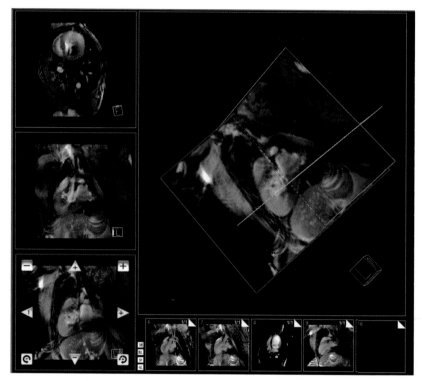

Fig. 18.3 Screen capture of the Siemens prototype Interactive Front End (IFE) graphical interface that enables real-time scan plane manipulation and serial acquisition of up to three imaging planes. An active injection catheter is colored to aid in transmyocardial injections of SPIO-labeled stem cells. Even with low-resolution imaging, the ability to visualize the myocardium is beneficial for directing injections. High-resolution viability images taken prior to cardiac catheterization can be used to select scan planes for targeting of the injections.

Limitations

Although direct labeling methods are simple and inexpensive methods for stem cell imaging, there are several potential limitations. As previously noted, should the label become detached from the donor cell, hypointensities on MRI may not indicate the engraftment and retention of cells. In fact, conflicting results have been presented as to whether the hypointensities at several weeks to months postadministration represent the donor cells in direct intracardiac injections of iron oxide-labeled stem cells, label alone, or hemorrhage (Figure 18.2) [58,59,61,76]. Potentially, using a combination of imaging techniques (e.g., T1-weighted, T2-weighted, proton density) distinctions can be made between intracardiac hemorrhage and iron oxide-labeled cells [77].

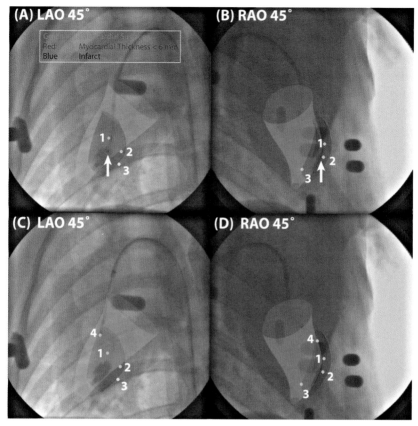

Fig. 18.4 X-ray fusion with MRI (XFM) targeting of endomyocardial injections according to infarct location (blue surface) and regional myocardial wall thickness (colored green for wall thickness greater than 6 mm and red for wall thickness less than or equal to 6 mm) in a chronic swine myocardial infarction. (A,B) These surfaces were overlaid on the x-ray in orthogonal projections. (C,D) Injections are only placed in regions with sufficient wall thickness. Previous injection locations (yellow spots, numbered 1 to 3) are also displayed to help avoid overlapping injections. From de Silva *et al.*, used with permission [75].

Another issue is that the magnetic susceptibility artifacts caused by iron oxide-labeled stem cells can be duplicated by many other things, such as calcification, motion, or metallic devices. Several groups have developed off-resonant imaging techniques that make these susceptibility artifacts appear hyperintense (Figure 18.5) [78–81]. Because off-resonant techniques cause a typically dipole pattern of hyperintensities, volume measurements may be useful for quantification of the amount of stem cells delivered. One can rest assured if the labeled cell

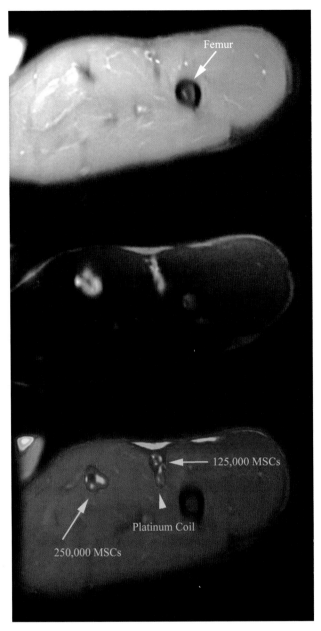

Fig. 18.5 Oblique axial fast-gradient echo image (top) of different concentrations of SPIO-labeled stem cells injected intramuscularly in a rabbit model of critical limb ischemia are difficult to visualize based on hypointensities. Inversion recovery with on-resonant water suppression (IRON) imaging, an off-resonant white marker technique, turns the hypointensities into hyperintense signals with suppression of the underlying anatomy (middle) [78]. A fused image of the gradient echo image (grayscale) and the positive enhanced IRON image shown (colorized) enables the rapid distinction of cell injections (arrows) from other magnetic susceptibility artifacts, such as a platinum coil (arrowhead).

magnetic resonance signal disappears with time, the cells have either vanished (i.e., died or migrated) or replicated to the extent that the signal is no longer detectable in the daughter cells. This sensitivity to detect a small number of cells will become important as it will differentiate cell removal and death from robust engraftment and differentiation [82]. Although some investigators have shown the ability to image single labeled cells in the brain, cardiac and respiratory motion limit detection in the heart to the order of 5×10^5 to 10×10^5 cells in practice [27,47,69,83]. However, initial results indicate that labeled microencapsulated cells, which allow for a higher concentration of the label, may enable the detection of a smaller quantity of cells [18].

An additional concern is that the process of exogenously labeling stem cells may alter the functional capacity of the cells. With iron oxide labeling, there are reports that in vitro differentiation of mesenchymal stem cells down a chondrogenic lineage is impaired. Fortunately, there have been no indications that the use of SPIO-labeled stem cells in animals adversely impairs the therapeutic response in cardiovascular applications [66,84]. Thus, a likely strategy in early clinical trials will be to label a portion of the cellular therapeutic to enable cell localization and tracking.

Conclusions

Despite these limitations, the advantages of labeled stem cells far outweigh the disadvantages. The ability to immediately confirm the success and anatomical placement of the injections could be very helpful in teasing out the discrepancies of the different therapeutic responses that have been seen in cardiovascular cellular clinical trials to date. A poignant example is in the first clinical trial using iron oxide-labeled dendritic cell vaccines where 50% of the patients failed to receive intranodal injections under ultrasound guidance, which were only detected due to the MRI [21]. As a first step, determination of the correct delivery of the therapy to the heart and the degree of stem cell engraftment will be critical for interpreting clinical trial results. Thus, in combination with the exquisite ability of MRI and CT to determine viability, perfusion, and function for prognostication, the future for designing cellular therapeutics based on noninvasive imaging is bright.

References

1 Rota, M., Kajstura, J., Hosoda, T., *et al.* (2007) Bone marrow cells adopt the cardiomyogenic fate in vivo. *Proc Natl Acad Sci USA* Nov 6 **104**(45): 17783–17788.

2 Weissleder, R., Lee, A.S., Fischman, A.J., *et al.* (1991) Polyclonal human immunoglobulin G labeled with polymeric iron oxide: antibody MR imaging. *Radiology* Oct **181**(1): 245–249.

3 McAteer, M.A., Schneider, J.E., Ali, Z.A., *et al.* (2007) Magnetic resonance imaging of endothelial adhesion molecules in mouse atherosclerosis using dual-targeted microparticles of iron oxide. *Arterioscler Thromb Vasc Biol* Oct 25.

4 Remsen, L.G., McCormick, C.I., Roman-Goldstein, S., *et al.* (1996) MR of carcinoma-specific monoclonal antibody conjugated to monocrystalline iron oxide nanoparticles: the potential for noninvasive diagnosis. *AJNR Am J Neuroradiol* **17**(3): 411–418.

5 Stark, D.D., Weissleder, R., Elizondo, G., *et al.* (1988) Superparamagnetic iron oxide: clinical application as a contrast agent for MR imaging of the liver. *Radiology* **168**: 297–301.

6 Gilad, A.A., McMahon, M.T., Walczak, P., *et al.* (2007) Artificial reporter gene providing MRI contrast based on proton exchange. *Nat Biotechnol* **25**(2): 217–219.

7 Weissleder, R., Moore, A., Mahmood, U., *et al.* (2000) In vivo magnetic resonance imaging of transgene expression. *Nat Med* **6**(3): 351–355.

8 Cohen, B., Ziv, K., Plaks, V., *et al.* (2007) MRI detection of transcriptional regulation of gene expression in transgenic mice. *Nat Med* **13**(4): 498–503.

9 Koretsky, A.P., Brosnan, M.J., Chen, L.H., *et al.* (1990) NMR detection of creatine kinase expressed in liver of transgenic mice: determination of free ADP levels. *Proc Natl Acad Sci USA* **87**(8): 3112–3116.

10 Auricchio, A., Zhou, R., Wilson, J.M., Glickson, J.D. (2001) In vivo detection of gene expression in liver by 31P nuclear magnetic resonance spectroscopy employing creatine kinase as a marker gene. *Proc Natl Acad Sci USA* **98**(9): 5205–5210.

11 Walter, G., Barton, E.R., Sweeney, H.L. (2000) Noninvasive measurement of gene expression in skeletal muscle. *Proc Natl Acad Sci USA* **97**(10): 5151–5155.

12 Gilad, A.A., Winnard, P.T., Jr., van Zijl, P.C., Bulte, J.W. (2007) Developing MR reporter genes: promises and pitfalls. *NMR Biomed* **20**(3): 275–290.

13 Heeschen, C., Lehmann, R., Honold, J., *et al.* (2004) Profoundly reduced neovascularization capacity of bone marrow mononuclear cells derived from patients with chronic ischemic heart disease. *Circulation* **109**(13): 1615–1622.

14 Walter, D.H., Haendeler, J., Reinhold, J., *et al.* (2005) Impaired CXCR4 signaling contributes to the reduced neovascularization capacity of endothelial progenitor cells from patients with coronary artery disease. *Circ Res* **97**(11): 1142–1151.

15 Pittenger, M.F., Martin, B.J. (2004) Mesenchymal stem cells and their potential as cardiac therapeutics. *Circ Res* **95**(1): 9–20.

16 Lim, F., Sun, A.M. (1980) Microencapsulated islets as bioartificial endocrine pancreas. *Science* **210**(4472): 908–910.

17 Dar, A., Shachar, M., Leor, J., Cohen, S. (2002) Optimization of cardiac cell seeding and distribution in 3D porous alginate scaffolds. *Biotechnol Bioeng* **80**(3): 305–312.

18 Barnett, B.P., Arepally, A., Karmarkar, P.V., *et al.* (2007) Magnetic resonance-guided, real-time targeted delivery and imaging of magnetocapsules immunoprotecting pancreatic islet cells. *Nat Med* **13**(8): 986–991.

19 Barnett, B.P., Kraitchman, D.L., Lauzon, C., *et al.* (2006) Radiopaque alginate microcapsules for x-ray visualization and immunoprotection of cellular therapeutics. *Molecular Pharmaceutics* **3**(5): 531–538.

20 Zhu, J., Zhou, L., XingWu, F. (2006) Tracking neural stem cells in patients with brain trauma. *N Engl J Med* **355**(22): 2376–2378.

21 de Vries, I.J., Lesterhuis, W.J., Barentsz, J.O., *et al.* (2005) Magnetic resonance tracking of dendritic cells in melanoma patients for monitoring of cellular therapy. *Nat Biotechnol* **23**(11): 1407–1413.

22 Simon, G.H., Bauer, J., Saborovski, O., *et al.* (2006) T1 and T2 relaxivity of intracellular and extracellular USPIO at 1.5 T and 3 T clinical MR scanning. *Eur Radiol* **16**(3): 738–745.

23 Thomsen, H.S. (2006) Nephrogenic systemic fibrosis: a serious late adverse reaction to gadodiamide. *Eur Radiol* **16**(12): 2619–2621.

24 Anderson, S.A., Lee, K.K., Frank, J.A. (2006) Gadolinium-fullerenol as a paramagnetic contrast agent for cellular imaging. *Invest Radiol* **41**(3): 332–338.

25 Vuu, K., Xie, J., McDonald, M.A., *et al.* (2005) Gadolinium-rhodamine nanoparticles for cell labeling and tracking via magnetic resonance and optical imaging. *Bioconjug Chem* **16**(4): 995–999.

26 Shen, T., Weissleder, R., Papisov, M., *et al.* (1993) Monocrystalline iron oxide nanocompounds (MION): physicochemical properties. *Magn Reson Med* **29**(5): 599–604.

27 Shapiro, E.M., Skrtic, S., Sharer, K., *et al.* (2004) MRI detection of single particles for cellular imaging. *Proc Natl Acad Sci USA* **101**(30): 10901–10906.

28 Hinshaw, W.S., Bottomley, P.A., Holland, G.N. (1977) Radiographic thin-section image of the human wrist by nuclear magnetic resonance. *Nature* **270**(5639): 722–723.

29 Partlow, K.C., Chen, J., Brant, J.A., *et al.* (2007) 19F magnetic resonance imaging for stem/progenitor cell tracking with multiple unique perfluorocarbon nanobeacons. *Faseb J* **21**(8): 1647–1654.

30 Bulte, J.W., Laughlin, P.G., Jordan, E.K., *et al.* (1996) Tagging of T cells with superparamagnetic iron oxide: uptake kinetics and relaxometry. *Acad Radiol* **3**(Suppl 2): S301–303.

31 Josephson, L., Tung, C.H., Moore, A., Weissleder, R. (1999) High-efficiency intracellular magnetic labeling with novel superparamagnetic-Tat peptide conjugates. *Bioconjug Chem* **10**(2): 186–191.

32 Weber, A., Pedrosa, I., Kawamoto, A., *et al.* (2004) Magnetic resonance mapping of transplanted endothelial progenitor cells for therapeutic neovascularization in ischemic heart disease. *Eur J Cardiothorac Surg* **26**(1): 137–143.

33 Bulte, J.W., Ma, L.D., Magin, R.L., *et al.* (1993) Selective MR imaging of labeled human peripheral blood mononuclear cells by liposome mediated incorporation of dextranmagnetite particles. *Magn Reson Med* **29**(1): 32–37.

34 Strable, E., Bulte, J.W.M., Moskowitz, B.M., *et al.* (2001) Synthesis and characterization of soluble iron oxide-dendrimer composites. *Chem Mater* **13**: 2201–2209.

35 Bulte, J.W., Douglas, T., Witwer, B., *et al.* (2001) Magnetodendrimers allow endosomal magnetic labeling and in vivo tracking of stem cells. *Nat Biotechnol* **19**(12): 1141–1147.

36 Frank, J.A., Miller, B.R., Arbab, A.S., *et al.* (2003) Clinically applicable labeling of mammalian and stem cells by combining superparamagnetic iron oxides and transfection agents. *Radiology* **228**: 480–487.

37 Frank, J.A., Zywicke, H., Jordan, E.K., *et al.* (2002) Magnetic intracellular labeling of mammalian cells by combining (FDA-approved) superparamagnetic iron oxide MR contrast agents and commonly used transfection agents. *Acad Radiol* **9**: S484–S487.

38 Kraitchman, D.L., Heldman, A.W., Atalar, E., *et al.* (2003) In vivo magnetic resonance imaging of mesenchymal stem cells in myocardial infarction. *Circulation* **107**(18): 2290–2293.

39 Bos, C., Delmas, Y., Desmouliere, A., *et al.* (2004) In vivo MR imaging of intravascularly injected magnetically labeled mesenchymal stem cells in rat kidney and liver. *Radiology* **233**(3): 781–789.

40 Terrovitis, J.V., Bulte, J.W., Sarvananthan, S., *et al.* (2006) Magnetic resonance imaging of ferumoxide-labeled mesenchymal stem cells seeded on collagen scaffolds — relevance to tissue engineering. *Tissue Eng* **12**: 2765–2775.

41 Verdijk, P., Scheenen, T.W., Lesterhuis, W.J., *et al.* (2007) Sensitivity of magnetic resonance imaging of dendritic cells for in vivo tracking of cellular cancer vaccines. *Int J Cancer* **120**(5): 978–984.

42 Daldrup-Link, H.E., Meier, R., Rudelius, M., *et al.* (2005) In vivo tracking of genetically engineered, anti-HER2/neu directed natural killer cells to HER2/neu positive mammary tumors with magnetic resonance imaging. *Eur Radiol* **15**(1): 4–13.

43 Walczak, P., Ruiz-Cabello, J., Kedziorek, D.A., *et al.* (2006) Magnetoelectroporation: improved labeling of neural stem cells and leukocytes for cellular magnetic resonance imaging using a single FDA-approved agent. *Nanomedicine* **2**(2): 89–94.

44 Kraitchman, D.L., Tatsumi, M., Gilson, W.D., *et al.* (2005) Dynamic imaging of allogeneic mesenchymal stem cells trafficking to myocardial infarction. *Circulation* **112**(10): 1451–1461.

45 Gao, J., Dennis, J.E., Muzic, R.F., *et al.* (2001) The dynamic in vivo distribution of bone marrow-derived mesenchymal stem cells after infusion. *Cell Tissues Organs* **169**: 12–20.

46 Vulliet, P.R., Greeley, M., Halloran, S.M., *et al.* (2004) Intra-coronary arterial injection of mesenchymal stromal cells and microinfarction in dogs. *Lancet* **363**(9411): 783–784.

47 Bulte, J.W., Kraitchman, D.L. (2004) Monitoring cell therapy using iron oxide MR contrast agents. *Curr Pharm Biotechnol* **5**(6): 567–584.

48 Limbourg, F.P., Ringes-Lichtenberg, S., Schaefer, A., *et al.* (2005) Haematopoietic stem cells improve cardiac function after infarction without permanent cardiac engraftment. *Eur J Heart Fail* **7**(5): 722–729.

49 Boyle, A.J., Schulman, S.P., Hare, J.M. (2006) Is stem cell therapy ready for patients? Stem cell therapy for cardiac repair—ready for the next step. *Circulation* **114**(4): 339–352.

50 Wollert, K.C., Meyer, G.P., Lotz, J., *et al.* (2004) Intracoronary autologous bone-marrow cell transfer after myocardial infarction: the BOOST randomised controlled clinical trial. *Lancet* **364**(9429): 141–148.

51 Janssens, S., Dubois, C., Bogaert, J., *et al.* (2006) Autologous bone marrow-derived stem-cell transfer in patients with ST-segment elevation myocardial infarction: double-blind, randomised controlled trial. *Lancet* **367**(9505): 113–121.

52 Bartunek, J., Vanderheyden, M., Vandekerckhove, B., *et al.* (2005) Intracoronary injection of CD133-positive enriched bone marrow progenitor cells promotes cardiac recovery after recent myocardial infarction: feasibility and safety. *Circulation* **112**(9 Suppl): I178–183.

53 Schachinger, V., Erbs, S., Elsasser, A., *et al.* (2006) Intracoronary bone marrow-derived progenitor cells in acute myocardial infarction. *N Engl J Med* **355**(12): 1210–1221.

54 Lunde, K., Solheim, S., Aakhus, S., *et al.* (2005) Autologous stem cell transplantation in acute myocardial infarction: the ASTAMI randomized controlled trial: intracoronary transplantation of autologous mononuclear bone marrow cells, study design and safety aspects. *Scand Cardiovasc J* **39**(3): 150–158.

55 Chen, S., Liu, Z., Tian, N., *et al.* (2006) Intracoronary transplantation of autologous bone marrow mesenchymal stem cells for ischemic cardiomyopathy due to isolated chronic occluded left anterior descending artery. *J Invasive Cardiol* **18**(11): 552–556.

56 Doyle, B., Kemp, B.J., Chareonthaitawee, P., *et al.* (2007) Dynamic tracking during intracoronary injection of 18F-FDG-labeled progenitor cell therapy for acute myocardial infarction. *J Nucl Med* **48**(10): 1708–1714.

57 Hou, D., Youssef, E.A., Brinton, T.J., *et al.* (2005) Radiolabeled cell distribution after intramyocardial, intracoronary, and interstitial retrograde coronary venous delivery: implications for current clinical trials. *Circulation* **112**(9 Suppl): I150–156.

58 Stuckey, D.J., Carr, C.A., Martin-Rendon, E., *et al.* (2006) Iron particles for noninvasive monitoring of bone marrow stromal cell engraftment into, and isolation of viable engrafted donor cells from, the heart. *Stem Cells* **24**(8): 1968–1975.

59 Ebert, S.N., Taylor, D.G., Nguyen, H.L., *et al.* (2007) Noninvasive tracking of cardiac embryonic stem cells in vivo using magnetic resonance imaging techniques. *Stem Cells* **25**(11): 2936–2944.

60 Tallheden, T., Nannmark, U., Lorentzon, M., *et al.* (2006) In vivo MR imaging of magnetically labeled human embryonic stem cells. *Life Sci* **79**(10): 999–1006.

61 Amsalem, Y., Mardor, Y., Feinberg, M.S., *et al.* (2007) Iron-oxide labeling and outcome of transplanted mesenchymal stem cells in the infarcted myocardium. *Circulation* **116**(Suppl I): I-38–45.

62 Hill, J.M., Dick, A.J., Raman, V.K., *et al.* (2003) Serial cardiac magnetic resonance imaging of injected mesenchymal stem cells. *Circulation* **108**(8): 1009–1014.

63 Garot, J., Unterseeh, T., Teiger, E., *et al.* (2003) Magnetic resonance imaging of targeted catheter-based implantation of myogenic precursor cells into infarcted left ventricular myocardium. *J Am Coll Cardiol* **41**(10): 1841–1846.

64 Rickers, C., Gallegos, R., Seethamraju, R.T., *et al.* (2004) Applications of magnetic resonance imaging for cardiac stem cell therapy. *J Interv Cardiol* **17**(1): 37–46.

65 Rickers, C., Kraitchman, D., Fischer, G., *et al.* (2005) Cardiovascular interventional MR imaging: a new road for therapy and repair in the heart. *Magn Reson Imaging Clin N Am* **13**(3): 465–479.

66 Amado, L.C., Salrais, A.P., Schuleri, K.H., *et al.* (2005) Cardiac repair with intramyocardial injection of allogeneic mesenchymal stem cells after myocardial infarction. *Proc Natl Acad Sci USA* **102**(32): 11474–11479.

67 Amado, L.C., Schuleri, K.H., Saliaris, A.P., *et al.* (2006) Multimodality noninvasive imaging demonstrates in vivo cardiac regeneration after mesenchymal stem cell therapy. *J Am Coll Cardiol* **48**(10): 2116–2124.

68 Zhang, H., Song, P., Tang, Y., *et al.* (2007) Injection of bone marrow mesenchymal stem cells in the borderline area of infarcted myocardium: heart status and cell distribution. *J Thorac Cardiovasc Surg* **134**(5): 1234–1240.

69 Dick, A.J., Guttman, M.A., Raman, V.K., *et al.* (2003) Magnetic resonance fluoroscopy allows targeted delivery of mesenchymal stem cells to infarct borders in swine. *Circulation* **108**(23): 2899–2904.

70 Saeed, M., Saloner, D., Weber, O., *et al.* (2005) MRI in guiding and assessing intramyocardial therapy. *Eur Radiol* **15**(5): 851–863.

71 Karmarkar, P.V., Kraitchman, D.L., Izbudak, I., *et al.* (2004) MR-trackable intramyocardial injection catheter. *Mag Reson Med* **51**(6): 1163–1172.

72 Krombach, G.A., Baireuther, R., Higgins, C.B., Saeed, M. (2004) Distribution of intramyocardially injected extracellular MR contrast medium: effects of concentration and volume. *Eur Radiol* **14**(2): 334–340.

73 Kraitchman, D.L., Gilson, W.D., Lorenz, C.H. (2008) Stem cell therapy: MRI guidance and monitoring. *J Magn Reson Imaging* **27**: 299–310.

74 Saeed, M., Lee, R., Martin, A., *et al.* (2004) Transendocardial delivery of extracellular myocardial markers by using combination x-ray/MR fluoroscopic guidance: feasibility study in dogs. *Radiology* **231**(3): 689–696.

75 de Silva, R., Gutierrez, L.F., Raval, A.N., *et al.* (2006) X-ray fused with magnetic resonance imaging (XFM) to target endomyocardial injections: validation in a swine model of myocardial infarction. *Circulation* **114**(22): 2342–2350.

76 van den Bos, E.J., Baks, T., Moelker, A.D., *et al.* (2006) Magnetic resonance imaging of haemorrhage within reperfused myocardial infarcts: possible interference with iron oxide-labelled cell tracking? *Eur Heart J* **27**(13): 1620–1626.

77 Kustermann, E., Roell, W., Breitbach, M., *et al.* (2005) Stem cell implantation in ischemic mouse heart: a high-resolution magnetic resonance imaging investigation. *NMR Biomed* **18**(6): 362–370.

78 Stuber, M., Gilson, W.D., Schär, M., *et al.* (2007) Positive contrast visualization of iron oxide-labeled stem cells using inversion recovery with ON-resonant water suppression (IRON). *Magn Reson Med* **58**: 1072–1077.

79 Mani, V., Saebo, K.C., Hskovich, V., *et al.* (2006) **GR**adient echo Acquisition for Supermagnetic particles with Positive contrast (GRASP): Sequence characterization in membrane and glass supermagnetic iron oxide phantoms at 1.5T and 3T. *Magn Reson Med* **55**: 126–135.

80 Cunningham, C.H., Arai, T., Yang, P.C., *et al.* (2005) Positive contrast magnetic resonance imaging of cells labeled with magnetic nanoparticles. *Magn Reson Med* **53**(5): 999–1005.

81 Seppenwoolde, J.H., Viergever, M.A., Bakker, C.J. (2003) Passive tracking exploiting local signal conservation: the white marker phenomenon. *Magn Reson Med* **50**(4): 784–790.

82 Walczak, P., Kedziorek, D.A., Gilad, A.A., *et al.* (2007) Applicability and limitations of MR tracking of neural stem cells with asymmetric cell division and rapid turnover: the case of the shiverer dysmyelinated mouse brain. *Magn Reson Med* **58**(2): 261–269.

83 Heyn, C., Bowen, C.V., Rutt, B.K., Foster, P.J. (2005) Detection threshold of single SPIO-labeled cells with FIESTA. *Magn Reson Med* **53**(2): 312–320.

84 Kedziorek, D.A., Gilson, W.D., Stuber, M., *et al.* (2007) Mesenchymal stem cell therapy in a rabbit hindlimb ischemia model. *J Am Coll Cardiol* **49**(9): 362A.

Chapter 19

Myocardial Imaging in CAD: Beyond Ischemia and Viability

Susan H. Kwon, Henry Wu, and Raymond Y. Kwong

Over the past decade, cardiac magnetic resonance (CMR) has emerged as the preeminent imaging technique for myocardial tissue characterization. The high spatial resolution and image contrast afforded by CMR is superior to many other existing imaging techniques, and can be further enhanced by the use of intravenous contrast agents. As discussed in Chapter 8, the use of an inversion pulse prior to image acquisition to null signals from normal myocardium has resulted in a marked improvement in the contrast noise ratio between normal and pathologic tissue [1]. This development has led to the development of the late gadolinium enhancement (LGE) CMR technique, which has the ability to detect necrotic areas that are smaller than 1% of the myocardial mass of the left ventricle [2]. As an example, CMR can delineate the infarct region at over 40-fold higher resolution than single photon emission computed tomography (SPECT) and has been shown to detect small subendocardial infarcts missed by the latter technique [3,4]. Moreover, by providing high tissue contrast, LGE can be used to evaluate various aspects of the infarcted myocardium throughout different stages of remodeling following myocardial infarction (MI). The use of CMR in quantifying infarct size and in determining myocardial viability has been extensively validated and discussed in Chapter 8. This chapter will focus on the potential role of CMR in characterizing the various myocardial tissue components after MI that may have important therapeutic and prognostic implications.

Novel Techniques for Imaging the Heart, 1st edition. Edited by M. Di Carli and R. Kwong.
© 2008 American Heart Association, ISBN: 9-781-4051-7533-3.

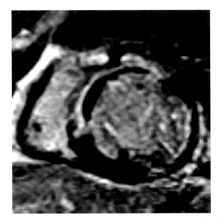

Fig. 19.1 Microvascular obstruction with large infarction. Note the large hypointense area surrounded by late enhanced myocardium, consistent with microvascular obstruction, in this patient with an acute occlusion of the proximal left anterior descending coronary artery. Successful revascularization of this coronary occlusion was not achieved due to delayed patient presentation.

The Role of CMR in Defining "Area at Risk" Post-MI

During acute MI, the extent of the hypoperfused myocardium during coronary occlusion is known as the *"area at risk."* The degree of myocardium that sustains reversible or irreversible injury depends on the duration of occlusion and presence of collateral vessels [5]. Histopathologically, the infarct zone is dynamic and heterogeneous. This region goes through an early endocardial necrotic phase followed by a fibrotic and remodeling phase, resulting in prolonged active collagen turnover and scar tissue contraction [6]. The area at risk can be conceptually classified into different territories: the periphery of the infarct zone is known as the *peri-infarct zone*, which is contained within a larger zone of myocardial edema that surrounds the infarct core [5,7–12]. In cases where perfusion cannot be completely restored at the tissue level despite epicardial coronary recanalization, a dark region within enhanced late enhancement representing microvascular obstruction can often be detected by contrast-enhanced CMR (Figure 19.1) [13–15].

Peri-infarct Zone

Histologically, the infarct portion of the myocardium is not uniformly composed of dense scar tissue. Instead, infarct myocardium is interspersed with bundles of viable myocytes, particularly in the border zones and periphery of the region [16]. Although scar formation resulting from MI has been well known to provide the critical substrate of reentrant ventricular arrhythmias, the importance of myocardial architecture in contributing to arrhythmia generation has

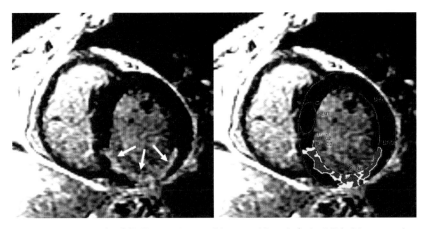

Fig. 19.2 An example of CMR in a 64-year-old man with an inferior MI (white arrows), preserved left ventricular systolic function (LVEF = 61%), and normal left ventricular systolic volume index. The MI of this patient was characterized by a substantial peri-infarct zone (yellow region), with a peri-infarct zone measuring 27% of the total LGE extent. This patient died suddenly 11 months after undergoing the CMR examination. From Yan *et al.*, used with permission [9].

only been recently appreciated. In animal models, a wealth of evidence has demonstrated that tissue heterogeneity within the infarct imparts nonuniform anisotropic properties that are requisite for the reentrant arrhythmias. These experimental data may help explain the adverse cardiovascular prognosis of patients found to have abnormal LGE by CMR. In patients with nonischemic cardiomyopathy, the transmural extent of fibrosis identified by LGE has been shown to predict inducible ventricular tachycardia by electrophysiological testing [10]. Moreover, among patients with a clinical suspicion of ischemic heart disease but without a history of MI, our group found that LGE involving even a very small myocardial extent imparts a high adverse cardiac risk [17]. Other investigators have reported consistent findings that quantification of infarct surface area and mass, as measured by LGE, were better predictors of inducibility than left ventricular ejection fraction (LVEF) [18].

More recently, our group evaluated LGE characteristics beyond infarct size that might be useful in predicting susceptibility to ventricular arrhythmias and adverse cardiovascular outcomes. This new application determines the degree of infarct tissue heterogeneity based on the variability of signal intensities within the infarct region. The core and peri-infarct regions are quantified by using a computer-assisted semiautomatic algorithm based on signal-intensity thresholds: an infarct core greater than three standard deviations above a remote non-infarct region and a peri-infarct zone between two and three standard deviations (Figure 19.2). Based on these criteria, the presence of the peri-infarct zones portends adverse cardiovascular outcomes. We found that the extent of the peri-infarct zone to be the strongest independent predictors of adverse cardiovascular outcomes, providing incremental prognostic value beyond LVEF or left ventricular systolic volume index [19]. Subsequently, using a similar technique but a different criteria for the peri-infarct zone, Schmidt *et al.* found that the extent of this peri-infarct zone is predictive of inducible ventricular arrhythmias in patients with left ventricular dysfunction [7]. Thus, evaluating the morphological features of the infarct zone by CMR holds promise in predicting sudden cardiac death after MI, and perhaps in identifying high-risk patients currently missed by ejection fraction criteria. Whether this novel CMR technique of infarct characterization can be used in guiding the decision of placement of an automatic implantable cardioverter and defibrillator (AICD) remains to be evaluated in prospective clinical studies.

Myocardial Edema

Myocardial edema during acute MI is well recognized, and prior animal studies reported a 25% increase in myocardial water content, regional swelling, and transmural distribution of edema [20,21]. Edema in the peri-infarct zone results from increased water content in both the extracellular and intracellular compartment volumes of viable myocardium. Inside acutely infarcted myocardium, cell lysis results in the conversion of intracellular space into extracellular space. Recently, studies have focused on assessing myocardial edema to differentiate acute from chronic irreversible myocardial injury [12]. Traditionally, SPECT imaging with technetium perfusion tracer injection during coronary occlusion has been used to directly measure myocardial salvage. However, logistics involving radioactive tracer availability and handling, a low spatial resolution, and an inability to differentiate infarcted myocardium are current limitations of SPECT applied in this setting [11].

In CMR, the signal intensity on T2-weighted (T2W) images are heavily influenced by the physical mobility of water protons. Thus, the area at risk appears hyperintense on T2W images because of the increased total water content and increased water mobility (Figure 19.3) [5,11]. Studies have shown elevated transmural T2W signal intensities in acute MI even though the myocardial necrosis involves only the subendocardial aspects of the injurious segments [12,22]. Furthermore, treatment of myocardial edema with mannitol resulted in a reduction of T2W signals, portraying that the T2W signal abnormality exceeds the scar and represents the reversible injury zone (area at risk) during acute MI [23]. Using a canine model of coronary artery occlusion, Aletras *et al.* demonstrated that T2W abnormality corresponds to the area at risk, and late gadolinium enhancement is confined to the area of necrosis (Figure 19.3). Using high-resolution (DENSE) systolic strain images, these investigators further confirmed the partial recovery of segmental function consistent with subendocardial infarction [5]. However, the low contrast-to-noise ratio between the area at risk and normal myocardium,

| Gd-DE | FISP-ED | T2W | DENSE |

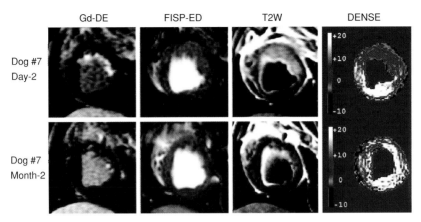

Fig. 19.3 Two days after infarct (top row), the T2 hyperintense area was essentially transmural and the infarcted region was subendocardial, as delineated by gadolinium delayed enhancement. The T2 hyperintense area more closely resembled the hypokinetic zone identified on the DENSE systolic strain maps (radial thickening). Two months later (bottom row), the left ventricular transmural T2W abnormality had largely resolved, and systolic strain had recovered. The color scale is calibrated from −10% to 20% strain, with zero strain at the transition from blue to green. Normal contraction is orange to white; the blue-green pixels represent severely hypokinetic to dyskinetic regions. From Aletras *et al.*, used with permission [5].

and the elimination of artifactual signal from the blood pool adjacent to the dysfunctional subendocardium, needs further technical improvement [11]. Abdul-Aty *et al.* demonstrated that edema post-MI resolves over one to two months and a T2W image can differentiate acute from chronic infarction [12]. Many have pointed out that strategies to quantify the myocardial salvage (area at risk without infarction) can affect the clinical management of patients who present with acute MI [11]. For instance, in patients who present late (more than 12 hours) after the onset of symptoms, if the infarction wavefront has not reached the epicardial border of the area at risk and thus there remains significant salvageable myocardium, it would conceivably be reasonable to perform late percutaneous coronary intervention (PCI) to restore coronary reperfusion in such selected patients. Also, T2W findings may contribute to decisions about adjunctive treatments to reperfusion therapies. These potential applications must be studied in prospective clinical trials.

Microvascular Obstruction and "No-Reflow" Phenomenon

The main goal of revascularization for acute MI is restoration of perfusion in the infarct-related artery (IRA). However, restoring patency to the IRA does not necessarily guarantee restoration of adequate perfusion to the ischemic myocardium [14]. Within the infarct core, myocytes and capillaries simultaneously undergo necrosis due to sustained ischemia. Capillaries become occluded by debris and blood cells such that even the restoration of blood flow will not promptly reperfuse the infarct core. This area of microvascular obstruction (MO) is called the *"no-flow" region* (Figure 19.1) [13]. This phenomenon is observed noninvasively by CMR after gadolinium-DTPA injection as dark subendocardial zones surrounded by hyperenchanced infarcted myocardium [15]. Wu *et al.* found that presence of MO was a prognostic marker of postinfarction complications and the risk increased with larger infarct size [13]. Taylor *et al.* demonstrated that CMR detects MO in acute MI patients despite successful PCI, which when severe is associated with a lack of wall motion recovery [14]. Hombach *et al.* found that post-MI cardiac death was associated with lower LVEF, larger infarcts, and a greater extent of MO than survivors. They concluded that MO was a better predictor of a major adverse cardiac event (MACE) than infarct size [15]. It is often difficult to determine by clinical factors alone if and when optimal reperfusion at the myocardial tissue level has occurred in patients who present with acute MI after PCI or thrombolytic therapy. Evidence from multicenter trials demonstrated that achievement of patent IRA does not necessarily translate into the best patient outcome when there is inadequate reperfusion at the tissue level [24–27]. Therefore, more aggressive medical management of patients with MO as identified by a noninvasive technique such as CMR may further improve patient management.

Manganese in Assessing Area at Risk

Manganese-based (Mn^{2+}) CMR contrast materials are intracellular agents that may offer unique advantages for characterizing myocardial pathology over gadolinium-based contrast media (Figure 19.4). Mn^{2+} is taken up by active cardiomyocytes via calcium channels and retained in the myocardium for several hours. This property of Mn^{2+} potentially allows for greater flexibility in scanning protocols with the administration of Mn^{2+} outside the scanner, imaging with a T1-weighted CMR technique at a high spatial resolution, and the quantification of myocardial Mn^{2+} contrast enhancement for up to several hours after contrast injection [28]. Using animal models, recent studies have demonstrated that the use of Mn^{2+}-based contrast agents enhance the myocardium and depict the area at risk post-MI [29–31]. These contrast agents are available in different formulations: mangafodipir trisodium (MnDPDP), which is the chelated form, has been FDA-approved at doses of 5 μmol/kg (0.1 ml/kg) with the injection given over 1 min; and $MnCl_2$ in the oral formulation only accumulates in the liver and bile [32]. The main issue regarding the use of Mn^{2+} (elemental form) was concern regarding cardiotoxicity [28]. At the approved dose, MnDPDP has demonstrated to be safe in liver imaging [32]. Different phase II and phase III clinical trials regarding efficacy and safety of Mn^{2+}-based contrast agents exhibited mainly minor side effects including nausea, headache, pruritus, flushing, and warmth [33–35]. Therefore, Mn^{2+}-based contrast agents have potentially

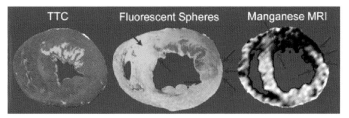

Fig. 19.4 Comparison of TTC-stained myocardium (left), myocardial area at risk demarcated by fluorescent microspheres (middle), and in vivo manganese-enhanced magnetic resonance image (right) corresponding anatomically to the two (left and middle) histopathologic slices. Left: On the TTC-stained specimen, the normal myocardium is stained red and the infarcted region appears as white subendocardial patches. Middle: Fluorescent microspheres injected at the time of the occlusion demarcate the perfused myocardium, which appears yellowish-green, and thus generate contrast between the normal myocardium and the area at risk (borders indicated by arrows). At 90 min of occlusion in these dogs, the infarcted region encompasses only a small percentage of the area at risk, which is largely transmural according to the region demarcated by the fluorescent microspheres. Right: In vivo manganese-enhanced phase-sensitive inversion-recovery fast-gradient recalled echo magnetic resonance image (7.8/3.4/350; voxel size, 1.0 × 0.9 × 8.0 mm) obtained in the short-axis plane at the midventricular level 2 hours after reperfusion, approximately 3 hours after $MnCl_2$ administration. The area at risk starts in the anterior septum and extends through the anterior and anterolateral walls (borders indicated by arrows). From Natanzon *et al.,* used with permission [29].

advantageous characteristics compared to gadolinium-based contrast agents in CMR. Clinical studies are necessary to further explore any emerging clinical applications of this class of CMR contrast agent. Another class of porphyrin-based MRI contrast agents has been classified as infarct-avid, and has been shown to accurately measure infarct size in animal models [36].

Conclusions

Despite significant advancements in the treatment of ischemic heart disease, coronary artery disease (CAD) and sudden cardiac death remain the leading causes of mortality in the United States [37,38]. Myocardial salvage from revascularization leads to decreased infarct size, preservation of left ventricular function, and improved survival [5,11]. However, important clinical questions regarding CAD management still remain a challenge: the optimal timing of late revascularization in acute coronary syndrome, correlation of coronary artery patency with myocardial tissue perfusion, as well as timing and cost-effective implantation of AICD post-MI for prevention of sudden cardiac death [39]. Thus, better characterization and understanding the role of this susceptible area at risk post-MI may generate novel therapeutic approaches and valuable prognostic information.

CMR is a powerful tool in characterizing myocardial tissue components post-MI with its high spatial and temporal resolution, high contrast-to-noise ratio, and accurate and reproducible assessment of left ventricular dimensions and function [14]. In addition to general morphologic and functional assessment, there are other emerging CMR techniques under investigation in evaluating the myocardium post-MI. The need for objective, reproducible assessment of regional ventricular function to assess myocardial deformation post-MI has placed interest in techniques such as magnetic resonance tagging, strain imaging, velocity-encoded imaging, and displacement-encoded imaging with stimulated echoes, or DENSE. Clinical validation of these strain-imaging techniques in the management of heart disease still must be defined [40]. Also, numerous investigators believe we may have reached a "therapeutic ceiling" with revascularization strategies. With promising data provided by cell-based techniques, the replenishment of myocardial cell population and angiogenesis are under investigation to determine its efficacy and safety in left ventricular remodeling post-MI. With its great accuracy and reproducibility, CMR serves as the main imaging modality to assess left ventricular function and dimension post-cell therapy. LGE is used to quantify infarct extent and microvascular obstruction, whereas perfusion imaging is performed to assess angiogenesis/arteriogenesis [41]. In our view, novel CMR techniques that characterize the myocardium hold promise for better understanding myocardial pathophysiology, and may lead to significant therapeutic and prognostic advancement.

References

1 Simonetti, O.P., *et al.* (2001) An improved MR imaging technique for the visualization of myocardial infarction. *Radiology* **218**(1): 215–223.

2 Wu, E., *et al.* (2001) Visualisation of presence, location, and transmural extent of healed Q-wave and non-Q-wave myocardial infarction. *Lancet* **357**(9249): 21–28.

3 Wagner, A., *et al.* (2003) Contrast-enhanced MRI and routine single photon emission computed tomography (SPECT) perfusion imaging for detection of subendocardial myocardial infarcts: an imaging study. *Lancet* **361**(9355): 374–379.

4 Ricciardi, M.J., *et al.* (2001) Visualization of discrete microinfarction after percutaneous coronary intervention associated with mild creatine kinase-MB elevation. *Circulation* **103**(23): 2780–2783.

5 Aletras, A.H., *et al.* (2006) Retrospective determination of the area at risk for reperfused acute myocardial infarction with T2-weighted cardiac magnetic resonance imaging: histopathological and displacement encoding with stimulated echoes (DENSE) functional validations. *Circulation* **113**(15): 1865–1870.

6 Sun, Y., *et al.* (2002) Infarct scar as living tissue. *Basic Res Cardiol* **97**(5): 343–347.

7 Schmidt, A., *et al.* (2007) Infarct tissue heterogeneity by magnetic resonance imaging identifies enhanced cardiac arrhythmia susceptibility in patients with left ventricular dysfunction. *Circulation* **115**(15): 2006–2014.

8 Klocke, F.J., Wu, E., Lee, D.C. (2006) "Shades of gray" in cardiac magnetic resonance images of infarcted myocardium: can they tell us what we'd like them to? *Circulation* **114**(1): 8–10.

9 Yan, A.T., *et al.* (2006) Characterization of the peri-infarct zone by contrast-enhanced cardiac magnetic resonance imaging is a powerful predictor of post-myocardial infarction mortality. *Circulation* **114**(1): 32–39.

10 Nazarian, S., *et al.* (2005) Magnetic resonance assessment of the substrate for inducible ventricular tachycardia in nonischemic cardiomyopathy. *Circulation* **112**(18): 2821–2825.

11 Pennell, D. (2006) Myocardial salvage: retrospection, resolution, and radio waves. *Circulation* **113**(15): 1821–1823.

12 Abdel-Aty, H., *et al.* (2004) Delayed enhancement and T2-weighted cardiovascular magnetic resonance imaging differentiate acute from chronic myocardial infarction. *Circulation* **109**(20): 2411–2416.

13 Wu, K.C., *et al.* (1998) Prognostic significance of microvascular obstruction by magnetic resonance imaging in patients with acute myocardial infarction. *Circulation* **97**(8): 765–772.

14 Taylor, A.J., *et al.* (2004) Detection of acutely impaired microvascular reperfusion after infarct angioplasty with magnetic resonance imaging. *Circulation* **109**(17): 2080–2085.

15 Hombach, V., *et al.* (2005) Sequelae of acute myocardial infarction regarding cardiac structure and function and their prognostic significance as assessed by magnetic resonance imaging. *Eur Heart J* **26**(6): 549–557.

16 Peters, N.S., Wit, A.L. (1998) Myocardial architecture and ventricular arrhythmogenesis. *Circulation* **97**(17): 1746–1754.

17 Kwong, R.Y., *et al.* (2006) Impact of unrecognized myocardial scar detected by cardiac magnetic resonance imaging on event-free survival in patients presenting with signs or symptoms of coronary artery disease. *Circulation* **113**(23): 2733–2743.

18 Bello, D., *et al.* (2005) Infarct morphology identifies patients with substrate for sustained ventricular tachycardia. *J Am Coll Cardiol* **45**(7): 1104–1108.

19 Yan, A.T., *et al.* (2006) Characterization of the peri-infarct zone by contrast-enhanced cardiac magnetic resonance imaging is a powerful predictor of post-myocardial infarction mortality. *Circulation* **114**(1): 32–39.

20 Garcia-Dorado, D., *et al.* (1993) Analysis of myocardial oedema by magnetic resonance imaging early after coronary artery occlusion with or without reperfusion. *Cardiovasc Res* **27**(8): 1462–1469.

21 Garcia-Dorado, D., Oliveras, J. (1993) Myocardial oedema: a preventable cause of reperfusion injury? *Cardiovasc Res* **27**(9): 1555–1563.

22 Nilsson, J.C., *et al.* (2001) Sustained postinfarction myocardial oedema in humans visualised by magnetic resonance imaging. *Heart* **85**(6): 639–642.

23 Miller, D.D., *et al.* (1989) Effect of hyperosmotic mannitol on magnetic resonance relaxation parameters in reperfused canine myocardial infarction. *Magn Reson Imaging* **7**(1): 79–88.

24 Gibson, C.M., *et al.* (2000) Relationship of TIMI myocardial perfusion grade to mortality after administration of thrombolytic drugs. *Circulation* **101**(2): 125–130.

25 Gibson, C.M., *et al.* (2002) Methodologic and clinical validation of the TIMI myocardial perfusion grade in acute myocardial infarction. *J Thromb Thrombolysis* **14**(3): 233–237.

26 Gibson, C.M., *et al.* (2002) The relationship of intracoronary stent placement following thrombolytic therapy to tissue level perfusion. *J Thromb Thrombolysis* **13**(2): 63–68.

27 Wong, G.C., *et al.* (2003) Time for contrast material to traverse the epicardial artery and the myocardium in ST-segment elevation acute myocardial infarction versus unstable angina pectoris/non-ST-elevation acute myocardial infarction. *Am J Cardiol* **91**(10): 1163–1167.

28 Wendland, M.F. (2004) Applications of manganese-enhanced magnetic resonance imaging (MEMRI) to imaging of the heart. *NMR Biomed* **17**(8): 581–594.

29 Natanzon, A., *et al.* (2005) Determining canine myocardial area at risk with manganese-enhanced MR imaging. *Radiology* **236**(3): 859–866.

30 Hu, T.C., *et al.* (2005) Manganese enhanced magnetic resonance imaging of normal and ischemic canine heart. *Magn Reson Med* **54**(1): 196–200.

31 Flacke, S., *et al.* (2003) Characterization of viable and nonviable myocardium at MR imaging: comparison of gadolinium-based extracellular and blood pool contrast materials versus manganese-based contrast materials in a rat myocardial infarction model. *Radiology* **226**(3): 731–738.

32 Bellin, M.F., *et al.* (2005) Safety of MR liver specific contrast media. *Eur Radiol* **15**(8): 1607–1614.

33 Torres, C.G., *et al.* (1997) MnDPDP for MR imaging of the liver: results from the European phase III studies. *Acta Radiol* **38**(4 Pt 2): 631–637.

34 Rummeny, E., *et al.* (1991) Manganese-DPDP as a hepatobiliary contrast agent in the magnetic resonance imaging of liver tumors: results of clinical phase II trials in Germany including 141 patients. *Invest Radiol* **26**(Suppl 1): S142–145; disc. S150–155.

35 Wang, C., *et al.* (1997) Diagnostic efficacy of MnDPDP in MR imaging of the liver: a phase III multicentre study. *Acta Radiol* **38**(4 Pt 2): 643–649.

36 Ni, Y., *et al.* (2005) Necrosis avid contrast agents: functional similarity versus structural diversity. *Invest Radiol* **40**(8): 526–535.

37 Rosamond, W., *et al.* (2007) Heart disease and stroke statistics — 2007 update: a report from the American Heart Association Statistics Committee and Stroke Statistics Subcommittee. *Circulation* **115**(5): e69–171.

38 Zipes, D.P., *et al.* (2006) ACC/AHA/ESC 2006 guidelines for management of patients with ventricular arrhythmias and the prevention of sudden cardiac death: a report of the American College of Cardiology/American Heart Association Task Force and the European Society of Cardiology Committee for Practice Guidelines (writing committee to develop guidelines for management of patients with ventricular arrhythmias and the prevention of sudden cardiac death): developed in collaboration with the European Heart Rhythm Association and the Heart Rhythm Society. *Circulation* **114**(10): e385–484.

39 Buxton, A.E. (2005) Sudden death after myocardial infarction — who needs prophylaxis, and when? *N Engl J Med* **352**(25): 2638–2640.

40 Castillo, E., Lima, J.A., Bluemke, D.A. (2003) Regional myocardial function: advances in MR imaging and analysis. *Radiographics* **23**(Spec No): S127–140.

41 Fuster, V., *et al.* (2006) The utility of magnetic resonance imaging in cardiac tissue regeneration trials. *Nat Clin Pract Cardiovasc Med* **3**(Suppl 1): S2–7.

Chapter 20

Technical Advances and the Future Prospects of High Field Strength MRI

Ahmed M. Gharib, Matthias Stuber, and Roderic I. Pettigrew

Cardiac magnetic resonance imaging (MRI) applications at high field strength is of growing interest, especially with the increasing availability of commercial 3T systems. The promise of increased signal-to-noise ratio (SNR) resulting from increased polarization of spins in a high-strength static magnetic field (B_0) opens many possibilities for improved image quality [1–3]. This potential enhancement of image quality can be directly appreciated as a more clear delineation of anatomic detail in clinical images or as improved spatial and temporal resolution derived from the higher SNR [4]. Simultaneously, the signal loss resulting from greater spatial resolution or from using parallel imaging is more tolerable [5,6].

An additional advantage of a high magnetic field strength for some applications is the associated increase in T1. This attribute has a practical benefit in myocardial tagging. The prolonged myocardial T1 values at higher field strengths prevent the premature fading of saturation bands commonly used for tagged images employed for the assessment of myocardial wall mechanics [7]. This prolonged T1 phenomena also makes spin labeling techniques an attractive alternative for coronary and possibly myocardial perfusion imaging without contrast agents because there is less decay of the labeled spins in concert with the inherently higher SNR [8]. Finally, the increase in chemical shift does not only facilitate fat saturation for imaging but in conjunction with the higher SNR, it also leads to an improved spectral resolution in cardiac spectroscopy [9].

Cardiac imaging at a higher magnetic filed strength also comes with many challenges. In addition to increased B_0 inhomogeneity (magnetic field susceptibility), transmit field (B_1) inhomogeneity also contributes to the degradation of image quality [1,3,8,10–12]. Further, the amplified magnetohydrodynamic effect

Novel Techniques for Imaging the Heart, 1st edition. Edited by M. Di Carli and R. Kwong.
© 2008 American Heart Association, ISBN: 9-781-4051-7533-3.

at high field strength can challenge reliable R-wave detection, which is essential for most cardiovascular applications [13]. Finally, the specific absorption rate (SAR) limitations pose an additional challenge for steady state free precision (SSFP) imaging and fast spin echo (FSE) imaging. This review will discuss the current and potential future applications of high magnetic field strength MRI.

Cardiac Function and Morphology

Cardiac wall motion and ventricular function are commonly assessed using SSFP-based techniques at 1.5 T. This technique provides an optimal contrast-to-noise ratio (CNR) between the myocardium and blood pool at a high SNR and is obtained in a relatively short breath-hold, allowing its practical application in the clinical setting [14,15]. Heart-lung interface induced B_0 inhomogeneity results in black-band artifacts commonly seen at 3 T [16]. Such artifacts can be reduced by improving B_0 homogeneity with localized linear or second-order shimming techniques and optimization of resonance frequency, in addition to minimizing the repetition time (TR) [7,17,18].

Michaely *et al.* demonstrated the feasibility of using both SSFP and segmented spoiled gradient echo (SGE) techniques at 3 T for cardiac function analysis with similar accuracy compared to 1.5 T [19]. In their study, 85.7% of all SSFP images at 3 T demonstrated off-resonance susceptibility artifacts at the heart-lung interface, all of which were eliminated on the repeat exams after using frequency scouts to determine the optimal frequency offset. They also concluded that SGE sequences benefited more from the higher magnetic field as a result of a 16% increase in CNR compared to 1.5 T, whereas with SSFP imaging potential benefits were reduced by the artifacts. Alternatively, Tyler *et al.* recommended the use of SSFP sequences because of the higher gain of SNR and CNR than SGE sequences at 3 T, therefore still yielding higher-quality images [20]. Undoubtedly, with the wider implementation of better shimming techniques, the technical challenges that inhibit the use of SSFP at 3 T will be overcome, allowing this to become the more commonly used cine technique at 3 T [17].

Parallel imaging is a generic group of techniques that enhances the efficiency of data acquisition by incorporating the spatial orientation of the surface coils used in data collection. This group of techniques can substantially accelerate data acquisition, and has been in routine clinical use at 1.5 T cardiac MRI. Although parallel imaging at an acceleration factor of two or more is often faced with artifacts or inadequate resultant SNR at 1.5 T, the inherent higher SNR at 3 T appears to compensate well for this SNR loss associated with parallel imaging. The benefits of parallel imaging at high field strength were demonstrated by Gutberlet *et al.*, whereby an acceleration factor of two improved data acquisition efficiency and reduced a scan time from 16 heart beats to 8 heart beats [7]. Despite this faster acquisition, the SNR at 3 T was superior to that at 1.5 T, both with and without parallel imaging. The use of parallel imaging resulted

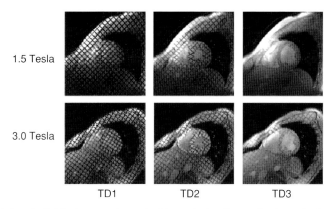

1.5 Tesla

3.0 Tesla

TD1 TD2 TD3

Fig. 20.1 Interindividual comparison of midventricular short-axis views obtained with gradient echo-based 2D cine tagging techniques for a healthy volunteer at 1.5 T (top) and 3.0 T (bottom) at the beginning of the cardiac cycle (trigger delay 1 = TD1), end-systole (TD2), and end-diastole (TD3). At 1.5 T, the saturation bands dissipated before the end of the cardiac cycle (TD3), and hence the tagging grids disappeared at approximately 75% of the R–R interval. At 3.0 T, the tags were present throughout the entire heart cycle (TD1 to TD3). From Gutberlet *et al.*, used with permission [11].

in only a 26% loss of SNR and 28% loss of CNR at 3 T compared to 37% and 38% at 1.5 T, respectively. The benefits of combining parallel imaging with high field strength additionally help counterbalance shortcomings associated with the increased radio-frequency power deposition. The shortening of scan time with less detrimental effect on image quality during cine breath-hold acquisitions promotes more reliable imaging due to abbreviated breath-hold durations. Additionally, more cine phases with less motion blurring can be acquired during a single breath-hold, allowing for added accuracy in the delineation of ventricular contours.

However, one of the major advantages of 3 T in assessing cardiac function is the improved myocardial tagging consequent to the prolonged longitudinal relaxation time at higher field strength [11]. With prolonged T1, the fading of the tags is reduced, thereby facilitating access to both systolic and diastolic phases of the cardiac cycle. It has been shown that in diastole, a significant increase in CNR (187%) and SNR (88%) can be obtained at 3 T when compared to 1.5 T [7]. These results are consistent with a more recent study (Figure 20.1) [11]. Therefore, myocardial tagging at higher magnetic field strength may become a valuable tool in the assessment of diastolic dysfunction, which is also important in the diagnosis of heart failure [21,22].

The use of T1- or T2-weighted techniques with inversion recovery (IR) preparation are also often used for cardiovascular applications. Although the sequences show improvement in SNR and CNR when applied at high field strength, the detrimental effect of B_1 and B_0 inhomogeneity affect uniformity of the IR preparation and can reduce image quality [11]. This problem can be overcome by using adiabatic pulses, which are less sensitive to such field inhomogeneities [23,24]. In addition to the potential spatial and temporal resolution benefits previously described, IR-prepared FSE techniques can also benefit from the synergy of parallel imaging at high field strength by reducing the number of phase-encoding steps and thereby power deposition [11]. An alternative technique to overcome the SAR limitations includes the use of variable flip angles and hyperechoes [25]. In principle, reducing the echo train length lengthens the scan time. However, if compensated by parallel imaging with acceleration factors that take advantage of the inherent signal reserve at high field strength, one can effectively contain the effects of image blurring due to shorter T2 at higher field strengths and still maintain sufficiently short acquisition times.

Infarction and Ischemia Imaging

One of the important uses of cardiac MRI at 1.5 T is in the detection of myocardial infarction using IR-prepared delayed-enhancement techniques. As discussed in Chapter 8, the differentiation of infarcted from hibernating myocardium with spatial resolution great enough to detect subendocardial infarcts is well-demonstrated at 1.5 T [26–28]. This image quality is further improved at 3 T as a result of increased SNR and CNR compared to 1.5 T [11,29]. The advantage of increased CNR is the result of prolonged longitudinal relaxation of unenhanced tissues with increased field strength, which leads to a higher sensitivity to injected gadolinium agents [29,30]. This relaxation may also allow for a reduction of the injected dose of the gadolinium agent. The prolonged T1 of myocardium necessitates the use of longer inversion times (TI) for the IR preparation (about 330 ms) at 3 T, compared to 260 ms for 1.5 T for optimal myocardial suppression [29]. Additionally, the lower T1 relaxation slope at 3 T compared to 1.5 T allows for a more exact determination of the inversion time, further improving the chances of optimal CNR and thereby supporting improved diagnostic image quality [29].

The most commonly used sequence for myocardial viability imaging is an IR-prepared spoiled gradient echo (IR-SGE) technique [31]. The use of high field strength scanners improves the CNR and SNR of this sequence, which can be exploited to shorten scan time by the complementary use of parallel imaging [11]. However, this T1-weighted sequence requires the individual predetermination of TI for adequate myocardial nulling to achieve the desired CNR effect after contrast administration. To avoid these pre-scans for accurate null-time determination (TI-scouts) and to achieve a consistent contrast, Kellman *et al.* proposed a phase-sensitive reconstruction at 1.5 T [32]. Huber *et al.* showed that such a technique can be implemented at 3 T and that it accurately depicts myocardial infarcts [33]. Furthermore, they used a single-shot readout that allows for

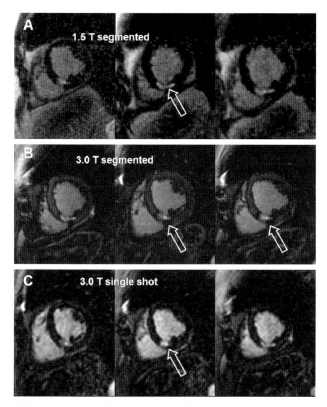

Fig. 20.2 A 67-year-old man with a subendocardial infarction in the perfusion territory of the right coronary artery and the circumflex artery. (a) The three upper images were acquired with a segmented IR turboFLASH at 1.5 T, (b) the middle images were acquired with a segmented IR turboFLASH sequence at 3.0 T, and (c) the three lower images were acquired with a single-shot IR turboFLASH sequence at 3.0 T. All images reveal hyperenhanced myocardium in the lateral, inferolateral, inferior, and inferoseptal segments corresponding to myocardial infarctions. From Bauner *et al.*, used with permission [34].

covering the entire left ventricle (nine slices) in a single breath-hold as opposed to a single slice per breath-hold for the more commonly used IR-SGE technique. The implementation of a single-shot readout results in a 22% CNR loss at 1.5 T. However, this readout technique at 3 T provides a significantly higher CNR compared to a similar technique and even the more conventional IR-SGE at 1.5 T. Therefore, despite shortening the scan time by using a single-shot readout and avoiding the required TI-scouts, there was a significant gain in CNR at 3 T. This advantage should be particularly useful for patients who cannot hold their breath well enough and patients with cardiac arrhythmias. This single-shot read-out method can be applied successfully at 3 T using both SGE (Figure 20.2) and

SSFP sequences with significant gain of CNR compared to similar techniques at 1.5 T [33,34].

Myocardial perfusion MRI during the administration of a contrast bolus is commonly used in many centers for the assessment of myocardial ischemia [35,36]. This method is substantially improved at 3 T [37]. Due to the acquisition speed required to capture the first-pass myocardial perfusion, a saturation recovery (SR) preparation is applied to either SSPF or SGE type sequences. This preparation provides the CNR desired for the detection of regional changes in myocardial perfusion during rest and stress, which in turn delineates the site of myocardial ischemia. However, in the attempt to obtain the best temporal resolution needed to better capture the passage of contrast bolus, the use of such SR prepared sequences has limited spatial resolution (2 to 3 mm in-plane). Image quality is also compromised by the use of parallel imaging and the relative decreased SNR at 1.5 T. Therefore, it is not surprising that perfusion imaging is significantly improved at a higher magnetic field strength [11,37–39]. As in viability imaging, this improvement is the result of both the increased SNR and prolonged T1 time of the myocardium.

Coronary Imaging

Coronary imaging by magnetic resonance is one of the more challenging applications at any field strength due to the small size of these vessels and the significant motion associated with breathing and intrinsic myocardial motion. Despite these challenges, coronary magnetic resonance angiography (MRA) at 1.5 T has been shown to be a tool capable of the routine imaging of coronary arteries in selected clinical settings and some limited assessment of coronary atherosclerotic disease (CAD) [40–42]. Early studies demonstrated the feasibility of coronary MRA at 3 T [3,43]. Compared to 1.5 T, the earliest use of 3 T did not show a significant improvement in sensitivity or specificity for the detection of CAD, although there was an increase in SNR [43]. However, the authors did not exploit the full potential of the stronger magnetic field by addressing some 3-T specific technical challenges that would allow pushing the limits of spatial or temporal resolution [43]. With the advent of coronary computed tomography angiography (CTA), which also provides high-quality images noninvasively, the limits of high field strength coronary MRA must be further investigated to offer a competitive alternative to CTA without the use of radiation or nephrotoxic contrast agents.

Coronary MRA at 1.5 T is most commonly performed using SSFP imaging sequences to maximize SNR and CNR [41]. Without the use of intravascular contrast agents, the desired CNR between oxygenated blood and the myocardium is achieved by using T2 preparatory (T2 Prep) pulses [44]. These techniques are implemented for both the whole-heart and targeted volume approaches [40–42,45,46]. Due to B_0 and B_1 inhomogeneities at stronger magnetic fields, the

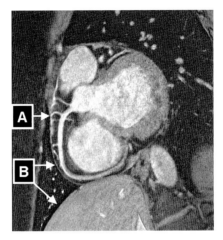

Fig. 20.3 Navigator-gated and navigator-corrected double-oblique 3D segmented k-space gradient-echo imaging sequence: 3 T, TR/TE = 7.5/2.3, $\alpha = 20°$, resolution = 0.35 × 0.35 × 1.5 mm, field of view = 270 × 216 mm, 800 × 610 matrix, scan duration = 906 sec, 12 radiofrequency excitations per R–R interval, acquisition time window T_{acq} = 90 msec, 10 slices (acquired), 20 slices (reconstructed), fat saturation. A high-resolution scan of a 23-year-old healthy man acquired at a trigger delay of 591 msec using FREEZE software, an automated tool for the identification of the period of minimal myocardial motion, shows (a) a highly visible interface in the region of coronary arteries (small-diameter branches) as well as (b) the pericardium and lung-liver interface. Together with ability to reveal small-diameter branching vessels, this result suggests excellent suppression of both intrinsic and extrinsic myocardial motion. From Ustun *et al.*, used with permission [48].

use of both SSFP and T2 Prep pose challenges. To address these challenges, the use of adiabatic T2 Prep in conjunction with SGE techniques is currently suggested [3,23].

The use of parallel imaging at 3 T improves temporal resolution, which allows for coronary MRA imaging using short acquisition windows. Despite the use of SGE sequences (as opposed to higher SNR allowed by SSFP used at 1.5 T), the SNR is sufficient to support imaging in the systolic quiescent period [47]. This result may provide an opportunity for coronary MRA imaging in patients with tachycardia who have contraindications to the use of beta blockers necessary for coronary CTA. Furthermore, high-resolution imaging of up to 350 μm^2 is possible at 3 T (Figure 20.3), which is similar to CTA resolution and currently not easily achievable at 1.5 T [48].

Although the previously mentioned advances were achieved using the targeted approach, a whole-heart technique similar to CTA is probably more desirable. This whole-heart approach is feasible at 3 T, as it is at 1.5 T, using either breath-holding or free-breathing navigator gated techniques [49–51]. Although the whole-heart technique at 3 T has been shown to be useful for the assessment of coronary artery anomalies, it has not been optimized and its use for CAD evaluation has not been evaluated [51]. Nonetheless, greater spatial and temporal resolution imaging using whole-heart techniques must be explored and more fully developed. Similarly, black-blood vessel wall imaging is feasible at 3 T, and is improved by using an adiabatic IR preparatory pulse [24]. However, the resolution limits and its application in CAD patients have not been exploited to date. The advantage of prolonged T1 time has also proven to be beneficial for contrast-enhanced coronary MRA at high magnetic field strength [49,50]. Further exploitation of this prolonged T1 time can potentially be used for spin-labeled coronary MRA as well [8].

Flow Assessment

Phase-contrast MRI is an accurate method of quantifying blood flow velocity and has been demonstrated to work well at 1.5 T [52–55]. Due to spatial and temporal resolution constraints, its implementation has been predominantly limited to large structures such as the ventricles, valves, or great vessels [56–59]. Similar accuracy and precision of blood velocity measurement is achievable at high (3 T) magnetic field strengths in potentially smaller vessels [11,60,61]. As a result of the increased SNR, a significantly higher velocity-to-noise ratio is possible at 3 T [11,60,61]. This reduction of noise allows more accurate velocity measurements at 3 T, especially for vessels with slower flow, where a smaller phase shift is expected. Additionally, the increased SNR at high field strength opens the opportunity for the assessment of three-dimensional velocity maps with three-directional velocity encoding [62–64]. This more comprehensive assessment of blood flow hemodynamics attainable at high field strength may allow for a better and more personalized understanding of congenital (see Figure 13.3 in Chapter 13) or acquired vascular disease and cardiac pathology. Furthermore, the exploitation of the higher SNR at 3 T also supports the assessment of coronary blood flow using the phase-contrast technique (Figure 20.4) with greater spatial and temporal resolution [65]. With coronary flow velocity measurements now possible, a true assessment of coronary flow reserve may be feasible in patients with coronary atherosclerosis.

Conclusions

The early experience is that cardiac MRI can benefit from the intrinsic advantages of a high magnetic field strength, specifically 3 T. However, continued technical development is required and several potential possibilities must be further defined and investigated, especially in targeted patient populations. Many of the challenges of imaging at high magnetic field strength have only been partially addressed. Further advances in sequence and coil design, such

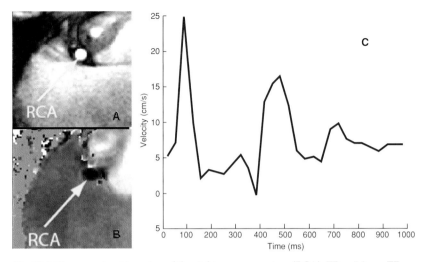

Fig. 20.4 Phase-contrast imaging of the right coronary artery (RCA); TR = 5.2 ms, TE = 2.8 ms, FOV = 280 mm, matrix = 368, V_{ENC} = 50 cm/s. (a) Magnitude image and (b) flow map through the RCA obtained at 3 T. (c) Through-plane blood velocity in the RCA measured during the cardiac cycle. Image courtesy of R. Nezafat and C. Stehning.

as phased-array coils with a larger number of coil elements, are expected and will undoubtedly support further improvements in cardiovascular imaging at 3 T. At the present time, it is unclear whether going to an even higher field strength (7 T) will further advance in vivo human cardiovascular MRI in general. The obstacles related to both B_0 and B_1 inhomogeneity, as well as those related to SAR and transmit coil design, may require many years of research and development. However, given the very promising early results obtained in brain imaging, it is likely that high-spatial resolution carotid MRI for the characterization of plaque is among the early beneficiaries of this high magnetic field strength.

References

1 Singerman, R.W., Denison, T.J., Wen, H., Balaban, R.S. (1997) Simulation of B1 field distribution and intrinsic signal-to-noise in cardiac MRI as a function of static magnetic field. *J Magn Reson* **125**: 72–83.

2 Noeske, R., Seifert, F., Rhein, K.H., Rinneberg, H. (2000) Human cardiac imaging at 3 T using phased array coils. *Magn Reson Med* **44**: 978–982.

3 Stuber, M., Botnar, R.M., Fischer, S.E., *et al.* (2002) Preliminary report on in vivo coronary MRA at 3 Tesla in humans. *Magn Reson Med* **48**: 425–429.

4 Dougherty, L., Connick, T.J., Mizsei, G. (2001) Cardiac imaging at 4 Tesla. *Magn Reson Med* **45**: 176–178.

5 Pruessmann, K.P., Weiger, M., Scheidegger, M.B., Boesiger, P. (1999) SENSE: sensitivity encoding for fast MRI. *Magn Reson Med* **42**: 952–962.

6 Sodickson, D.K., Manning, W.J. (1997) Simultaneous acquisition of spatial harmonics (SMASH): fast imaging with radiofrequency coil arrays. *Magn Reson Med* **38**: 591–603.

7 Gutberlet, M., Schwinge, K., Freyhardt, P., *et al.* (2005) Influence of high magnetic field strengths and parallel acquisition strategies on image quality in cardiac 2D CINE magnetic resonance imaging: comparison of 1.5 T vs. 3.0 T. *Eur Radiol* **15**: 1586–1597.

8 Stuber, M., Weiss, R.G. (2007) Coronary magnetic resonance angiography. *J Magn Reson Imaging* **26**: 219–234.

9 Schar, M., Kozerke, S., Boesiger, P. (2004) Navigator gating and volume tracking for double-triggered cardiac proton spectroscopy at 3 Tesla. *Magn Reson Med* **51**: 1091–1095.

10 Bottomley, P.A., Andrew, E.R. (1978) RF magnetic field penetration, phase shift and power dissipation in biological tissue: implications for NMR imaging. *Phys Med Biol* **23**: 630–643.

11 Gutberlet, M., Noeske, R., Schwinge, K., *et al.* (2006) Comprehensive cardiac magnetic resonance imaging at 3.0 Tesla: feasibility and implications for clinical applications. *Invest Radiol* **41**: 154–167.

12 Nayak, K.S., Cunningham, C.H., Santos, J.M., Pauly, J.M. (2004) Real-time cardiac MRI at 3 Tesla. *Magn Reson Med* **51**: 655–660.

13 Fischer, S.E., Wickline, S.A., Lorenz, C.H. (1999) Novel real-time R-wave detection algorithm based on the vectorcardiogram for accurate gated magnetic resonance acquisitions. *Magn Reson Med* **42**: 361–370.

14 Plein, S., Bloomer, T.N., Ridgway, J.P., *et al.* (2001) Steady-state free precession magnetic resonance imaging of the heart: comparison with segmented k-space gradient-echo imaging. *J Magn Reson Imaging* **14**: 230–236.

15 Thiele, H., Nagel, E., Paetsch, I., *et al.* (2001) Functional cardiac MR imaging with steady-state free precession (SSFP) significantly improves endocardial border delineation without contrast agents. *J Magn Reson Imaging* **14**: 362–367.

16 Atalay, M.K., Poncelet, B.P., Kantor, H.L., *et al.* (2001) Cardiac susceptibility artifacts arising from the heart-lung interface. *Magn Reson Med* **45**: 341–345.

17 Schar, M., Kozerke, S., Fischer, S.E., Boesiger, P. (2004) Cardiac SSFP imaging at 3 Tesla. *Magn Reson Med* **51**: 799–806.

18 Duerk, J.L., Lewin, J.S., Wendt, M., Petersilge, C. (1998) Remember true FISP? A high SNR, near 1-second imaging method for T2-like contrast in interventional MRI at 0.2 T. *J Magn Reson Imaging* **8**: 203–208.

19 Michaely, H.J., Nael, K., Schoenberg, S.O., *et al.* (2006) Analysis of cardiac function—comparison between 1.5 Tesla and 3.0 Tesla cardiac cine magnetic resonance imaging: preliminary experience. *Invest Radiol* **41**: 133–140.

20 Tyler, D.J., Hudsmith, L.E., Petersen, S.E., *et al.* (2006) Cardiac cine MR-imaging at 3 T: FLASH vs SSFP. *J Cardiovasc Magn Reson* **8**: 709–715.

21 Stuber, M., Scheidegger, M.B., Fischer, S.E., *et al.* (1999) Alterations in the local myocardial motion pattern in patients suffering from pressure overload due to aortic stenosis. *Circulation* **100**: 361–368.

22 Chinnaiyan, K.M., Alexander, D., Maddens, M., McCullough, P.A. (2007) Curriculum in cardiology: integrated diagnosis and management of diastolic heart failure. *Am Heart J* **153**: 189–200.

23 Nezafat, R., Stuber, M., Ouwerkerk, R., *et al.* (2006) B1-insensitive T2 preparation for improved coronary magnetic resonance angiography at 3 T. *Magn Reson Med* **55**: 858–864.

24 Priest, A.N., Bansmann, P.M., Kaul, M.G., *et al.* (2005) Magnetic resonance imaging of the coronary vessel wall at 3 T using an obliquely oriented reinversion slab with adiabatic pulses. *Magn Reson Med* **54**: 1115–1122.

25 Busse, R.F. (2004) Reduced RF power without blurring: correcting for modulation of refocusing flip angle in FSE sequences. *Magn Reson Med* **51**: 1031–1037.

26 Ansari, M., Araoz, P.A., Gerard, S.K., *et al.* (2004) Comparison of late enhancement cardiovascular magnetic resonance and thallium SPECT in patients with coronary disease and left ventricular dysfunction. *J Cardiovasc Magn Reson* **6**: 549–556.

27 Hunold, P., Brandt-Mainz, K., Freudenberg, L., *et al.* (2002) Evaluation of myocardial viability with contrast-enhanced magnetic resonance imaging — comparison of the late enhancement technique with positron emission tomography. *Rofo* **174**: 867–873.

28 Kim, R.J., Fieno, D.S., Parrish, T.B., *et al.* (1999) Relationship of MRI delayed contrast enhancement to irreversible injury, infarct age, and contractile function. *Circulation* **100**: 1992–2002.

29 Klumpp, B., Fenchel, M., Hoevelborn, T., *et al.* (2006) Assessment of myocardial viability using delayed enhancement magnetic resonance imaging at 3.0 Tesla. *Invest Radiol* **41**: 661–667.

30 Rinck, P.A., Muller, R.N. (1999) Field strength and dose dependence of contrast enhancement by gadolinium-based MR contrast agents. *Eur Radiol* **9**: 998–1004.

31 Kim, R.J., Wu, E., Rafael, A., *et al.* (2000) The use of contrast-enhanced magnetic resonance imaging to identify reversible myocardial dysfunction. *N Engl J Med* **343**: 1445–1453.

32 Kellman, P., Arai, A.E., McVeigh, E.R., Aletras, A.H. (2002) Phase-sensitive inversion recovery for detecting myocardial infarction using gadolinium-delayed hyperenhancement. *Magn Reson Med* **47**: 372–383.

33 Huber, A., Bauner, K., Wintersperger, B.J., *et al.* (2006) Phase-sensitive inversion recovery (PSIR) single-shot TrueFISP for assessment of myocardial infarction at 3 tesla. *Invest Radiol* **41**: 148–153.

34 Bauner, K.U., Muehling, O., Wintersperger, B.J., *et al.* (2007) Inversion recovery single-shot TurboFLASH for assessment of myocardial infarction at 3 Tesla. *Invest Radiol* **42**: 361–371.

35 Al-Saadi, N., Nagel, E., Gross, M., *et al.* (2000) Noninvasive detection of myocardial ischemia from perfusion reserve based on cardiovascular magnetic resonance. *Circulation* **101**: 1379–1383.

36 Nagel, E., Klein, C., Paetsch, I., *et al.* (2003) Magnetic resonance perfusion measurements for the noninvasive detection of coronary artery disease. *Circulation* **108**: 432–437.

37 Cheng, A.S., Pegg, T.J., Karamitsos, T.D., *et al.* (2007) Cardiovascular magnetic resonance perfusion imaging at 3-Tesla for the detection of coronary artery disease: a comparison with 1.5-Tesla. *J Am Coll Cardiol* **49**: 2440–2449.

38 Ruan, C., Yang, S.H., Cusi, K., *et al.* (2007) Contrast-enhanced first-pass myocardial perfusion magnetic resonance imaging with parallel acquisition at 3.0 Tesla. *Invest Radiol* **42**: 352–360.

39 Theisen, D., Wintersperger, B.J., Huber, A., *et al.* (2007) Myocardial perfusion imaging with gadobutrol: a comparison between 3 and 1.5 Tesla with an identical sequence design. *Invest Radiol* **42**: 499–506.

40 Kim, W.Y., Danias, P.G., Stuber, M., *et al.* (2001) Coronary magnetic resonance angiography for the detection of coronary stenoses. *N Engl J Med* **345**: 1863–1869.

41 Sakuma, H., Ichikawa, Y., Chino, S., *et al.* (2006) Detection of coronary artery stenosis with whole-heart coronary magnetic resonance angiography. *J Am Coll Cardiol* **48**: 1946–1950.

42 Sakuma, H., Ichikawa, Y., Suzawa, N., *et al.* (2005) Assessment of coronary arteries with total study time of less than 30 minutes by using whole-heart coronary MR angiography. *Radiology* **237**: 316–321.

43 Sommer, T., Hackenbroch, M., Hofer, U., *et al.* (2005) Coronary MR angiography at 3.0 T versus that at 1.5 T: initial results in patients suspected of having coronary artery disease. *Radiology* **234**: 718–725.

44 Brittain, J.H., Hu, B.S., Wright, G.A., *et al.* (1995) Coronary angiography with magnetization-prepared T_2 contrast. *Magn Reson Med* **33**: 689–696.

45 Stuber, M., Botnar, R.M., Danias, P.G., *et al.* (1999) Double-oblique free-breathing high resolution three-dimensional coronary magnetic resonance angiography. *J Am Coll Cardiol* **34**: 524–531.

46 Weber, O.M., Martin, A.J., Higgins, C.B. (2003) Whole-heart steady-state free precession coronary artery magnetic resonance angiography. *Magn Reson Med* **50**: 1223–1228.

47 Gharib, A.M., Herzka, D.A., Ustun, A.O., *et al.* (2007) Coronary MR angiography at 3 T during diastole and systole. *JMRI* **268**: 921–926.

48 Ustun, A., Desai, M., Abd-Elmoniem, K.Z., *et al.* (2007) Automated identification of minimal myocardial motion for improved image quality on MR angiography at 3 T. *AJR* **188**: W283–290.

49 Bi, X., Li, D. (2005) Coronary arteries at 3.0 T: Contrast-enhanced magnetization-prepared three-dimensional breathhold MR angiography. *J Magn Reson Imaging* **21**: 133–139.

50 Bi, X., Park, J., Larson, A.C., *et al.* (2005) Contrast-enhanced 4D radial coronary artery imaging at 3.0 T within a single breath-hold. *Magn Reson Med* **54**: 470–475.

51 Gharib, A.M., Ho, V.B., Rosing, D.R., *et al.* (2007) Coronary artery anomalies and variants: of assessment with coronary MR angiography at 3T technical feasibility study. *Radiology* **247**: 220–227.

52 Moran, P.R., Moran, R.A., Karstaedt, N. (1985) Verification and evaluation of internal flow and motion. True magnetic resonance imaging by the phase gradient modulation method. *Radiology* **154**: 433–441.

53 Zananiri, F.V., Jackson, P.C., Goddard, P.R., *et al.* (1991) An evaluation of the accuracy of flow measurements using magnetic resonance imaging (MRI). *J Med Eng Technol* **15**: 170–176.

54 Oshinski, J.N., Ku, D.N., Bohning, D.E., Pettigrew, R.I. (1992) Effects of acceleration on the accuracy of MR phase velocity measurements. *J Magn Reson Imaging* **2**: 665–670.

55 Pettigrew, R.I., Dannels, W., Galloway, J.R., *et al.* (1987) Quantitative phase-flow MR imaging in dogs by using standard sequences: comparison with in vivo flow-meter measurements. *AJR* **148**: 411–414.

56 Globits, S., Higgins, C.B. (1995) Assessment of valvular heart disease by magnetic resonance imaging. *Am Heart J* **129**: 369–381.

57 Globits, S., Pacher, R., Frank, H., *et al.* (1995) Comparative assessment of right ventricular volumes and ejection fraction by thermodilution and magnetic resonance imaging in dilated cardiomyopathy. *Cardiology* **86**: 67–72.

58 Maier, S.E., Meier, D., Boesiger, P., *et al.* (1989) Human abdominal aorta: comparative measurements of blood flow with MR imaging and multigated Doppler US. *Radiology* **171**: 487–492.

59 Chatzimavroudis, G.P., Oshinski, J.N., Franch, R.H., *et al.* (2001) Evaluation of the precision of magnetic resonance phase velocity mapping for blood flow measurements. *J Cardiovasc Magn Reson* **3**: 11–19.

60 Lotz, J., Doker, R., Noeske, R., *et al.* (2005) In vitro validation of phase-contrast flow measurements at 3 T in comparison to 1.5 T: precision, accuracy, and signal-to-noise ratios. *J Magn Reson Imaging* **21**: 604–610.

61 Pai, V.M. (2007) Phase contrast using multiecho steady-state free precession. *Magn Reson Med* **58**: 419–424.

62 Frydrychowicz, A., Bley, T.A., Dittrich, S., *et al.* (2007) Visualization of vascular hemodynamics in a case of a large patent ductus arteriosus using flow sensitive 3D CMR at 3T. *J Cardiovasc Magn Reson* **9**: 585–587.

63 Frydrychowicz, A., Harloff, A., Jung, B., *et al.* (2007) Time-resolved, 3-dimensional magnetic resonance flow analysis at 3 T: visualization of normal and pathological aortic vascular hemodynamics. *J Comput Assist Tomogr* **31**: 9–15.

64 Markl, M., Harloff, A., Bley, T.A., *et al.* (2007) Time-resolved 3D MR velocity mapping at 3 T: improved navigator-gated assessment of vascular anatomy and blood flow. *J Magn Reson Imaging* **25**: 824–831.

65 Nezafat, R., Stehning, C., Gharib, A.M., *et al.* (2005) Improved spatial-temporal resolution MR coronary blood flow imaging at 3 T. *J Cardiovasc Magn Reson* **7**: 199–200.

Chapter 21

Technical Advances in MDCT for Imaging Coronary Artery Stenoses and Physiology

Humberto Wong, Elsie T. Nguyen, and Geoffrey D. Rubin

Tremendous technological advances have been made in the field of computed tomography (CT) over the past 15 years. The development of helical CT made CT angiography (CTA) possible [1–3]. Early attempts at applying single-row helical CT angiography to the coronary vascular tree were limited by insufficient temporal and spatial resolution [4]. Over the subsequent years, advances in temporal resolution and spatial resolution as well as increased axial volume coverage, decreased radiation exposure, and advanced postprocessing techniques have made coronary CTA a viable clinical examination (Table 21.1).

With the introduction of four-row multidetector CT (MDCT) in 1998, improved cardiac imaging studies were enabled by three key features: increased volume coverage, decreased CT gantry rotation times, and electrocardiographic (ECG) triggering or gating [5–9]. Both prospective ECG triggering and retrospective ECG gating were used to synchronize the acquisition of CT images with the patient's ECG tracing and reconstruct images of the entire heart registered to user-specified time points within the R–R interval.

Temporal Resolution

In the early 1990s, single-row helical CT had gantry rotation times of approximately 1 sec. Gantry rotation times were reduced to 0.5 sec with four-row MDCT, and were capable of achieving an effective temporal resolution of 250 ms using a half-scan reconstruction algorithm. Faster gantry rotation times of 0.375 sec were introduced with 16-row MDCT systems in 2001 [10]. This technology led to more robust clinical results and allowed the introduction of ECG gated coronary CTA

Novel Techniques for Imaging the Heart, 1st edition. Edited by M. Di Carli and R. Kwong.
© 2008 American Heart Association, ISBN: 9-781-4051-7533-3.

Table 21.1 Performance Characteristics of CT in Comparison from 1972 to 2004 (modified with permission from Kalender) [10]

	1972	1980	1990	2004
Minimum scan time	300 sec	5–10 sec	1–2 sec	0.33–0.5 sec
Data per 360° scan	57.6 kB	1 MB	1–2 MB	10–100 MB
Data per spiral scan	—	—	24–48 MB	200–4000 MB
Image matrix	80 × 80	256 × 256	512 × 512	512 × 512
Power	2 kW	10 kW	40 kW	60–100 kW
Slice thickness	13 mm	2–10 mm	1–10 mm	0.5–1 mm
Spatial resolution	3 Lp/cm	8–12 Lp/cm	10–15 Lp/cm	12–25 Lp/cm
Contrast resolution	5 mm/5 HU/ 50 mGy	3 mm/3 HU/ 30 mGy	3 mm/3 HU/ 30 mGy	3 mm/3 HU/ 30 mGy

into mainstream clinical practice. The use of 16-row MDCT scanners in coronary CTA led to a decrease in the number of nonassessable coronary segments and increased lesion detection [11–15]. Multiple studies have demonstrated a high negative predictive value of coronary CTA for the detection of significant stenoses in coronary segments with a diameter of at least 1.5 or 2 mm [11–13,15–21]. The introduction of 64-row CT systems in 2004, which featured decreased CT gantry rotation times as low as 330 ms, resulted in increased robustness and facilitated analysis of the entire coronary tree [22]. The recent introduction in late 2005 of dual-source CT (DSCT) scanning has provided substantial further improvements in temporal resolution [23].

The time needed to freeze cardiac motion in systole is on the order of 50 ms for heart rates under 70 bpm, which can be achieved with conventional angiography. The DSCT system described by Flohr and colleagues has two x-ray tubes mounted at a 90° angle and two sets of detectors (Figure 21.1) [23]. Simulating heart rates of 70 and 90 bpm, Flohr *et al.* demonstrated a temporal resolution of 83 ms using single-segment reconstruction with the DSCT [23]. In comparison, single-row CT using two-segment reconstruction resulted in 140 and 160 ms of temporal resolution for simulated heart rates of 70 and 90 bpm, respectively. Further experiments have established improved visualization of coronary plaques at high heart rates by DSCT [24].

Further improvements in temporal resolution present substantial technical challenges. Modern scanners with gantry rotation times in the range of 300 ms generate forces of up to 30 g. Using a single source CT, a reduction in rotation time to less than 0.2 sec is required to achieve a heart rate-independent temporal

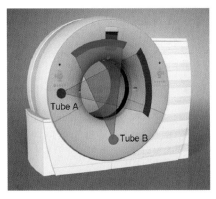

Fig. 21.1 Schematic of the dual-source CT with two x-ray tubes mounted at a 90° angle and two sets of detectors (courtesy of Thomas Flohr).

resolution of less than 100 ms, which led to estimates that such increases in gantry rotation speed could generate mechanical forces greater than 75 g, which is beyond current mechanical limits [23,25]. By combining technology used in a single-source CT, the DSCT is a current solution that achieves heart rate-independent temporal resolution of under 100 ms. However, while it is possible that CT systems with more than two sources can further reduce effective scan times, Kalender suggests that this approach would be more technically demanding without providing additional useful clinical information [10].

Volume Coverage

With a 1-cm axial detector coverage, four-row CT systems were able to decrease overall scan times and make breath-hold imaging an achievable goal. Scan times for coronary CTA have decreased from 40 sec (4-row MDCT) to 15–20 sec (16-row MDCT) to approximately 5–15 sec (64-row MDCT). However, in clinical settings where many patients are short of breath or have tachycardia, the relatively long breath-hold times for four-row scanners introduced motion artifacts, which led to approximately 30% of coronary segments being nondiagnostic [26,27].

Single-source 64-row CT is now available from all the major vendors. Extensive clinical data regarding CT imaging of the heart has been derived from these systems. With the widespread adoption of these single-source CT systems, cardiac imaging is now moving beyond the early trial stage. Meta-analyses of the performance of increasing the number of detector rows have concluded that with the newer generations of multidetector CT scanners, the diagnostic performance for the assessment of coronary artery disease has significantly improved, and the proportion of nonassessable segments has decreased [28–30].

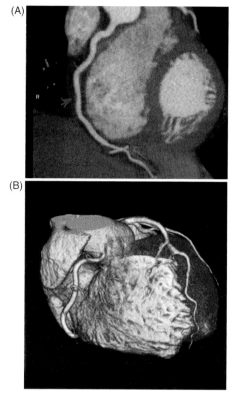

Fig. 21.2 (A) Curved planar reformation of a prospective (70% to next R interval) ECG-Gated Coronary CT angiogram completed on a 320-row MDCT scanner in a 48-year-old man with a history of hypertension, smoking, atypical chest pain, and a normal Sestamibi scan. Note the non-calcified plaque (arrow) in the distal right coronary artery causing approximately 10% stenosis, which may be an incidental finding unrelated to te chest pan. Calcium score was zero. Using half scan reconstruction, and one heart beat, the total radiation dose, including the calcium score scan, was 11.2 mSv, which is at least 50% lower than the dose on a 64-row MDCT scanner using multisegment reconstruction. (B) 3D volume-rendered image of the heart acquired on a 256 MDCT (courtesy of Kazuhiro Katada).

Current state-of-the-art 64-row CT provides 20 to 40 mm of longitudinal coverage per single gantry rotation. This resolution limits the evaluation of volumetric cine imaging by introducing misregistration secondary to the multiple heart beats required to cover the entire heart. Prototype 256-row CT systems have demonstrated increases in volume coverage to 12.8 cm, raising the possibility of non-ECG gated evaluation of entire organs including the heart and brain (Figure 21.2A and 21.2B) [31,32]. Mori and colleagues were the first to develop a 256-row detector prototype that uses a wide-area cylindrical 2D detector mounted on a 16-row detector CT gantry frame [33]. From one heart beat, sufficient data can be acquired during one 0.5-sec rotation at 0.5-mm row thickness through the entire volume of the heart. The 256-row CT prototype has 912 (transverse) and 256 (cranio-caudal) elements, each approximately 0.5×0.5 mm at the center of rotation. A 128-mm total beam width allows for approximately 100 mm of cranio-caudal coverage per rotation. The current limitation in craniocaudal coverage is due to the geometry of cone-beam CT using the Feldkamp algorithm [33]. Because the imaging volume is a cylinder with two cones at each end, the effective imaging volume is determined by the height of the cylinder (see figure 21.1 in Mori *et al.* [33]). With the 256-detector CT prototype, four scanning modes are possible: contiguous axial mode to acquire a volume greater than the detector width, a volumetric cine imaging mode to perform CT subtraction angiography (CTSA), a fluoroscopic imaging mode for interventional procedures, and a helical mode [33,34].

Multirow scanners in current clinical use require that CT data are acquired with simultaneous ECG gating for 4D functional information. Because the 256-row CT can acquire the 128-mm scan range, the entire cardiac volume can be scanned with a single rotation. This feature has allowed for non-ECG gated cardiac CTA in both experimental settings as well as with human subjects [32,35]. The preliminary results with the 256-row CT are based on five subjects [32]. The technique included imaging of the whole heart in approximately 1.5 sec to cover one cardiac cycle during a single breath-hold without ECG gating. A half-scan reconstruction algorithm was used (with an effective temporal resolution of 250 ms) to generate 0.5-mm thick axial images reconstructed at 50 ms intervals for a total of 26 data sets. With a 1.5-sec acquisition time, the entire cardiac cycle can be imaged if the heart rate is greater than 48 bpm, or an R–R interval less than or equal to 1.25 sec. Using this system, 90.9% of the coronary arteries were assessable, a rate better than that reported for traditional MDCT systems with comparable 250-ms temporal resolution. They attribute the improved assessability of the coronary arteries to the isophasic data, which is acquired in one cardiac cycle. They also speculate that with acquisition of approximately 5 sec of data, it may be possible to obtain simultaneous coronary angiography as well as perfusion data.

A promising application of 256-row CT is volumetric whole-organ perfusion imaging. A significant challenge to performing CTSA with the 256-row CT is the large amount of data produced by a ten-rotation volumetric cine scan. It is estimated that a ten-rotation volumetric cine scan with 0.1-sec reconstruction increments would generate 100 phases, corresponding to 25,600 transverse sections. To decrease the calculation time required for volumetric CTSA, a raw projection data subtraction method known as *raw data-based CTSA* has been developed. Compared to image-based CTSA, the advantage of this system is that it allows for a significant reduction in the calculation time by subtracting raw data rather than reconstructed images. Raw data-based CTSA subtracts unenhanced raw data from individual pixel values for contrast-enhanced raw data along the time axis [36]. In one animal study, raw data-based CTSA images required 8.4 min to reconstruct, compared to an image-based CTSA reconstruction time of 76 min.

Three hundred and twenty-row MDCT scanners have been introduced very recently. With heart rates less than 65 bpm, half scan reconstruction can be used and effective temporal resolution is approximately 225 ms (350 ms full gantry rotation speed, therefore, temporal resolution is 175 ms plus fan angle) to acquire images of the entire heart (128 mm of coverage) in less than 1 sec and using one heart beat. This translates into radiation dose savings compared to the 64 row MDCT scanners. One study comparing radiation dose based on 25 healthy male volunteers scanned on a 320 MDCT compared with a clinical cohort (matched to body mass index) scanned on a 64 MDCT demonstrated a 70% dose reduction using the 320 MDCT [37].

Spatial Resolution

Current state-of-the-art for heart rate-independent resolution is achieved with the DSCT, which can achieve 0.5-mm transverse and 0.4-mm longitudinal resolution using the thinnest slice width and edge enhancing, sharp reconstruction kernels [23]. Increases in spatial resolution are typically accompanied by the need for increased x-ray power to maintain the signal-to-noise ratio. This results in increased radiation exposure to the patient unless compensating algorithms and scan approaches are developed to mitigate against a radiation dose increase. One approach that would increase the resolution of CT reconstructions without requiring truncation of the display field-of-view would be a transition from a 512×512 display matrix to a 1024×1024 display matrix. This transition has many implications for storage, display, and processing of CT data but would seem to be an inevitable development if the transverse resolution of CT scanners improves.

Radiation Dose Reduction in Coronary CTA

One of the main obstacles in applying coronary CTA, particularly in women and children, is the high radiation dose that is deposited with current 64-slice single-source CT. The mean radiation dose for a retrospectively ECG gated helical coronary CTA has been reported at 18.4 mSv with a range of 10 to 21 mSv [38–42]. The high radiation dose is in large part caused by the use of retrospective ECG gating, requiring a low pitch to avoid gaps in anatomic coverage. The use of radiation during portions of the cardiac cycle where the coronary arteries are not well visualized also increases the radiation dose without a gain in diagnostic information. A variety of dose-reduction strategies have helped decrease the cardiac CT dose, including autoexposure control systems that modulate tube current longitudinally as well as angular current modulation, targeted field-of-view cardiac beam-shaping filters, increased pitch values for faster heart rates, and ECG-based tube current modulation, and prospective axial gating

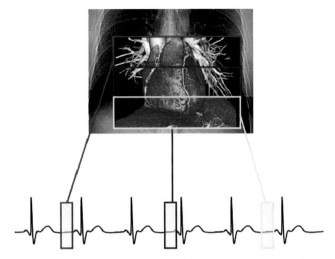

Fig. 21.3 Prospective axial gating uses a step-and-shoot approach and is demonstrated with 4-cm longitudinal coverage imaging the entire volume of the heart in three to five heart beats (image courtesy of James P. Earls).

(Figure 21.3) [38,43]. Chapter 3 includes a detailed discussion of dose-reduction techniques.

Workstations and Visualization

Advanced postprocessing has allowed for novel and more efficient interactions with the large data sets acquired by faster and more complex MDCT scanners. Multiplanar reformations, volume rendering, and curved planar reformations can be very valuable. In particular, curved planar reformations, created either with or without automated centerline extraction tools, can be extremely useful in determining the degree of coronary stenosis, particularly in small or tortuous coronary arteries. Volume renderings are helpful to delineate the course of the coronary arteries and to provide a roadmap, demonstrating normal and variant coronary artery origins and course. Opacity transfer functions and other display settings can be adjusted to emphasize different cardiac structures based on their CT number. Algorithms have been developed to segment coronary arteries, identify plaque, and facilitate plaque characterization (noncalcified versus calcified) and assessment of luminal stenosis. However, validation of these algorithms by comparing the degree of stenosis or plaque characterization with conventional angiography or pathologic specimens has not been published to our knowledge. Functional analyses for assessing ventricular and valvular function are becoming automated and are increasingly available on workstations. End-diastolic and systolic volumes and ejection fractions can be calculated with results comparable to that of echocardiography or magnetic resonance imaging (MRI).

Conclusions

CT development has progressed at an astonishingly rapid pace over the past 15 years, with substantial gains in temporal and spatial resolution and radiation dose reduction. The recent introduction of dual-source CT, 320-row, wide-area detectors and wide cone-angle sources, as well as novel detector and source designs, will encourage continued improvement in cardiac CT scan quality and safety while also allowing myocardial perfusion imaging, improved functional assessment, and greater resolution coronary angiography to become a reality.

References

1 Napel, S., *et al.* (1992) CT angiography with spiral CT and maximum intensity projection. *Radiology* **185**(2): 607–610.

2 Rubin, G.D., *et al.* (1992) Spiral CT creates 3-D neuro, body angiograms. *Diagn Imaging (San Franc)* **14**(8): 66–74.

3 Rubin, G.D., *et al.* (1999) Computed tomographic angiography: historical perspective and new state-of-the-art using multidetector-row helical computed tomography. *J Comput Assist Tomogr* **23**(Suppl 1): S83–90.

4 Kachelriess, M., Kalender, W.A. (1998) Electrocardiogram-correlated image reconstruction from subsecond spiral computed tomography scans of the heart. *Med Phys* **25**(12): 2417–2431.

5 Achenbach, S., *et al.* (2000) Noninvasive coronary angiography by retrospectively ECG-gated multislice spiral CT. *Circulation* **102**(23): 2823–2828.

6 Becker, C.R., *et al.* (2000) Imaging of noncalcified coronary plaques using helical CT with retrospective ECG gating. *AJR* **175**(2): 423–424.

7 Kachelriess, M., Ulzheimer, S., Kalender, W.A. (2000) ECG-correlated imaging of the heart with subsecond multislice spiral CT. *IEEE Trans Med Imaging* **19**(9): 888–901.

8 Ohnesorge, B., *et al.* (2000) Cardiac imaging by means of electrocardiographically gated multisection spiral CT: initial experience. *Radiology* **217**(2): 564–571.

9 Taguchi, K., Anno, H. (2000) High temporal resolution for multislice helical computed tomography. *Med Phys* **27**(5): 861–872.

10 Kalender, W.A. (2005) *Computed Tomography: Fundamentals, System Technology, Image Quality, Applications*. Wiley-VCH, Berlin.

11 Nieman, K., *et al.* (2002) Reliable noninvasive coronary angiography with fast submillimeter multislice spiral computed tomography. *Circulation* **106**(16): 2051–2054.

12 Ropers, D., *et al.* (2003) Detection of coronary artery stenoses with thin-slice multidetector row spiral computed tomography and multiplanar reconstruction. *Circulation* **107**(5): 664–666.

13 Kuettner, A., *et al.* (2005) Diagnostic accuracy of noninvasive coronary imaging using 16-detector slice spiral computed tomography with 188 ms temporal resolution. *J Am Coll Cardiol* **45**(1): 123–127.

14 Kuettner, A., *et al.* (2005) Coronary vessel visualization using true 16-row multi-slice computed tomography technology. *Int J Cardiovasc Imaging* **21**(2–3): 331–337.

15 Mollet, N.R., *et al.* (2004) Multislice spiral computed tomography coronary angiography in patients with stable angina pectoris. *J Am Coll Cardiol* **43**(12): 2265–2270.

16 Achenbach, S., *et al.* (2005) Detection of coronary artery stenoses using multi-detector CT with 16 × 0.75 collimation and 375 ms rotation. *Eur Heart J* **26**(19): 1978–1986.

17 Hoffmann, U., *et al.* (2004) Predictive value of 16-slice multidetector spiral computed tomography to detect significant obstructive coronary artery disease in patients at high risk for coronary artery disease: patient versus segment-based analysis. *Circulation* **110**(17): 2638–2643.

18 Hoffmann, U., *et al.* (2006) Noninvasive assessment of plaque morphology and composition in culprit and stable lesions in acute coronary syndrome and stable lesions in stable angina by multidetector computed tomography. *J Am Coll Cardiol* **47**(8): 1655–1662.

19 Morgan-Hughes, G.J., *et al.* (2005) Highly accurate coronary angiography with submillimetre, 16-slice computed tomography. *Heart* **91**(3): 308–313.

20 Schuijf, J.D., *et al.* (2007) Assessment of left ventricular volumes and ejection fraction with 16-slice multi-slice computed tomography; comparison with 2D-echocardiography. *Int J Cardiol* **116**(2): 201–205.

21 Schuijf, J.D., *et al.* (2005) Noninvasive coronary imaging and assessment of left ventricular function using 16-slice computed tomography. *Am J Cardiol* **95**(5): 571–574.

22 Flohr, T., *et al.* (2004) Performance evaluation of a 64-slice CT system with z-flying focal spot. *Rofo* **176**(12): 1803–1810.

23 Flohr, T.G., *et al.* (2006) First performance evaluation of a dual-source CT (DSCT) system. *Eur Radiol* **16**(2): 256–268.

24 Reimann, A.J., *et al.* (2007) Dual-source computed tomography: advances of improved temporal resolution in coronary plaque imaging. *Invest Radiol* **42**(3): 196–203.

25 Flohr, T.G., Schoepf, U.J., Ohnesorge, B.M. (2007) Chasing the heart: new developments for cardiac CT. *J Thorac Imaging* **22**(1): 4–16.

26 Achenbach, S., *et al.* (2001) Detection of coronary artery stenoses by contrast-enhanced, retrospectively electrocardiographically gated, multislice spiral computed tomography. *Circulation* **103**(21): 2535–2538.

27 Nieman, K., *et al.* (2001) Coronary angiography with multi-slice computed tomography. *Lancet* **357**(9256): 599–603.

28 Vanhoenacker, P.K., *et al.* (2007) Diagnostic performance of multidetector CT angiography for assessment of coronary artery disease: meta-analysis. *Radiology* **244**(2): 419–428.

29 Stein, P.D., *et al.* (2006) Multidetector computed tomography for the diagnosis of coronary artery disease: a systematic review. *Am J Med* **119**(3): 203–216.

30 Schuijf, J.D., *et al.* (2006) Meta-analysis of comparative diagnostic performance of magnetic resonance imaging and multislice computed tomography for noninvasive coronary angiography. *Am Heart J* **151**(2): 404–411.

31 Mori, S., *et al.* (2005) Volumetric cine imaging for cardiovascular circulation using prototype 256-detector row computed tomography scanner (4-dimensional computed

tomography): a preliminary study with a porcine model. *J Comput Assist Tomogr* **29**(1): 26–30.

32 Kido, T., *et al.* (2007) Cardiac imaging using 256-detector row four-dimensional CT: preliminary clinical report. *Radiat Med* **25**(1): 38–44.

33 Mori, S., *et al.* (2006) Properties of the prototype 256-row (cone beam) CT scanner. *Eur Radiol* **16**(9): 2100–2108.

34 Mori, S., *et al.* (2005) Clinical potentials of the prototype 256-detector row CT-scanner. *Acad Radiol* **12**(2): 148–154.

35 Mizuno, N., *et al.* (2007) Utility of 256-slice cone beam tomography for real four-dimensional volumetric analysis without electrocardiogram gated acquisition. *Int J Cardiol* **120**(2): 262–267.

36 Mori, S., Endo, M. (2007) Candidate image processing for real-time volumetric CT subtraction angiography. *Eur J Radiol* **61**(2): 335–341.

37 Paul, N., *et al. Low Dose CT Coronary Angiography with 320-row MDCT in Annual Meeting and Scientific Assembly of the Radiological Society of North America.* 2008: Chicago, IL.

38 Earls, J., Urban, B., Curry, C. (2006) Prospectively gated axial coronary CT angiography; a comparison with retrospectively gated helical CT angiography. In *Annual Meeting and Scientific Assembly of the Radiological Society of North America.* Chicago, IL.

39 Earls, J., *et al.* Prospectively gated axial coronary CT angiography: improved image quality and reduced radiation dose as compared to retrospectively gated helical technique. *Radiology* (in press).

40 Gallagher, M.J., *et al.* (2007) The diagnostic accuracy of 64-slice computed tomography coronary angiography compared with stress nuclear imaging in emergency department low-risk chest pain patients. *Ann Emerg Med* **49**(2): 125–136.

41 Leber, A.W., *et al.* (2004) Accuracy of multidetector spiral computed tomography in identifying and differentiating the composition of coronary atherosclerotic plaques: a comparative study with intracoronary ultrasound. *J Am Coll Cardiol* **43**(7): 1241–1247.

42 Mollet, N.R., *et al.* (2005) High-resolution spiral computed tomography coronary angiography in patients referred for diagnostic conventional coronary angiography. *Circulation* **112**(15): 2318–2323.

43 McCollough, C.H., *et al.* (2007) Dose performance of a 64-channel dual-source CT scanner. *Radiology* **243**(3): 775–784.

Chapter 22

Imaging of Myocardial Mechanics

Hiroshi Ashikaga and Elliot R. McVeigh

Magnetic resonance imaging (MRI) is sensitive to motion, and thus provides data from which myocardial mechanics can be evaluated [1]. The motion of myocardial tissue can be described by strain and strain rate. *Strain* measures deformation, or a change in shape, of an object relative to its original shape. Strains of a three-dimensional (3D) object can be calculated from 3D displacement, or movement, of material points within the solid. In 3D, six independent strain components completely describe the deformation of an object: three normal strains describe stretching or shortening along each of the three initially orthogonal axes, and three shear strains describe angle changes between pairs of the coordinate axes. *Strain rate* is a temporal derivative of strain; therefore there are six independent strain rates in 3D (Figure 22.1a).

In describing myocardial mechanics, the local cardiac coordinate system is used to calculate strains over the cardiac cycle where three mutually orthogonal axes are defined at a given region: radial (R), longitudinal (L), and circumferential (C) axes (Figure 22.1b) [2]. The R-axis points from endocardium to epicardium. The L-axis is a projection of the left ventricular (LV) long axis, defined by the LV apex and the left aortic valve commissure (the position between the center of the mitral valve and the aortic valve), and is perpendicular to the R-axis.

Whereas three normal strains (E_{cc}, E_{ll}, and E_{rr}) and three shear strains (E_{cl}, E_{lr}, and E_{rc}) can be calculated to describe 3D deformation in the local cardiac coordinate system, only normal strains are usually of physiological interest, where the change in length in each direction is expressed in a percentage (Figure 22.1c). By convention, a positive strain indicates stretching

Novel Techniques for Imaging the Heart, 1st edition. Edited by M. Di Carli and R. Kwong.
© 2008 American Heart Association, ISBN: 9-781-4051-7533-3.

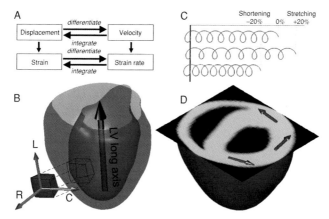

Fig. 22.1 (a) Relationship between displacement, velocity, strain, and strain rate. (b) Local cardiac coordinate system. R, radial axis; L, longitudinal axis; C, circumferential axis. (c) Normal strain indicates stretching or shortening along a coordinate axis, where the change in length is expressed in percentage. A positive strain indicates stretching (e.g., +20%), whereas a negative strain indicates shortening (e.g., −20%). (d) Mid-wall circumferential directions in an LV short-axis plane, where E_{cc} can be calculated from 2D displacements.

(e.g., +20%), whereas a negative strain indicates shortening (e.g., −20%). In magnetic resonance-based analysis, the circumferential strain (E_{cc}) at the mid-wall is mainly used because the myofibers run predominantly in the circumferential direction in the mid-wall, thus E_{cc} can be considered a measure of myofiber stretch or shortening [2]. To reduce overall image acquisition time, E_{cc} can also be calculated from 2D displacements, instead of 3D, in appropriately selected LV short-axis planes (Figure 22.1d).

Magnetic Resonance Techniques for Myocardial Mechanics

Tagging

Magnetic resonance *tagging*, or placing marks in deformable objects, can quantify complex myocardial deformations [3–4]. The most commonly used tagging technique is the spatial modulation of magnetization (SPAMM), which creates a periodic appearance of dark bands seen as parallel stripe tags or *grid tags*, where magnetization is saturated [5]. Because the tags reflect magnetization patterns encoded in the tissue, they track the motion of the heart and deform as the underlying tissue deforms (Figure 22.2).

From the tagged images, the underlying myocardial motion can be assessed qualitatively or quantitatively. Quantitative strain analysis requires image processing techniques that consist of tag detection, estimation of displacement of the myocardium, and the calculation of strains. To perform 3D strain analysis of

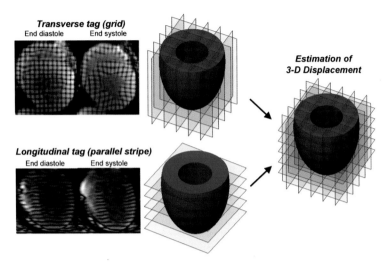

Fig. 22.2 Example images of tagged MRI are shown, where grid tags in the transverse direction and parallel stripe tags in the longitudinal direction are encoded. The tags track the motion of the heart and deform from end-diastole to end-systole. Each tag line can be considered as a plane (shown in gray) that deforms as the underlying tissue deforms. From the displacement of the tag planes in three orthogonal directions, 3D displacement of the myocardium at any point in space can be estimated.

the myocardium, images with parallel stripe tags in three mutually orthogonal directions are required (e.g., grid transverse tags and parallel longitudinal tags; Figure 22.2) [6,7]. When quantifying only in-plane strain components, mainly the circumferential strain (E_{cc}) in LV short-axis images, a rapid postprocessing method called the harmonic phase (HARP) imaging technique can be used [8]. HARP imaging derives the motion information from the noncentral spectral peaks in the k-space, and can provide close to real-time strain analysis at a user-defined myocardial region.

DENSE

The *displacement-encoding of stimulated echo* (DENSE) is an evolved form of a magnetic resonance-based mechanical analysis technique [9]. The fundamental principle is similar to that of tagging, but the DENSE technique uses a stimulated echo to encode the net displacement of tissue with signal phase [10]. The signal intensity in the DENSE phase image at each voxel is proportional to the displacement along one direction, thus 3D displacement of the myocardium can be calculated from DENSE acquisitions in three orthogonal directions (Figure 22.3). The DENSE technique achieves pixel-by-pixel spatial resolution and direct extraction of displacement data, and it requires much less user input for postprocessing compared with other techniques such as tagging.

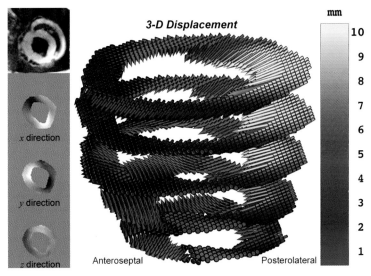

Fig. 22.3 The left panel shows example images of DENSE in a canine heart with anteroseptal MI. The top is a magnitude image, and the other three are phase images from three separate acquisitions. The signal intensity in the phase images at each voxel is proportional to the displacement along the x-, y-, and z-direction, from top to bottom. Based on the phase information, the 3D displacement of each voxel can be calculated. The right panel shows 3D displacement vectors of each voxel in the same heart. The arrow tail indicates the location of each voxel at end-diastole, which moves to a new location (arrow head) at end-systole. The color of each vector indicates the magnitude of the displacement. Note the magnitude of displacement in the MI region (anteroseptal wall) is diminished (shown in blue) compared with that of the lateral wall (yellow). Modified from Ashikaga *et al.*, used with permission [16].

Clinical Applications

Intraventricular Conduction Delay

Cardiac resynchronization therapy (CRT) improves cardiac function in moderate-to-severe heart failure associated with an intraventricular conduction delay, most commonly of a left bundle branch block (LBBB) type [11]. Nevertheless, 20 to 30% of patients who receive CRT do not respond [12]. Quantitative assessment of mechanical dyssynchrony may provide new metrics to improve the patient selection process and reduce the number of the nonresponders [13–15].

Figure 22.4 illustrates the effects of CRT by showing the time series of quantitative strain analysis using tagged MRI in a canine heart with LBBB and tachycardia-induced heart failure. The circumferential strains (E_{cc}) at each region of the LV and the corresponding tagged images are shown at each time point. With right atrial pacing (Figure 22.4a; video clips 26 and 27),

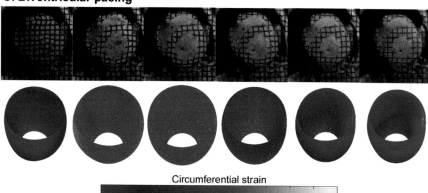

A. Right atrial pacing

End diastole → End systole

Posterior
Base
Apex
Anterior
Septum
Lateral

B. LV lateral wall pacing

C. Biventricular pacing

Circumferential strain

-10%
Shortening

0%

+10%
Stretching

Fig. 22.4 Time series of quantitative strain analysis using tagged MRI in a canine heart with left bundle branch block (LBBB) and tachycardia-induced heart failure. The circumferential strains (E_{cc}) at each region of the LV and the corresponding tagged images are shown at each time point. (a) Right atrial pacing. (b) LV lateral wall pacing. (c) Biventricular pacing. The reference configuration of the circumferential strains is end-diastole, and the temporal resolution of each series is 14 ms. See text for details.

intraventricular mechanical dyssynchrony is immediately obvious during late diastole; substantial septal shortening (blue) and lateral stretching occur simultaneously as a consequence of LBBB, when most of the regions still undergo normal stretching (red) due to ventricular filling. After end-diastole, lateral shortening (blue) occurs prior to shortening of other regions of the LV toward end-systole. In contrast, with LV lateral wall pacing (Figure 22.4b; video clips 28 ⬬ and 29 ⬬), substantial lateral shortening and septal stretching are observed. Although a little delay of shortening is observed in the septal region, other regions underwent relatively synchronous contraction compared with right atrial pacing, presumably due to fusion of electrical conduction from the intact His-Purkinje system. With biventricular pacing (Figure 22.4c; video clips 30 ⬬ and 31 ⬬), intraventricular dyssynchrony improves; both ventricular filling during diastole and contraction during systole are synchronous, indicated by homogeneous circumferential shortening (blue) across the LV.

Ischemic Heart Disease

The assessment of not just global function (e.g., ejection fraction) but mechanical function at each ventricular region is critically important in evaluating patients with ischemic heart disease. Quantitative mechanical analysis can play an important role, along with viability and perfusion imaging, in evaluating myocardial viability to predict recovery of function after revascularization.

Figure 22.5 (video clips 32 ⬬ and 33 ⬬) shows the time series of quantitative strain analysis using DENSE in a swine heart with chronic anteroseptal myocardial infarction (MI) during normal sinus rhythm, where the region circumscribed by the solid yellow line indicates MI. The viable myocardium undergoes relatively homogeneous systolic deformation (blue), whereas the apical MI region undergoes systolic stretch (red). In addition, abnormal stretch (yellow) appears in the viable myocardium opposite to the MI (lateral wall), which subsides toward end-systole. This diagram visually demonstrates substantial dyssynchrony of LV contraction in ischemic heart disease.

Conclusions

Magnetic resonance-based imaging of mechanics is a noninvasive method that allows the objective quantification and visualization of myocardial mechanics in not only a particular region but the whole heart. Improvement of the spatiotemporal resolution with fast MRI techniques continues to reveal new information about the highly sophisticated nature of myocardial mechanics in ischemic heart disease, heart failure, congenital heart disease, and various cardiomyopathies. The imaging of mechanics will continue to evolve as a reliable guide for diagnosis and treatment for patients with cardiovascular disease.

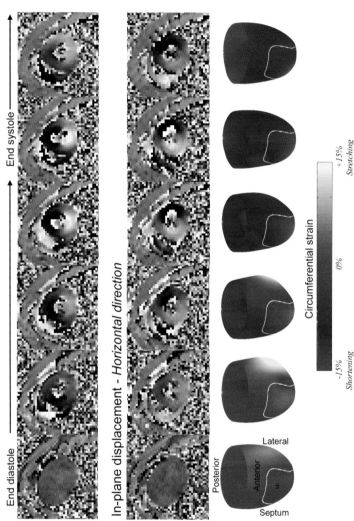

Fig. 22.5 Quantitative strain analysis using DENSE in a swine heart with chronic anteroseptal myocardial infarction (MI). The circumferential strains (E_{cc}) at each region of the LV and the corresponding DENSE images are shown at each time point. The region circumscribed by the solid yellow line indicates MI. The reference configuration of the circumferential strains is end-diastole, and the temporal resolution is 9 ms. See text for details.

Acknowledgments

This work was supported by a grant from the National Heart, Lung, and Blood Institute (Z01-HL004609 to McVeigh). The authors would like to thank Han Wen, Daniel B. Ennis, Bruce Hopenfeld, J. Andrew Derbyshire, Owen Faris, and David A. Kass for their contributions.

References

1 Axel, L. (2002) Biomechanical dynamics of the heart with MRI. *Ann Rev Biomed Eng* **4**: 321–347.

2 Streeter, D.D., Jr., *et al.* (1969) Fiber orientation in the canine left ventricle during diastole and systole. *Circ Res* **24**(3): 339–347.

3 Morse, O.C., Singer, J.R. (1970) Blood velocity measurements in intact subjects. *Science* **170**(956): 440–441.

4 Zerhouni, E.A., *et al.* (1988) Human heart: tagging with MR imaging—a method for noninvasive assessment of myocardial motion. *Radiology* **169**(1): 59–63.

5 Axel, L., Dougherty, L. (1989) MR imaging of motion with spatial modulation of magnetization. *Radiology* **171**(3): 841–845.

6 Ozturk, C., Derbyshire, J.A., McVeigh, E.R. (2003) Estimating motion from MRI data. *Proc IEEE* **91**(10): 1627–1648.

7 McVeigh, E., Ozturk, C. (2001) Imaging myocardial strain. *IEEE Sign Proc* **18**(6): 44–56.

8 Osman, N.F., *et al.* (1999) Cardiac motion tracking using CINE harmonic phase (HARP) magnetic resonance imaging. *Magn Reson Med* **42**(6): 1048–1060.

9 Aletras, A.H., *et al.* (1999) DENSE: displacement encoding with stimulated echoes in cardiac functional MRI. *J Magn Reson* **137**(1): 247–252.

10 Caprihan, A., Griffey, R.H., Fukushima, E. (1990) Velocity imaging of slow coherent flows using stimulated echoes. *Magn Reson Med* **15**(2): 327–333.

11 Kass, D.A. (2007) Does cardiac resynchronization therapy reduce the long-term mortality risk in patients with heart failure? *Nat Clin Pract Cardiovasc Med* **4**(4): 190–191.

12 Kass, D.A. (2003) Ventricular resynchronization: pathophysiology and identification of responders. *Rev Cardiovasc Med* **4**(Suppl 2): S3–S13.

13 Leclercq, C., *et al.* (2002) Systolic improvement and mechanical resynchronization does not require electrical synchrony in the dilated failing heart with left bundle-branch block. *Circulation* **106**(14): 1760–1763.

14 Helm, R.H., *et al.* (2005) Cardiac dyssynchrony analysis using circumferential versus longitudinal strain: implications for assessing cardiac resynchronization. *Circulation* **111**(21): 2760–2767.

15 Bader, H., *et al.* (2004) Intra-left ventricular electromechanical asynchrony: a new independent predictor of severe cardiac events in heart failure patients. *J Am Coll Cardiol* **43**(2): 248–256.

16 Ashikaga, H., *et al.* (2005) Electromechanical analysis of infarct border zone in chronic myocardial infarction. *Am J Physiol Heart Circ Physiol* **289**(3): H1099–H1105.

Chapter 23

Cardiovascular Interventional MRI

Colin Berry and Robert J. Lederman

Interventional cardiovascular magnetic resonance (iCMR) imaging represents a new attempt to harness the tissue imaging capabilities of magnetic resonance imaging (MRI) to guide therapeutic catheter procedures. By making small compromises in spatial or temporal resolution, and with minor modifications to commercial high-performance MRI systems, images can be acquired and displayed almost instantaneously to physicians manipulating catheter devices. This technique may be useful to avoid ionizing radiation during conventional catheter-based procedures, especially in children. More importantly, iCMR may enable more advanced procedures not otherwise possible without open surgical exposure.

Equipping an iCMR Laboratory

Commercial MRI systems can be adapted to guide investigational cardiovascular interventional procedures. Typical configurations use adjoining x-ray fluoroscopy and MRI systems separated by doors that permit the two to be used independently or together. Most vendors offer tables that safely move instrumented patients under sterile conditions. Invasive clinical hemodynamic recording systems are not yet commercially available. Instead, investigators either install laboratory physiologic recording equipment or adapt clinical (low-resolution) monitoring systems to display rhythm and hemodynamics data inside the scanner room. Headsets are available to permit staff and patients to communicate despite the audio noise generated by MRI gradient systems during scanning.

Novel Techniques for Imaging the Heart, 1st edition. Edited by M. Di Carli and R. Kwong.
© 2008 American Heart Association, ISBN: 9-781-4051-7533-3.

Shielded LCD displays or projectors can present monitoring, real-time images, and scanner information to the operators inside the MRI room.

MRI scanners are usually configured for efficient image acquisition followed by off-line image interpretation after the studies are completed. Commercial options are available for real-time imaging, which means low-latency data acquisition and nearly instantaneous image construction and display. Several laboratories have successfully employed low-resolution real-time MRI at 5 to 20 frames per second and acquisition-to-display latency of less than 250 ms to guide preclinical or clinical interventional procedures.

Steady state free precession (SSFP) MRI pulse sequences are used for most iCMR procedures because of the efficient use of magnetization. During typical procedures, operators alternate real-time SSFP (rtSSFP) for catheter manipulation and segmented (non-real-time) SSFP pulse sequences for more detailed evaluation of results. This technique is analogous to x-ray interventional operators' use of low-dose fluoroscopy alternating with high-dose cineangiography.

Our laboratories and others have developed interventional work stations to control the scanner and provide additional functionality for iCMR [1–5]. Enhancements include multiple interleaved real-time slices; simultaneous 3D rendering of these multiplanar acquisitions; parallel imaging capabilities such as SENSE; temporal image filtering (averaging) to increase signal-to-noise as needed; interactive magnetization preparation such as nonselective water or fat saturation to alter image contrast and permit, for example, dynamic tissue inspection and target selection; and interactive electrocardiographic (ECG) gating to "freeze" motion. We find individual adjustment and the colorized display of signals detected from "active" antenna-catheter devices to be crucial to permit the operator to unambiguously distinguish devices from tissue during navigation [6]. We also found a "projection-mode" feature useful during catheter manipulations within target slices [7]. When parts of catheter devices move outside these selected slices, they appear "lost." By toggling to a projection mode (which switches to sliceless imaging), the catheter can be "found" and manipulated back into the target slice (Figure 23.1).

Interventional Catheter Devices

X-ray catheter devices are unsuitable for iCMR because they incorporate ferrous materials to enhance mechanical performance, are inconspicuous under proton MRI, or they contain long conductive wires that heat inductively during MRI radiofrequency excitation. Indeed, the chief remaining limitation to clinical development of interventional cardiovascular MRI is the availability of clinical-grade catheter devices.

"Passive" designs exploit the material properties of the catheters to make them conspicuous and safe for iCMR. One way is to incorporate small ferrous or superparamagnetic markers on the catheters to create "blooming" susceptibility

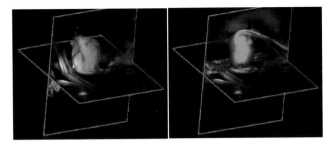

Fig. 23.1 Multislice imaging and projection mode. Two slices are acquired together and "rendered" in 3D. Left panel: An active myocardial injection catheter (green) is positioned in the heart, but its tip is outside the selected slice and therefore not visible. Right panel: "Projection mode" shows the entire length of the injection catheter. From Dick *et al.*, used with permission [6].

artifacts (large black spots) in images. Several teams have developed off-resonance pulse sequences to make these black spots appear bright, although this may limit visibility depending on device orientation with regard to the static magnetic field, and may compromise soft-tissue imaging [8]. Other laboratories use large devices devoid of protons, such as CO_2-filled balloons. Still others have coated catheters with T1-shortening agents such as gadolinium hydro-gels [9]. These approaches suffer from volume averaging or the nonspecifity of black spots on magnetic resonance images. We find passively visualized devices inadequate for the purposes of high-risk interventional procedures (Figure 23.2).

Instead, we favor "active" catheter devices, which incorporate receiver elements or antennae and which connect directly to the MRI scanner hardware. Active devices can be fitted with "tracking" receiver coils to detect a 3D position

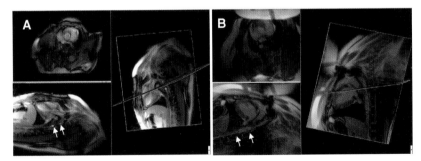

Fig. 23.2 Coarctation stenting over (a) passive and (b) active guidewires. Each panel contains two slices (left top and bottom) and a 3D rendering. The stent is crimped on a gadolinium-filled balloon (white arrows). The devices and procedures are more conspicuous using the active guidewire (see video clips 34 ⊙ and 35 ⊙). From Raval *et al.*, used with permission [10].

using short nonimaging pulse sequences acquired between images. Synthesized position markers are superimposed on images. "Profiling" active devices are used with ordinary imaging pulse sequences and display a length or profile of the catheter device that brightens nearby blood or tissue to make it conspicuous. Active and passive approaches can be combined, for example, to brighten a balloon filled with dilute gadolinium contrast used over an active profiling guidewire antenna (Figure 23.2) [10].

Active catheter devices require special efforts to prevent their long conductive transmission lines from heating [11,12]. An alternative is to make active devices couple inductively with external MRI coils to brighten nearby tissue wirelessly [13].

Potential Clinical Applications

Suitable and Unsuitable Applications

iCMR is well suited to manipulate large structures with discrete borders — great vessels and myocardium are good examples. iCMR is not well suited for targets that are small and highly mobile. Meaningful coronary artery iCMR procedures are not likely attainable barring an unforeseen technical advance.

Diagnostic Cardiovascular Catheterization

Cardiac catheterization remains important to characterize complex congenital heart defects in children. Schalla *et al.* conducted comprehensive clinical-style invasive hemodynamic characterization of pigs with atrial septal defect using active-tracking catheter devices [14]. Razavi *et al.* conducted diagnostic catheterization of children and adults with congenital heart disease using passive CO_2-filled catheters [15]. Others have characterized pulmonary vascular disease in humans [16,17].

Vascular Angioplasty, Stenting, and Endograft Therapy

Arterial angioplasty and stenting have been performed in animal models using iCMR and either passive or active methods [18]. Renal artery interventions have been reported and might benefit from online assessment of the parenchymal impact of these procedures [19,20].

Our group treated aortic coarctation in pigs using platinum stents deployed over active guidewires [10]. iCMR permitted interactive sizing of the stent during deployment, which may prove useful in this abnormality where a true reference vessel caliber is unknown. Perhaps more importantly, intentional aortic perforation was immediately evident, providing an extra safety margin for operators to respond to life-threatening emergencies. Eggebrecht *et al.* used iCMR to deploy aortic endografts in porcine thoracic aortic dissection [21]. Even using passive devices, iCMR distinguished "true" from "false" aortic lumen and guided the obliteration of dissections (Figure 23.3). Our group excluded

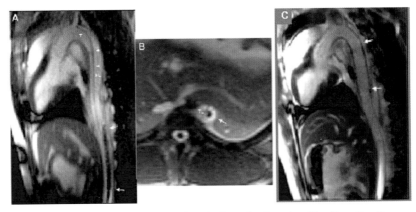

Fig. 23.3 iCMR endograft treatment of aortic dissection in swine. The dissection flap (arrowheads) separates true lumen (TL) and false lumen (FL). (a, b) The passive endograft (arrows) has entered the false lumen and thereafter is redirected. (c) Following endograft deployment, the false lumen is obliterated (see video clips 36 👁, 37 👁, and 38 👁). From Eggebrecht *et al.*, used with permission [21].

abdominal aortic aneurysm using temporarily active tube endografts and rescued catastrophic aortic rupture [22].

iCMR might prove useful for chronic total arterial occlusion. X-ray does not visualize the occluded artery, and occluded lumens cannot fill with contrast. Raval *et al.* used iCMR to recanalize complex total peripheral artery occlusions while remaining within the borders of the target artery [23].

Preliminary human endovascular treatments have been reported using iCMR. Krueger *et al.* performed balloon dilatations of aortic coarctation [24]. The Regensburg team performed iliac stenting and femoropopliteal angioplasties in patients [25,26].

Myocardial, Congenital, and Valve Disease

Passively visualized nitinol-occluder devices have been deployed under iCMR to treat porcine models of atrial septal defect and thereafter to assess hemodynamics using phase-contrast MRI [27–29]. Kuehne *et al.* implanted a prosthetic nitinol aortic valve using iCMR from a transfemoral approach [30]. Horvath *et al.* implanted a prosthetic aortic valve in beating hearts using minimally invasive transapical surgery [31].

Our laboratories and others have used iCMR to deliver cells and other materials into normal and infarcted animal hearts [6,32–35]. Targets can be chosen based on wall motion or contrast enhancement. iCMR can depict the intramyocardial dispersion of the injected materials, which can confirm successful delivery, assure uniform or confluent treatment, or avoid overlapping injections (Figure 23.4).

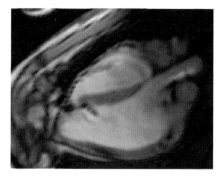

Fig. 23.4 Endomyocardial injection of mesenchymal stromal cells (black spots) labeled with iron into the borders of a small myocardial infarction. The active injection catheter is green and the needle tip is red (see video clip 39 👁). From Dick *et al.*, used with permission [6].

Image-Guided Cardiac Electrophysiology

Image-guided myocardial ablation to treat rhythm disorders is already conducted under direct surgical exposure; iCMR might provide comparable "exposure" for catheter-based treatment. iCMR may depict the extent and continuity of tissue ablation [36]. The group at Johns Hopkins has developed custom catheters that permit iCMR electro-anatomic mapping [37]. The teams at Massachusetts General Hospital and General Electric have positioned electrophysiology catheters in an MRI system overlaid onto high-resolution cardiac MRI [38].

Transseptal and Extra-anatomic Communications

iCMR may permit treatments outside of normal lumen spaces. The first steps have been taken by Arepally *et al.* and others, who conducted atrial septal puncture under iCMR to connect adjacent vascular chambers [39,40]. The Stanford team conducted human transjugular intrahepatic portosystemic shunting (TIPS) using a special dual x-ray and MRI system [41]. Arepally *et al.* created a catheter-based mesocaval shunt outside the liver capsule in animals [42].

Transitional Technology: X-ray Fused with MRI

MRI roadmaps may enhance conventional x-ray procedures using standard clinical-grade catheter devices. Such x-ray fused with MRI (XFM) requires registration of 3D MRI and 2D x-ray projection data. Approaches include assuming that a patient is immobilized on a table common to two modalities; attaching fiducial markers to the patient and warping the images so that the fiducial markers correspond; using endogenous fiducial markers, such as bones or vessel bifurcations; and using image similarity to make them correspond.

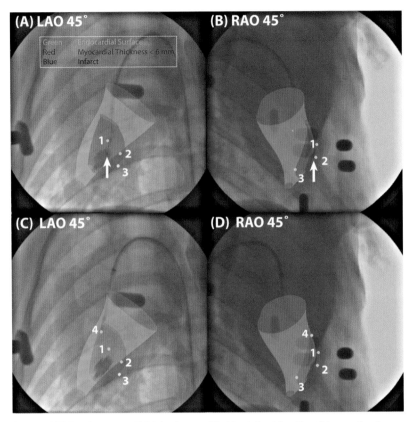

Fig. 23.5 XFM endomyocardial injections guided by infarct location (blue surface) and regional myocardial wall thickness (colored green for wall thickness greater than 6 mm, and red for wall thickness less than or equal to 6 mm) in an animal (see video clip 40 👁). From de Silva *et al.*, used with permission [43].

The King's College London group used the common-table approach for electrophysiology procedures in patients immobilized under general anesthesia [15]. We use external fiducial markers taped to subjects' skin to register the two imaging modalities, and thereafter automatically correct for gantry rotation, table panning, magnification changes, and even phases of the cardiac cycle. We used this approach to target cell delivery to infarct borders and to avoid dangerously thinned myocardium (Figure 23.5) [43].

Conclusions

iCMR exploits soft-tissue imaging to guide catheter procedures, including some not readily attainable without surgery. The chief remaining obstacle to clinical translation is the development of clinical-grade catheter devices. We can expect considerable progress in the near future.

References

1 Guttman, M.A., Ozturk, C., Raval, A.N., *et al.* Interventional cardiovascular procedures guided by real-time MR imaging: an interactive interface using multiple slices, adaptive projection modes and live 3D renderings. *J Magn Reson Imaging* (in press).

2 Kerr, A.B., Pauly, J.M., Hu, B.S., *et al.* (1997) Real-time interactive MRI on a conventional scanner. *Magn Reson Med* **38**(3): 355–367.

3 Zhang, Q., Wendt, M., Aschoff, A.J., *et al.* (2000) Active MR guidance of interventional devices with target-navigation. *Magn Reson Med* **44**(1): 56–65.

4 Quick, H.H., Kuehl, H., Kaiser, G., *et al.* (2003) Interventional MRA using actively visualized catheters, TrueFISP, and real-time image fusion. *Magn Reson Med* **49**(1): 129–137.

5 Bock, M., Muller, S., Zuehlsdorff, S., *et al.* (2006) Active catheter tracking using parallel MRI and real-time image reconstruction. *Magn Reson Med* **55**(6): 1454–1459.

6 Dick, A.J., Guttman, M.A., Raman, V.K., *et al.* (2003) Magnetic resonance fluoroscopy allows targeted delivery of mesenchymal stem cells to infarct borders in swine. *Circulation* **108**(23): 2899–2904.

7 Peters, D.C., Lederman, R.J., Dick, A.J., *et al.* (2003) Undersampled projection reconstruction for active catheter imaging with adaptable temporal resolution and catheter-only views. *Magn Reson Med* **49**(2): 216–222.

8 Seppenwoolde, J.H., Viergever, M.A., Bakker, C.J. (2003) Passive tracking exploiting local signal conservation: the white marker phenomenon. *Magn Reson Med* **50**(4): 784–790.

9 Unal, O., Li, J., Cheng, W., *et al.* (2006) MR-visible coatings for endovascular device visualization. *J Magn Reson Imaging* **23**(5): 763–769.

10 Raval, A.N., Telep, J.D., Guttman, M.A., *et al.* (2005) Real-time magnetic resonance imaging-guided stenting of aortic coarctation with commercially available catheter devices in swine. *Circulation* **112**(5): 699–706.

11 Ladd, M.E., Quick, H.H. (2000) Reduction of resonant RF heating in intravascular catheters using coaxial chokes. *Magn Reson Med* **43**(4): 615–619.

12 Weiss, S., Vernickel, P., Schaeffter, T., *et al.* (2005) Transmission line for improved RF safety of interventional devices. *Magn Reson Med* **54**(1): 182–189.

13 Quick, H.H., Zenge, M.O., Kuehl, H., *et al.* (2005) Interventional magnetic resonance angiography with no strings attached: wireless active catheter visualization. *Magn Reson Med* **53**(2): 446–455.

14 Schalla, S., Saeed, M., Higgins, C.B., *et al.* (2003) Magnetic resonance—guided cardiac catheterization in a swine model of atrial septal defect. *Circulation* **108**(15): 1865–1870.

15 Razavi, R., Hill, D.L., Keevil, S.F., *et al.* (2003) Cardiac catheterisation guided by MRI in children and adults with congenital heart disease. *Lancet* **362**(9399): 1877–1882.

16 Kuehne, T., Yilmaz, S., Schulze-Neick, I., *et al.* (2005) Magnetic resonance imaging guided catheterisation for assessment of pulmonary vascular resistance: in vivo validation and clinical application in patients with pulmonary hypertension. *Heart (Br Card Soc)* **91**(8): 1064–1069.

17 Muthurangu, V., Atkinson, D., Sermesant, M., *et al.* (2005) Measurement of total pulmonary arterial compliance using invasive pressure monitoring and MR flow quantification during MR-guided cardiac catheterization. *Am J Physiol Heart Circ Physiol* **289**(3): H1301–1306.

18 Buecker, A., Neuerburg, J.M., Adam, G.B., *et al.* (2000) Real-time MR fluoroscopy for MR-guided iliac artery stent placement. *J Magn Reson Imaging* **12**(4): 616–622.

19 Omary, R.A., Gehl, J.A., Schirf, B.E., *et al.* (2006) MR imaging versus conventional x-ray fluoroscopy-guided renal angioplasty in swine: prospective randomized comparison. *Radiology* **238**(2): 489–496.

20 Elgort, D.R., Hillenbrand, C.M., Zhang, S., *et al.* (2006) Image-guided and -monitored renal artery stenting using only MRI. *J Magn Reson Imaging* **23**(5): 619–627.

21 Eggebrecht, H., Kuhl, H., Kaiser, G.M., *et al.* (2006) Feasibility of real-time magnetic resonance-guided stent-graft placement in a swine model of descending aortic dissection. *Eur Heart J* **27**(5): 613–620.

22 Raman, V.K., Karmarkar, P., Dick, A.J., *et al.* (2004) Real-time MRI guidance for endograft delivery in a porcine model of abdominal aortic aneurysm. *Circulation.* Ref Type: Abstract.

23 Raval, A.N., Karmarkar, P.V., Guttman, M.A., *et al.* (2006) Real-time magnetic resonance imaging-guided endovascular recanalization of chronic total arterial occlusion in a swine model. *Circulation* **113**(8): 1101–1107.

24 Krueger, J.J., Ewert, P., Yilmaz, S., *et al.* (2006) Magnetic resonance imaging-guided balloon angioplasty of coarctation of the aorta: a pilot study. *Circulation* **113**(8): 1093–1100.

25 Manke, C., Nitz, W.R., Djavidani, B., *et al.* (2001) MR imaging-guided stent placement in iliac arterial stenoses: a feasibility study. *Radiology* **219**(2): 527–534.

26 Paetzel, C., Zorger, N., Bachthaler, M., *et al.* (2005) Magnetic resonance-guided percutaneous angioplasty of femoral and popliteal artery stenoses using real-time imaging and intra-arterial contrast-enhanced magnetic resonance angiography. *Invest Radiol* **40**(5): 257–262.

27 Buecker, A., Spuentrup, E., Grabitz, R., *et al.* (2002) Magnetic resonance-guided placement of atrial septal closure device in animal model of patent foramen ovale. *Circulation* **106**(4): 511–515.

28 Rickers, C., Jerosch-Herold, M., Hu, X., *et al.* (2003) Magnetic resonance image-guided transcatheter closure of atrial septal defects. *Circulation* **107**(1): 132–138.

29 Schalla, S., Saeed, M., Higgins, C.B., *et al.* (2005) Balloon sizing and transcatheter closure of acute atrial septal defects guided by magnetic resonance fluoroscopy: assessment and validation in a large animal model. *J Magn Reson Imaging* **21**(3): 204–211.

30 Kuehne, T., Yilmaz, S., Meinus, C., *et al.* (2004) Magnetic resonance imaging-guided transcatheter implantation of a prosthetic valve in aortic valve position: feasibility study in swine. *J Am Coll Cardiol* **44**(11): 2247–2249.

31 McVeigh, E.R., Guttman, M.A., Lederman, R.J., *et al.* (2006) Real-time interactive MRI-guided cardiac surgery: aortic valve replacement using a direct apical approach. *Magn Reson Med* **56**(5): 958–964.

32 Corti, R., Badimon, J., Mizsei, G., *et al.* (2005) Real time magnetic resonance guided endomyocardial local delivery. *Heart (Br Card Soc)* **91**(3): 348–353.

33 Karmarkar, P.V., Kraitchman, D.L., Izbudak, I., *et al.* (2004) MR-trackable intramyocardial injection catheter. *Magn Reson Med* **51**(6): 1163–1172.

34 Krombach, G.A., Pfeffer, J.G., Kinzel, S., *et al.* (2005) MR-guided percutaneous intramyocardial injection with an MR-compatible catheter: feasibility and changes in T1 values after injection of extracellular contrast medium in pigs. *Radiology* **235**(2): 487–494.

35 Saeed, M., Lee, R., Martin, A., *et al.* (2004) Transendocardial delivery of extracellular myocardial markers by using combination x-ray / MR fluoroscopic guidance: feasibility study in dogs. *Radiology* **231**(3): 689–696.

36 Dickfeld, T., Kato, R., Zviman, M., *et al.* (2007) Characterization of acute and subacute radio-frequency ablation lesions with nonenhanced magnetic resonance imaging. *Heart Rhythm* **4**(2): 208–214.

37 Susil, R.C., Yeung, C.J., Halperin, H.R., *et al.* (2002) Multifunctional interventional devices for MRI: a combined electrophysiology/MRI catheter. *Magn Reson Med* **47**(3): 594–600.

38 Reddy, V., Malchano, Z., Dukkipati, S., *et al.* (2005) Interventional MRI: electroanatomical mapping using real-time MR tracking of a deflectable catheter. *Heart Rhythm* **2**(15): S279–S280. Ref Type: Abstract.

39 Arepally, A., Karmarkar, P.V., Weiss, C., *et al.* (2005) Magnetic resonance image-guided trans-septal puncture in a swine heart. *J Magn Reson Imaging* **21**(4): 463–467.

40 Raval, A.N., Karmarkar, P.V., Guttman, M.A., *et al.* (2006) Real-time MRI guided atrial septal puncture and balloon septostomy in swine. *Catheter Cardiovasc Interv* **67**(4): 637–643.

41 Kee, S.T., Ganguly, A., Daniel, B.L., *et al.* (2005) MR-guided transjugular intrahepatic portosystemic shunt creation with use of a hybrid radiography/MR system. *J Vasc Interv Radiol* **16**(2 Pt 1): 227–234.

42 Arepally, A., Karmarkar, P.V., Weiss, C., Atalar, E. (2006) Percutaneous MR imaging-guided transvascular access of mesenteric venous system: study in swine model. *Radiology* **238**(1): 113–118.

43 de Silva, R., Gutierrez, L.F., Raval, A.N., *et al.* (2006) X-ray fused with magnetic resonance imaging (XFM) to target endomyocardial injections: validation in a swine model of myocardial infarction. *Circulation* **114**(22): 2342–2350.

Table 14.1 Classification of the severity of heart valve disease in adults, based partly on the 2006 ACC/AHA Guidelines (Reference 1), which refer mainly to echocardiographic indices.

Aortic Stenosis

	Mild	Moderate	Severe
Peak jet velocity (m/s)	<3	3–4	>4
Orifice area (cm²)	>1.5	1.0–1.5	<1.0
Orifice area index (cm² per m²)			<0.6
Additional features			LV hypertrophy, post stenotic dilatation of the ascending aorta
			Sub-aortic stenosis and coarctation should be considered and excluded

Pulmonary Stenosis

	Mild	Moderate	Severe
Peak jet velocity (m/s)	<3	3–4	>4.0
Valve orifice area (cm²)			<1.0
Additional features			RV hypertrophy, post stenotic dilatation of the MPA and LPA
			Sub-pulmonary and pulmonary artery stenosis should be excluded

Mitral Stenosis

	Mild	Moderate	Severe
Peak jet velocity	<1.2	1.2–2.2	>2.2
Valve orifice area (cm²)	>1.5	1–1.5	<1.0
Additional features		Possible evidence of pulmonary hypertension	

Tricuspid Stenosis

	Mild	Moderate	Severe
Valve orifice area (cm²)			<1.0

Aortic Regurgitation

	Mild	Moderate	Severe
Regurgitant volume (ml per beat)	<30	30–60	>60
Regurgitant fraction	<30%	30–50%	>50% (CMR flow measurements tend to underestimate AR, unless corrected for aortic root motion)
Regurgitant orifice area (cm²)	<0.1	0.1–0.3	>0.3

(continued)

Table 14.1 (*continued*)

Pulmonary Regurgitation (assuming near normal pulmonary resistance)

	Mild	Moderate	"Free" or "Almost Free" (but may be well tolerated)
Regurgitant jet or stream width	narrow, <2 mm	moderate 2–5 mm	Unobstructed reversed stream, >6 mm across.
Valve leaflet appearances	mobile, coapting	partly coapting	Ineffective leaflets with wide failure of coaptation.
Regurgitant volume (ml per beat)	<30	30–40	>40
Regurgitant fraction	<25%	20–35%	>35%, but modified by up- and down-stream factors.
Additional features			Free PR occurs mainly in the first half of diastole, typically followed by late diastolic forward flow if the right ventricle is full and conduit-like when the atrium contracts.

Mitral Regurgitation

	Mild	Moderate	Severe
Regurgitant jet width	Narrow, <1.0 mm No visible jet core	1.0–2 mm Narrow core	>2 mm, with extensive jet or swirling LA flow Bright jet core >2 mm width
Regurgitant volume (ml per beat)	<30	30–60	>60
Regurgitant fraction	<30%	30–50%	>50%
Regurgitant orifice area (cm^2)	<0.2	0.2–0.4	>0.4
Additional features			Dilated left atrium and pulmonary veins Systolic flow reversal in pulmonary veins

Tricuspid Regurgitation (assuming near normal pulmonary resistance)

	Mild	Moderate	Severe
Regurgitant jet width	narrow, <2 mm	2–6 mm	>6 × 6 mm, measured on a through plane velocity map.
Additional features			Dilated right atrium and caval veins.

Measurements by CMR should generally be comparable to those by echo. They can be more accurate than echo where measurements of flow volume and/or ventricular volume are used to quantify regurgitation, particularly pulmonary regurgitation. But CMR may not measure the peak velocity of a narrow or fragmented jet as accurately as Doppler echo. These jet velocities anyway depend on the rate of flow as well as the amount of area reduction. Direct planimetry may be feasible by CMR, but only in cases where the jet core, immediately downstream of an orifice, is coherent and of suitable size, shape and location relative to the image voxels for clear delineation.

Index

(Author Disclosure Table)

Working group member	Employment	Research grant	Other research support	Speakers bureau/ honoraria	Expert witness	Ownership interest	Consultant/ advisory board	Other
Abbara	Massachusetts General Hospital	NIH+	None	None	None	Amirsys*	Ezem*, Perceptive Informatics*	None
Aggarwal	Wake Forest University Baptist Medical Center	None	None	None	None	None	None	None
Ashikaga	National Institutes of Health	None	None	None	None	None	None	None
Axel	NYU Langone Medical Center	None	None	None	None	None	None	None
Beller	University of Virginia	None	None	None	None	None	None	None
Berry	University of Glasgow	None	None	None	None	None	None	None
Bluemke	Johns Hopkins University	None	None	None	None	None	General Electric+	None
Bonow	Northwestern University	None	None	None	None	None	None	None
Carr	Northwestern University	None	None	None	None	None	None	None
Edelman	Northwestern University	None	None	None	None	None	None	None

Working group member	Employment	Research grant	Other research support	Speakers bureau/ honoraria	Expert witness	Ownership interest	Consultant/ advisory board	Other
Garcia	Mount Sinai Hospital	Philips Medical+	None	Vital Images*	None	None	Philips Medical*	None
Gerber	None	None	None	None	None	None	None	None
Gharib	National Institutes of Health	None	None	None	None	None	None	None
Gottlieb	Johns Hopkins University	None	None	None	None	None	None	None
Hachamovitch	None	GE Healthcare+, Bracco+, Astellas+	Siemens Healthcare+	GE Healthcare*	None	None	King Pharmaceuticals*, BMS Medical Imaging*	None
Halperin	Johns Hopkins University	Zoll Circulation+	None	None	None	None	Phillips, Imricor, Boston Scientific, Zoll Circulation, Cardiac Concepts, Inc*	None
Hansalia	Mount Sinai Medical Center	None	None	None	None	None	None	None
Hundley	Wake Forest University School of Medicine	NIH+	None	None	None	Prova, Inc*	None	None
Kalra	Massachusetts General Hospital	None	None	None	None	None	None	None

Name	Institution							
Karamitsos	University of Oxford	None	None	None	None	None	None	None
Kilner	Royal Brompton Hospital	None	None	None	None	None	None	None
Kim (Danny)	NYU Medical Center	None	None	None	None	None	None	None
Kim (Han)	Duke University	None	None	None	None	None	None	None
Kim (Raymond)	Duke University	None	None	None	None	None	None	Raymond Kim is one of the inventors of a patent on Delayed Enhancement MRI which is owned by Northwestern University
Kraitchman	Johns Hopkins University	None	Boston Scientific Corporation* Bayer Pharma Healthcare*	None	None	None	None	None
Kramer	University of Virginia Health System	GE Healthcare+, Astellas+	Siemens Medical Solutions+, Merck+	None	None	None	Novartis*	None
Kwon	Brigham and Women's Hospital	None	None	None	None	None	None	None
Lederman	National Institutes of Health	None	None	None	None	None	None	None

Working group member	Employment	Research grant	Other research support	Speakers bureau/honoraria	Expert witness	Ownership interest	Consultant/advisory board	Other
Li	Northwestern University	None	None	None	None	None	None	None
Libby	Brigham and Women's Hospital	Donald Reynolds Foundation+	Donald Reynolds Foundation+	None	None	None	None	None
Lima	Johns Hopkins University	None	Toshiba, Astellas, Bracco*	None	None	None	None	None
Liu	Northwestern University	None	None	None	None	None	None	None
McVeigh	Johns Hopkins University	None	None	None	None	None	None	None
Mordini	Evanston Northwestern Healthcare	None	None	None	None	None	None	None
Nazarian	Johns Hopkins University	None	None	None	None	None	None	None
Nguyen	Not Applicable	None	None	None	None	None	None	None
Ntim	Wake Forest University School of Medicine	None	None	None	None	None	None	None
Patel	University of Virginia	NIH+	None	None	None	None	None	None

Pettigrew	National Institutes of Health	None	None	None	None	None
Rubin	Stanford University	None	None	None	None	None
Selvanayagam	Flinders Medical Center	None	None	None	None	None
Salerno	Duke University Medical Center	None	None	None	None	None
Stuber	Johns Hopkins University+	NIHI NHLBI Coronary MRI+	None	None	None	Philips Medical Systems*	None
Taylor	US Army	None	None	None	None	None
Wong	Stanford University Medical Center	None	None	None	None	None
Wu	Brigham and Women's Hospital	None	None	None	None	None

*Modest

+Significant

This table represents the relationships of writing group members that may be perceived as actual or reasonably perceived conflicts of interest as reported on the Disclosure Questionnaire which all writing group members are required to complete and submit. A relationship is considered to be "Significant" if (a) the person receives $10,000 or more during any 12 month period, or 5% or more of the person's gross income; or (b) the person owns 5% or more of the voting stock or share of the entity, or owns $10,000 or more of the fair market value of the entity. A relationship is considered to be "Modest" if it is less than "Significant" under the preceding definition.

The AHA Clinical Series

SERIES EDITOR • ELLIOTT ANTMAN

Biomarkers in Heart Disease
James A. de Lemos
9781405175715

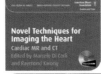
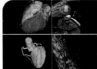

Novel Techniques for Imaging the Heart
Marcelo Di Carli & Raymond Kwong
9781405175333

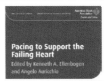
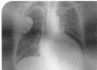

Pacing to Support the Failing Heart
Kenneth A. Ellenbogen
& Angelo Auricchio
9781405175340

Metabolic Risk for Cardiovascular Disease
Robert H. Eckel
9781405181044

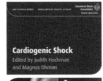
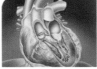

Cardiogenic Shock
Judith Hochman
& E. Magnus Ohman
9781405179263

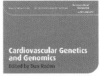

Cardiovascular Genetics and Genomics
Dan Roden
9781405175401

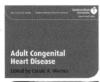
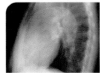

Adult Congenital Heart Disease
Carole A. Warnes
9781405178204

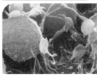

Antiplatelet Therapy In Ischemic Heart Disease
Stephen Wiviott
9781405176262

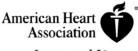